The Type 2 Diabetic Woman

Other books by M. Sara Rosenthal:

The Thyroid Sourcebook, 3d edition

The Gynecological Sourcebook, 3d edition

The Pregnancy Sourcebook, 2d edition

The Fertility Sourcebook, 2d edition

The Breastfeeding Sourcebook, 2d edition

The Breast Sourcebook, 2d edition

The Gastrointestinal Sourcebook

Managing Your Diabetes: The Only Complete Guide to Type 2 Diabetes for Canadians

Managing Diabetes for Women: The Only Canadian Women's Guide to Type 2 Diabetes

The Type 2 Diabetic Woman

M. Sara Rosenthal

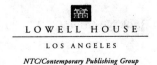

LOWELL HOUSE

LOS ANGELES

NTC/Contemporary Publishing Group

Important Notice

The purpose of this book is to educate. It is sold with the understanding that the author and publisher shall have neither liability nor responsibility for any injury caused or alleged to be caused directly or indirectly by the information contained in this book. While every effort has been made to ensure its accuracy, the book's contents should not be construed as medical advice. Each person's health needs are unique. To obtain recommendations appropriate to your particular situation, please consult a qualified health care provider.

Library of Congress Cataloging-in-Publication Data

Rosenthal, M. Sara.
    The type 2 diabetic woman / M. Sara Rosenthal
      p   cm.
    ISBN 07373-0078-7 (pbk.)
    1. Diabetes in woman Popular works. 2. Diabetes in pregnancy
    Popular works. 3. Non-insulin-dependent diabetes Popular works.
    I. Title.

RC662.18.R66	1999
616.4'62'0082—dc21	99-13013
	CIP

Published by Lowell House, a division of NTC/Contemporary Publishing Group, Inc., 4255 West Touhy Avenue, Lincolnwood, Illinois 60646-1975 U.S.A.

Design by Andrea Reider

Printed and bound in the United States of America

International Standard Book Number: 0-7373-0078-9
10 9 8 7 6 5 4 3

For Andrea

CONTENTS

Acknowledgments   ix

Introduction   xi

Chapter 1   What Is Type 2 Diabetes and Why Should I Worry
About It?   1
What's in a Name?   1
Risk Factors You Can Change   6
Risk Factors You Can't Change   13
When Your Doctor Says "You Have Diabetes"   22

Chapter 2   Women, Weight, and Type 2 Diabetes   43
The "Good Times Disease"   44
Psychological Roles of Fat   56
The Act of Getting Fat: Compulsive Eating   59
Biological Causes of Obesity   64
Teaching Children Good Eating Habits   68

Chapter 3   The Estrogen Connection   71
The Estrogen Refresher Course   72
Birth Control and Diabetes   76
Hormone Replacement Therapy and Diabetes   100

Chapter 4   Type 2 Diabetes, Fertility, and Pregnancy   117
Getting Pregnant   118
Being Pregnant   126
Gestational Diabetes   129
Special Delivery   135
After the Baby Is Born   138

Chapter 5   Type 2 Diabetes and the Menopausal Woman   141
Natural Menopause   142

Surgical Menopause   152

Long-Term Effects of Estrogen Loss: Postmenopausal
Symptoms   154

Other Postmenopausal Concerns   162

Chapter 6   Women, Exercise, and Type 2 Diabetes   171

What Does Exercise *Really* Mean?   172

Let's Get Physical   182

Chapter 7   How Sweet It Is: Counting Sugar, Planning
Meals   187

A Few Good Foods   187

Going Shopping   195

Sweeteners   202

At the Liquor Store   205

Chapter 8   Diabetes Doctors and Diabetes Medications   209

The Right Primary Care Doctor   213

Your Diabetes Specialist   218

Self-Service   223

What the Doctor Orders   225

When Your Doctor Tells You to Take a Pill   229

When Your Doctor Prescribes Insulin   239

Chapter 9   Women Down the Diabetes Road   251

Macro Versus Micro   251

From Head to Toe   254

Preventing Complications   275

Chapter 10   Prevention: Low-Fat and Healthful Eating   279

The Skinny on Fat   281

The Incredible Bulk   286

Food Pills   288

Changing Your Diet   And Helping the Environment,
Too!   290

Glossary   301

Appendix A   Chronology: Diabetes to Date   311

Appendix B   Resources   319

Bibliography   329

Index   347

ACKNOWLEDGMENTS

I wish to thank the following people (listed alphabetically) for their commitment, hard work, and guidance, which helped to frame so much of the content of this book:

Brenda Cook, R.D., University of Alberta Hospitals; Tasha Hamilton, Ba.Sc., R.D., Diabetes Educator-Dietitian, Tri-Hospital Diabetes Education Centre; Stuart Harris, M.D., M.P.H., C.C.F.P., A.B.P.M., Assistant Professor, Departments of Family Medicine and Epidemiology and Biostatistics, University of Western, Ontario, and former Medical Director, University of Toronto Sioux Lookout Program; Anne Kenshole, M.B., B.S., F.R.C.P.C., F.A.C.P., Medical Director of TRIDEC, Professor of Medicine, University of Toronto; Anne Levin, B.Sc.P.T., M.C.P.A., Physiotherapist and Certified Hydrotherapist, Baycrest Centre for Geriatric Care, Coordinator, Arthritis Education and Exercise Program, and Lecturer, Physical Therapy, Faculty of Medicine, University of Toronto; Barbara McIntosh, R.N., B.Sc.N., C.D.E., Nurse Coordinator, Adult Diabetes Education Program, Grand River Hospital, Kitchener, Ontario; James McSherry, M.B., Ch.B, F.C.F.P., F.R.C.G.P., F.A.A.F.P., F.A.B.M.P., Medical Director, Victoria Family Medical Centre, Chief of Family Medicine, The London Health Sciences Centre; Robert Panchyson, B.Sc.N., R.N., Nurse Clinician, Diabetes Educator, Hamilton Civic Hospitals, Hamilton

General Division; Diana Phayre, Clinical Nurse Specialist, Diabetes Education Centre, The Doctor's Hospital; Robert Silver, M.D., F.R.C.P.C., Endocrinologist, Division of Endocrinology and Metabolism, Toronto Hospital.

Special thanks to Gary May, M.D., F.R.C.P., Clinical Assistant Professor of Medicine, Department of Medicine, Division of Gastroenterology, University of Calgary, who provided some of the groundwork for this text through his role as medical advisor on a past work.

Gillian Arsenault, M.D., C.C.F.P., I.B.C.L.C., F.R.C.P., Simon Fraser Health Unit, served as a consultant on two past works, and has never stopped advising me and sending valuable information. Irving Rootman, Ph.D., Director, Centre for Health Promotion, University of Toronto, put me in touch with several experts, and always encourages my interest in primary prevention and health promotion issues.

I also wish to thank the following people for advising me on previously published women's health books, which has helped to frame so much of the material in this book: Suzanne Pratt, M.D., F.A.C.O.G; Susan R. George, M.D., F.R.C.P. (C), F.A.C.P.; Michelle Long, M.D.; and Masood A. Khatamee, M.D., F.A.C.O.G., Executive Director, Fertility Research Foundation.

My editorial assistant, Larissa Kostoff, worked hard to make this edition come to fruition. I would also like to thank Claudia McCowan, Project Editor; Suzie DeFazio; Maria Magallanes, Managing Editor; and Bud Sperry, Senior Editor, for their patience and expertise.

To all the women interviewed for this book: your stories, struggles, and important suggestions regarding content for this volume were very much appreciated.

In the moral support department—Thanks to my husband, Gary S. Karp, and all the relatives and friends who cheered me on.

In 1978, my obese and physically inactive grandmother, who had Type 2 diabetes, dropped dead from a massive heart attack at the age of sixty-two. She was survived by her own mother by a full decade. I have still never quite recovered from this loss, because it was such an untimely death. To this day, I dream of her. In a recurring dream, she is alive and well, but I know that her heart will give out at any moment. The feeling that she will "die again" always interferes with my fantasy visits; even in the dream world, my time with her is limited. My grandfather, a family physician who died in 1989, used to say that my grandmother "ate herself to death." The more I learn about Type 2 diabetes, the more I understand what he meant by this comment.

Sixty-five to 70 percent of those diagnosed with Type 2 diabetes are women; according to some experts, about 95 percent of women with Type 2 diabetes are obese. My grandmother was a textbook case. In her midforties, she developed *late onset diabetes mellitus,* known today as Type 2 diabetes. (All diabetes-related terms will be explained in chapter 1.) My grandmother was an out-of-control diabetic who outlived her baby sister, who also died from complications of Type 2 diabetes. (My aunt, too, was obese.) Despite her little sister's fate, my grandmother never made any effort to adjust her own eating habits. My grandmother used to coax my mother, who has spent most of her adult life battling obesity, into eating rich desserts with comments such as, "It's a sin not to eat it."

Indeed, my grandmother's great character flaw was her appetite. She could never pass up rich, tasty foods. Part of the reason is the hard times she experienced coming of age in the Prairies during the Depression. She developed heart disease, and apparently spent most of her forties and fifties as a very unwell woman, continuously plagued with one health problem after another. Given this information, you're probably not surprised that she died early. After all, the woman was a "walking time bomb." The funny thing is, everyone who loved her was shocked by her death. My great-grandmother suffered the terrible fate of outliving almost all her children; most of them died from complications related to Type 2 diabetes.

This is the book I wish my grandmother had read. I not only want to prevent you from undergoing my grandmother's fate; I want to give you the information my grandmother should have had, and might have used—if it had been available to her.

Why are women more prone to Type 2 diabetes than men? Women have more body fat than men because they require more weight to protect their reproductive organs, tend to gain weight during pregnancy and after childbirth, and lose 25 percent of their metabolic efficiency after menopause.

Roughly 12 million Americans have diabetes. By 2004, one in four North Americans over the age of forty-five will be diagnosed with Type 2 diabetes. These statistics have a staggering impact on women's health, considering the fact that 52 percent of these "one in four" North Americans are women, while more than 70 percent of all patients in the health care system are female. Since diabetes affects women's gynecological and overall health, it's crucial to understand how to manage Type 2 diabetes in a woman's body. For example, diabetes is often more difficult to monitor during menstruation, while estrogen has an effect on insulin resistance. This means that decisions regarding birth control, hormone replacement therapy, and pregnancy must all be carefully weighed for women with diabetes. After menopause, issues such as fluctuating blood sugar levels, heart disease, osteoporosis, and even breast cancer risk can factor into diabetes management decisions.

Unless you live in a large city, you may not have immediate (or any!) access to the proper health care professionals. Millions of Americans have no health insurance; and many of those uninsured have Type 2 diabetes. Take heart—there are other ways to get the information you need to manage your disease. Every manufacturer of a diabetes product, be it a glucose meter, an insulin pen, or a diabetes medication, has a 1-800 customer care line. These are excellent sources of information. Of course, the American Diabetes Association (ADA) should be the first place you call once you're diagnosed. You can also get a lot of information through the Internet. Check the back of this book for useful numbers and Web sites.

As I'll stress again and again in this book, Type 2 diabetes is a genetic disease; but by modifying your lifestyle and diet, you may be able to delay or even prevent its onset.

CHAPTER 1

What Is Type 2 Diabetes and Why Should I Worry About It?

You've just come home from your doctor's office. You can't remember anything she said other than those three horrible words: "You have diabetes." What does this mean? How will your life change? You've never been any good at diets, meal plans, or exercising. And since you can't stand the sight of blood, how can you be expected to prick your finger every day (or however often necessary) to monitor your blood sugar?

Whether you've just been diagnosed with Type 2 diabetes, or you've been living with it for years, this is a difficult disease to understand. Part of the problem is that there are so many names for this one disease, and so many *other* types of diabetes, which also have more than one name. It's easy to get mixed up about what kind of diabetes you have. So I'm going to begin this chapter by clearing up all this confusion regarding names, labels, and definitions; this is the first step in managing Type 2 diabetes.

WHAT'S IN A NAME?

It has long been known that there was a "milder" kind of diabetes and a more severe form. But diabetes wasn't officially labeled "Type 1" and "Type 2" until 1979. Type 2 diabetes means that your pancreas is functioning. You are making plenty of insulin. In fact, you are probably making too much insulin, a condition called *hyperinsulinemia* ("too much insulin"). Insulin is a hormone made by your *beta cells,* the insulin-producing cells within the *islets of Langerhans*—small islands of cells afloat in your pancreas. The *pancreas* is a bird-beak-shaped gland situated behind the stomach.

Insulin is a major player in our bodies. One of its most important functions is to regulate blood sugar levels. It does this by acting as a sort of courier, "knocking" on the cell's door, and announcing, "Sugar's here; come and get it!" Your cells then open the door to let in sugar from your bloodstream. That sugar is absolutely vital to your health, and provides you with the energy you need to function.

But what happens if the cells don't answer the door? Two things: First, the sugar in your bloodstream will accumulate, having nowhere to go. It's like the kind of situation that develops when your newspapers pile up on your porch when you're away. Second, your pancreas will keep sending out more couriers to try to get your cells to open that door and take in the "newspapers." The result of the cell's not complying is a pile of newspapers *and* a lineup of unsuccessful couriers by your door. When the cell doesn't answer the door, this is called *insulin resistance*; the cell is resisting insulin. Why this is happening is discussed further on. The end result, however, is *diabetes*, which means "high blood sugar." A synonym for diabetes is *hyperglycemia*, which also means "high blood sugar." If insulin resistance goes on for too long, the pancreas can become overworked and eventually may not make enough, or any, insulin. In effect, it's like a courier strike. And finally, the liver, being the good neighbor that it is, will lend a "bowl or two" of sugar to the sugar-deprived cell (see below). But this can exacerbate existing high blood sugar.

Type 2 diabetes, a genetic disease, is a completely different disease than Type 1 diabetes, an autoimmune disease. In Type 1, the immune system attacks the beta cells in the pancreas, caus-ing them to be impaired or defective. The result is that no insulin is produced by the pancreas at all. That means no couriers are sent to knock at the cell's door. In this case, the result is a pile of newspapers *without* the lineup of couriers.

Type 1 diabetes is usually diagnosed before age thirty, often in childhood. For this reason, Type 1 diabetes was once known as *juvenile diabetes,* or *juvenile-onset diabetes.* Because people with Type 1 diabetes depend on insulin injections to live, it was also called *insulin-dependent diabetes mellitus* (IDDM). The word *mellitis* comes from the Greek word meaning "sweet," a leftover term from the days when diabetes was diagnosed by "urine tasters"; the urine becomes sweet when blood sugar is danger-ously high, something that doesn't usually occur in Type 2. Only 10 percent of all people with diabetes have Type 1 diabetes.

Type 2: The Topic of *This* Book

Type 2 diabetes, on the other hand, accounts for 90 percent of all people with diabetes. Since Type 2 diabetes doesn't usually develop until after age forty-five, it was once known as *mature-onset diabetes* or *adult-onset diabetes.* In rare cases, when Type 2 develops before age thirty, it is called *mature-onset diabetes in the young* (MODY). Since Type 2 diabetes is a disease of insulin resistance, rather than no insulin, it often can be managed through diet and exercise, without insulin injections. For this rea-son, Type 2 diabetes was also known as *non-insulin-dependent diabetes mellitis* (NIDDM).

Here's where it gets really confusing! When you are told that you have non-insulin-dependent diabetes, it's logical to con-clude that you will never need to have an insulin injection. But this just isn't so. In fact, about one-third of all people with Type 2 diabetes will eventually need to begin insulin therapy, for rea-sons I explain on page 240. Does this mean you now have insulin dependent diabetes, or Type 1? After all, if you need insulin, aren't you now insulin-dependent, which, by definition, means Type 1? This is a logical conclusion, *but it's wrong.* As stated above, Type 2 diabetes is a genetic disease; Type 1 diabetes is an autoimmune disease. Type 2 diabetes cannot "turn into" Type 1 diabetes any more than an apple can turn into a banana. So what do you call it when someone with Type 2 diabetes requires insulin? This is *insulin-requiring Type 2 diabetes.*

Something else you need to understand about Type 2 diabetes is that the high blood sugar that results from insulin resistance can lead to a number of other diseases, including cardiovascular disease (heart disease and stroke) and peripheral vascular disease (PVD), which means that the blood doesn't flow properly to various parts of your body. This can create a number of problems, discussed in chapter 9. Many women who suffer a heart attack or stroke have Type 2 diabetes.

Screening studies show that Type 2 diabetes is prevalent all over the world, particularly in countries that are becoming Westernized. Especially disturbing is that Type 2 diabetes is increasing in the developed world at an annual rate of about 6 percent, while the number of people with Type 2 diabetes doubles every fifteen years. Roughly 6 percent of all Caucasian adults have Type 2 diabetes; however, the disease affects African North Americans at a rate of 12 to 15 percent, Hispanics at a rate of 20 percent, and Native (aboriginal) North Americans at a rate exceeding 30 percent. In some Native American communities, up to 70 percent of adults have Type 2 diabetes.

"Full-Blown" Type 2

Many women with Type 2 diabetes aren't diagnosed until they have "full-blown Type 2," meaning that the disease has progressed to the point where they are experiencing complications (what I call "Type 2–defining illnesses." This situation is analogous to the "HIV-positive" status versus "full-blown AIDS" story. You should be worried about Type 2 diabetes because of what the disease most often leads to—cardiovascular disease and peripheral vascular disease. People with Type 2 diabetes are four times more likely to develop heart disease and five times more likely to suffer a stroke than people without Type 2 diabetes.

Who's at Risk?

If you consume a diet higher in fat than carbohydrates, and low in fiber, you increase your risk of developing Type 2 diabetes (if you are genetically predisposed to the disease). If you weigh at least 20 percent more than you should for your height and age (the definition of "obese"), are sedentary, and are over age forty-five, you are considered at high risk for Type 2 diabetes. Your risk further increases if you are

- of Native or aboriginal descent (this is true for aboriginal peoples all over the world, from Australia to North America; in the United States, the Pima Indians and Pacific Islanders are at highest risk);
- of African or Hispanic descent;
- of Asian descent;
- have a family history of Type 2 diabetes;
- are obese (73 percent of all women with diabetes are obese— discussed more in chapter 2);
- are pregnant (one in twenty women will develop gestational diabetes by their third trimester; this number increases with age, and gestational diabetes can predispose you to Type 2 diabetes later in life—see chapter 4 for more details).

There are several cofactors that contribute to your risk profile, which can change your risk from higher to lower. The purpose of this section is to give you a clear idea of where you fit into this risk puzzle. That way, you'll be more aware of early warning signs of the disease, making it easier for you to get an accurate diagnosis.

RISK FACTORS YOU CAN CHANGE

Type 2 diabetes could be considered an epidemic. In 1985, the World Health Organization (WHO) estimated that roughly 30 million people globally had Type 2 diabetes. By 1993, that number jumped to 98.9 million people, and it's estimated that 250 million people worldwide will have Type 2 diabetes by 2020.

One in four North Americans over the age of forty-five will be diagnosed with diabetes by 2004. And unless more people modify their risk factors, that number is likely to increase by 2020.

Thirty-two percent of people with diabetes have at least three of the risk factors that can *double* their chances of developing Type 2 diabetes, while 89 percent of people with the disease have at least one *modifiable* risk factor. That means you can lower your risk of developing diabetes by changing your lifestyle and/or diet.

Calculating your risk of developing a particular disease is a very tricky business. To simplify matters, I've divided this "risk section" into two: modifiable risk factors—risk factors you can change; and risk markers—risk factors you cannot change, such as your age or genes. It's also crucial to understand that risk estimates are only guesses that are not based on you personally, but on people *like* you, who share your physical characteristics or lifestyle patterns. It's like betting on a horse. You look at the age of the horse, its vigor and shape, its breeding, its training, and where the race is being run. Then you come up with odds. If you own the horse, you can't change your horse's color or breeding, but you can change its training, its diet, its jockey, and ultimately, where, when, and how often it's being raced. Chance, of course, plays a role in horse racing. You can't control acts of God. But you can decide whether you're going to tempt fate by racing your horse during a thunderstorm.

Obesity

For women, the most important modifiable risk factor is obesity. The topic of obesity and women is complex, and is not limited to biology, "fat genes," or dieting. It involves many sociological and psychological issues, which are explored in detail in chapter 2. Unfortunately, obesity can lead to many of the health problems discussed in this section.

High Cholesterol

Cholesterol is a whitish, waxy fat made in vast quantities by the liver. That's why liver is high in cholesterol! Cholesterol is needed to make hormones as well as cell membranes. If you have high cholesterol, the excess cholesterol in your blood can lead to narrowed arteries, which can cause a heart attack. Saturated fat, discussed in detail in chapter 10, is often a culprit when it comes to high cholesterol. But the highest levels of cholesterol are due to a genetic defect in the liver. Since people with diabetes are four times more likely to develop heart disease and five times more likely to suffer a stroke, lowering your cholesterol, especially if you're already at risk for Type 2 diabetes, is a good idea.

Insulin's role in "fat control"

Insulin not only keeps blood sugar in check, it also keeps the levels of "good" cholesterol (HDL—high-density lipoproteins), "bad" cholesterol (LDL—low-density lipoproteins), and triglycerides in check. When you're not making enough insulin or your body isn't using insulin efficiently, your LDL levels and your triglycerides rise; more important, *your HDL levels fall,* which can lead to heart disease. When diabetes is in control, cholesterol levels will return to normal, which will cut your risk of heart disease and stroke.

Checking your cholesterol

Cholesterol levels are checked through a simple blood test. You can also ask your pharmacist about the availability of home cholesterol tests. The magic number is 200 milligrams per deciliter (200 mg/dl) or lower. At this level, you can have your cholesterol levels checked every five years.

If your blood cholesterol is between 200 and 239 mg/dl, so long as you don't smoke, are not obese, have normal blood pressure, are a premenopausal female, and do not have a family history of heart disease—you're fine! But chances are you do not meet all these criteria. In this case, discuss with your doctor how often you need to have your cholesterol levels checked.

A high cholesterol reading should always be followed up with an HDL–LDL analysis. If your LDL number is below 130 mg/dl, you're fine, but if LDL levels are between 130 and 160 mg/dl, you are considered a "borderline" case of high cholesterol. Once your LDL levels reach 160, you should definitely be on a treatment plan to lower your cholesterol.

Hypertension (High Blood Pressure)

About 12 percent of North American adults suffer from hypertension, or high blood pressure. What is blood pressure? The blood flows from the heart into the arteries (blood vessels), pressing against the artery walls. The simplest way to explain this is to think about a liquid soap dispenser. When you want soap, you need to get it out by pressing down on the little dispenser pump, the "heart" of the dispenser. The liquid soap is the "blood" and the little tube through which the soap flows is the "artery." The pressure that's exerted on the wall of the tube is the "blood pressure."

When the tube is hollow and clean, you needn't pump very hard to get the soap; it comes out easily. But when the tube gets narrower as a result of old, hardened, gunky liquid soap blocking it, you have to pump down much harder to get any soap, while the force the soap exerts against the tube is increased. Obviously, this is a simplistic explanation of a very complex problem, but essentially, the narrowing of the arteries created by higher blood pressure forces your heart to work harder to pump the blood. If this goes on too long, your heart muscle enlarges and becomes weaker, which can lead to a heart attack. Higher pressure can also weaken the walls of your blood vessels, which can cause a stroke.

The term hyper*tension* refers to the tension or force exerted on your artery walls. (Hyper means "too much," as in "too much tension.") Blood pressure is measured in two readings: X over Y. The X is the systolic pressure, which is the pressure that occurs during the heart's contraction. The Y is the diastolic pressure, which is the pressure that occurs when the heart rests between contractions. In "liquid soap" terms, the systolic pressure occurs when you press the pump down; the diastolic pressure occurs when you release your hand from the pump and allow it to rise back to its "resting" position.

Normal blood pressure readings are 120 over 80 (120/80). Readings of 140/90 or higher are generally considered borderline, although for some people this is still considered a normal reading. For the general population, 140/90 is "lecture time," when your doctor will begin to counsel you about dietary and lifestyle habits. By 160/100, many people are prescribed a drug designed to lower blood pressure.

Let's examine some of the causes of hypertension. The same factors that put you at risk for Type 2 diabetes, such as obesity, can also put you at risk for hypertension. Hypertension is also exacerbated by tobacco and alcohol consumption, and too much sodium, or salt in the diet. (People of African descent tend to be more salt sensitive.)

If high blood pressure runs in your family, you're at greater risk of developing hypertension. High blood pressure can also be caused by kidney disorders (which may be initially caused by diabetes) or pregnancy (known as pregnancy-induced hypertension). Medications are also common culprits. Estrogen-containing medications (such as oral contraceptives); nonsteroidal anti-inflammatory drugs (NSAIDs, such as ibuprofen), nasal decongestants, cold remedies, appetite suppressants, certain antidepressants, and other drugs can all increase blood pressure. Be sure to check with your pharmacist.

How to lower your blood pressure without drugs

- Change your diet and begin exercising.
- Limit alcohol consumption to no more than 2 oz of liquor or 8 oz of wine or 24 oz of beer per day (and lower still for "liver health").
- Limit your salt intake to about 1½ teaspoons per day. Cut out all foods high in sodium, such as canned soups, pickles, and soy sauce. Some canned soups contain 1,000 mg of sodium. That's a lot!
- Increase your intake of calcium or dairy products and potassium (such as bananas). Some still-unproven studies suggest that people with hypertension are calcium and potassium deficient.
- Lower your stress levels. Studies show that by lowering your stress, your blood pressure decreases.

Sedentary Lifestyle

What's the definition of sedentary? *Not moving!* If you have a desk job or spend most of your time at a computer, in your car, or watching television (even if it *is* PBS or CNN), you are a sedentary person. If you do roughly twenty minutes of exercise less than once a week, you're relatively sedentary. You need to incorporate some sort of movement into your daily schedule in order to be considered active. That movement can be anything: aerobic exercise, brisk walks around the block, or walking your dog. If you lead a sedentary lifestyle, and are obese, you are at significant risk of developing Type 2 diabetes in your forties (if you are genetically predisposed). If you are not obese, as a woman, your risk is certainly lowered, but you are then predisposed to a number of other problems. Chapter 6 discusses exercise and Type 2 diabetes in detail.

Smoking

Smoking and diabetes is a toxic combination. You already know that smoking leads to heart attacks. But what you might not know is that if you have Type 2 diabetes, you are *already* four times more likely to have a heart attack than a person without diabetes even if you are a nonsmoker. If you smoke *and* have Type 2 diabetes, you have an even greater risk of having a heart attack than nonsmokers without diabetes.

Smoking and obesity

Smoking and obesity often coexist. Women begin to smoke in their teens as a way to lose weight. A 1997 study by the Department of Psychology and Preventive Medicine at the University of Memphis in Tennessee shows that this approach doesn't work. Smoking teens are just as likely to become obese as nonsmokers. In fact, the heavier the person, the more cigarettes he or she smoked. In the long run, smokers often wound up weighing more than nonsmokers because they substituted food for nicotine when they quit or attempted to quit.

Sleep Deprivation or Sleep Disorders

There are studies linking obesity, and hence, Type 2 diabetes, to lack of sleep, snoring, loss of REM sleep, and a range of other sleep disorders. When you don't sleep well or get enough sleep—particularly REM sleep (rapid eye movement, which occurs in deep sleep)—you will be irritable and drowsy during the day. That means you'll eat more and will likely crave fast-energy foods high in sugar or starch. By visiting a sleep disorder clinic or, in some cases, by going to a time management seminar, you should be able to improve the quality of your sleep.

Vitamin Deficiency

Blood samples from people with diabetes show a tendency toward "oxidative stress," meaning that people with diabetes tend to be antioxidant deficient. Antioxidants are vitamins found in colored (nongreen) fruits and vegetables, discussed in more detail in chapter 7.

Many people make the mistake of cutting out nutrients along with the fat in their diets. Experts recommend that to meet all vitamin needs through food alone, females need 1,200 calories per day and males need 1,500 calories per day (unless you need more or less vitamins due to a medical condition). Studies reveal that when diets fall to 1,000 calories, intake of essential vitamins drop to approximately 60 percent of recommended levels. This is where vitamin supplements, meal replacement drinks, or health bars come in. They're designed to supply your daily requirement of vitamins and minerals. If you're on a low-fat diet, make sure that you're not cutting out all protein, calcium, or carbohydrates. You do need some of these! (See chapter 10.)

Studies also show that approximately 25 percent of North Americans skip breakfast, while an additional 38 percent skip lunch. Eating breakfast will help you lower your fat intake because it reduces impulsive snacking in the late afternoon and actually improves your nutrient absorption.

Age can also interfere with vitamin intake. Research shows that seniors (over age sixty-five) tend to be deficient in vitamins A, C, D, protein, and calcium, yet these nutrients boost the immune system and improve bone density and cardiovascular health.

RISK FACTORS YOU CAN'T CHANGE

By *modifying* any of the factors noted above, you can help to off-set your chances of developing Type 2 diabetes if you have any of the following risk markers. While you can't change your genetic makeup, medical history, or age, you can significantly reduce the odds of these factors predisposing you to Type 2 diabetes.

Age

The risk of developing Type 2 diabetes increases with age. Perhaps at no other time in history have we seen so many people over age forty-five—the so-called baby boom generation. This may, in part, account for the increase in Type 2 diabetes, as well as other age-related diseases. The lifestyle and dietary habits you practice before age forty-five count either against you or for you, however. By changing your diet and becoming more active before middle age, though you may not be able to prevent your genetic fate, you may certainly be able to delay it. And in the event that you develop Type 2 diabetes, a healthy diet and active lifestyle will go a long way in controlling the disease.

It's crucial to keep in mind that studies regarding diet, lifestyle, and Type 2 diabetes are still unclear; however, experts agree that there is a strong relationship between genetic markers for diabetes and environmental factors, such as activity levels, weight, and diet.

Menopause

When women reach menopause, estrogen loss can lead to well-documented problems, such as osteoporosis (because estrogen helps to maintain calcium levels) and heart disease (because estrogen raises HDL levels, or "good" cholesterol, which protects premenopausal women from heart disease). Menopause also carries special concerns for women with Type 2 diabetes. Therefore, chapter 5 is devoted to this topic.

Genes

Type 2 diabetes is a genetic disease, which means you have the "wiring" installed for Type 2 diabetes at birth. Fortunately, we do understand some of the outside factors that can trip the Type 2 switch. Body shape, diet, and activity levels are strong switch-trippers. On the other hand, if you don't have any Type 2 diabetes genes (in other words, you're not "wired" for this disease), these outside factors cannot, by themselves, cause you to develop Type 2 diabetes. For instance, there are plenty of obese and sedentary people who do not have and will not develop Type 2 diabetes.

When underdeveloped populations become urbanized and adopt a Western lifestyle, there is an explosion in Type 2 diabetes. But the genes must be present in order to allow for the disease in the first place. This is more proof that there is a genetic-environmental combination at work when it comes to this disease. The question is, What aspect of Westernization triggers Type 2 diabetes in these regions? "Western" means many things, including a higher-fat diet, less physical activity, and access to medical care (which means populations are living longer).

In addition, what role does earlier screening and better detection of Type 2 diabetes play in the global increase of the disease? As one doctor put it, "When you don't look for it, you don't find it." More and more evidence points to the fact that Type 2 diabetes has been around for a long time.

What are the odds?

Type 2 diabetes is caused by multiple factors. The odds of developing it relate to a genetic predisposition interacting with environmental factors. Obesity, excess calories, deficient calorie expenditure, and aging can all lead to insulin resistance. If you remove the environmental risks, however, you can probably modify the risk of Type 2 diabetes.

Who are you?

As discussed earlier, aboriginal cultures, such as Native Americans, develop Type 2 diabetes at far higher rates than other North Americans. On some reservations, Type 2 diabetes is present in 70 percent of the adult population. (See the separate section, Diabetes and Native Americans, on page 16.)

Approximately 15 percent of African North American adults have Type 2 diabetes, while about 20 percent of all North American Hispanics have Type 2 diabetes.

The "thrifty gene" is thought to be responsible for the higher rates of Type 2 diabetes in the Native and African North American populations. The more recently your culture has lived indigenously or nomadically (that is, living off the land and eating seasonally), the more efficient your metabolism is. Unfortunately, it is also more sensitive to nutrient excess. If you're a Native North American, only about one hundred years have passed since your ancestors lived indigenously. This is an exceedingly short amount of time for thousands of years of hunter-gatherer genes to adjust to a Western diet. If you're African North American, your ancestors haven't lived here any longer than about four hundred years; prior to that they were living a tribal, nomadic lifestyle. Again, four hundred years is *not* a long time.

As for Hispanic or other immigrant populations, many come from families who have spent generations in poverty. Their metabolisms adjusted to long periods of famine, and are often overloaded by Western foods. The other problem is low economic levels in North America. Native, African, and Hispanic populations tend to have much lower incomes, and are therefore eating lower-quality food, which, combined with the "thrifty gene," can trigger Type 2 diabetes.

What about Eastern populations?

Type 2 diabetes seems to occur in Southeast Asian populations at Western rates even when the diet is Eastern. East Indians, in particular, have very high rates of heart disease. In fact, India has the largest Type 2 population in the world. Urbanization is cited as a major factor.

Multiracial North Americans

Your risk of developing Type 2 diabetes depends on your mix of genes and your current and past lifestyle and diet. If you are part Native American and part European, for example, you will probably need to be more conscientious about your diet than if you were part Asian and part European. Studying your family tree and family history of Type 2 diabetes is the best way to assess your odds and make the necessary changes in your own diet and lifestyle to lower them.

Other medical conditions

There are certain diseases, such as Prader-Willi, Down's syndrome, Turner's syndrome, Cushing's disease, or acromegaly (large face, long arms and hands) that can lead to diabetes in the long term. In this case, diabetes is a presenting feature of the disorder. Many diseases occur together; this is another example.

Diabetes and Native Americans

The terms *aboriginal* or *native people* refer to those whose ancestors are indigenous to North America. Native Americans (including American Indians, Alaskan Natives, and Pacific Islanders) comprise more than 545 Indian tribes, bands, pueblos, and villages. These communities, for the most part, have tribal governments organized under the Indian Reorganization Act, Oklahoma Indian Welfare Act, and Alaska Native Act, and have adopted written constitutions approved by the Secretary of the Interior. Many of these tribes, however, operate traditional governments based on tribal customs rather than written constitutions.

According to conservative estimates, diabetes is four to eight times more common in aboriginal cultures than in the general population. For example, the Pima Indians on the Gila River Reservation have the highest rates of diabetes in the world. For Pacific Islanders (Native Hawaiians), the death rate from diabetes is 222 percent higher than that of the general population. On many reservations, *more than 75 percent of residents older than thirty-five have diabetes,* up from 50 percent in 1989, while in some Native American communities, up to half of *all* adults have diabetes. Because the symptoms of diabetes can be vague and develop slowly, many aboriginal people have the disease but do not realize it. For every known case of diabetes among aboriginal people, at least one goes undiagnosed. And when you consider that Type 2 diabetes was not a recognized health problem in this community until the 1940s, this is a staggering increase.

Native Americans also suffer more end-stage renal disease (ESRD), a common complication of diabetes (discussed in chapter 9) than the general population. For example, in Navajo communities, end-stage renal disease from diabetes is ten times higher than that of the general U.S. population.

Two hundred years is an exceedingly short amount of time for our immune systems and metabolisms to adjust to new lifestyles. Aboriginal people have not built up an immunity to "overnutrition" the way many nonnative North Americans have. Europeans, for the most part, haven't lived nomadically for thousands of years, and have therefore developed metabolisms that can adjust to sedentary lifestyles in response to urbanized living.

This is why aboriginal people have an inherited tendency toward diabetes. Because aboriginal people lived seasonally, on indigenous diets, for so many centuries, their bodies still function as though they were living in precolonial North America.

Prior to contact with Europeans, North America's aboriginal people were leading the kind of healthy lifestyle that may ultimately prevent diabetes from developing in the first place. At that time, aboriginal people enjoyed good health: infections were rare, fevers were unheard of, and mental, emotional, and physical vigor was the norm. Before being exposed to European food, aboriginal people lived on an ideal diet of seasonal foods native to North America.

As European ships arrived in North America, they brought with them a smorgasbord of strange and new bacteria and viruses, causing terrible epidemics among indigenous populations. In a sense, the result was genocide: Native Americans died by the thousands during the eighteenth and nineteenth centuries.

Thus began an incredible transformation: Healthy people became more and more unhealthy as Europeans continued to emigrate to North America. Sources of food and clothing from the land diminished, while centuries of a traditional economy dissolved. Worst of all, once mobile, active people were confined to small plots of land with limited natural resources and poor sanitation. *Fit people became unfit.*

The impact of pollution

As waters became polluted and environmental raping of resources continued, the diseases changed from infectious to chronic. "Country food," traditional food indigenous to North America, such as wild game, fish, root vegetables, fruit, and whale meat and blubber (protective foods now known to contain omega-3 oils, linked to low levels of heart disease and cholesterol) became inherently unavailable, forcing aboriginal people to eat the Europeans' processed, refined foods. Cut off from their habitat and exposed to infections, alcohol, and overprocessed foods high in fat and sugar, aboriginal people developed poor eating habits and became obese and inactive. As noted, the main risk factors for Type 2 diabetes are obesity, poor eating habits, and physical inactivity.

Cash crops further deteriorated indigenous food supplies. By the early twentieth century, chemical agriculture and factory farming revolutionized food production, increasing the detrimental effect on the traditional aboriginal diet.

Today's eating habits, coupled with a sedentary lifestyle, are shown not only to extend the incidence of obesity and hence, diabetes, but to increase blood pressure and exacerbate dental problems. Aboriginal people also suffer from heart disease, cancer, and infant morbidity and mortality more frequently than the general population.

Impaired Glucose Tolerance (IGT)

Prior to September 1998, many people with Type 2 diabetes were told they had *impaired glucose tolerance* (IGT), more widely known as "borderline diabetes." For the record, there is no such thing as borderline diabetes. In light of new guidelines announced in 1998, however, many people once diagnosed with IGT will now be diagnosed with diabetes.

IGT was what many doctors referred to as the "gray zone" between normal blood sugar levels and full-blown diabetes. Normal fasting blood sugar levels (before you've eaten) are between 60 milligrams per deciliter (mg/dl) and 90 mg/dl or, in the metric system, 3 to 5 millimoles per liter—mmol/L. (To convert "mg/dl" to "mmol/L," simply divide by 18; you may need to know this when traveling in Canada or Europe.)

In the past, three fasting blood glucose levels between 90 mg/dl (5 mmol/L) and 140 mg/dl (7.8 mmol/L) meant that you had IGT. A fasting blood glucose level over 140 mg/dl (7.8 mmol/L) or a random (any time of day) blood glucose level greater than 200 mg/dl (or 11.1 mmol/L) meant that you had diabetes.

But that's all changed. Today, anyone with a fasting blood sugar level higher than 126 mg/dl (7.0 mmol/L) is considered to be in the diabetic range, and is officially diagnosed with Type 2 diabetes. A new term, *impaired fasting glucose* (IFG), has also been introduced, which refers to blood glucose levels between 110 mg/dl and less than 126 mg/dl (6.1 mmol/L and 6.9 mmol/L). The term *IGT* is now used only when describing people who have a blood glucose level between 140 mg/dl and 200 mg/dl (7. 8 and 11.1 mmol/L) *two hours after an oral glucose tolerance test.* Take a look at Table 1.1 for more details.

It's also possible to have abnormally low blood glucose levels, called *hypoglycemia* (discussed in detail further on).

Pancreatitis

Diabetes can be caused by a condition known as pancreatitis, which means inflammation of the pancreas. This occurs when the pancreas's digestive enzymes turn on you and attack your own pancreas. This can cause the gland to bleed, as well as cause serious tissue damage, infection, and cysts. (Other organs, such as your heart, lungs, and kidneys can be affected in severe cases.) Pancreatitis is most often chronic, caused by years of alcohol abuse. In fact, 90 percent of all chronic pancreatitis affects men between the ages of thirty and forty. In rare cases, chronic pancreatitis is inherited, but experts are not sure why. People with chronic pancreatitis tend to have three main symptoms: pain, weight loss (due to poor food absorption and digestion), and diabetes (the type depends on how much damage was done to your islet, or insulin-producing cells).

The treatment is to first stop drinking. Then you will need to be managed like any other diabetes patient: blood glucose monitoring, meal planning, and possibly, insulin injections.

Table 1.1 Definitions of Diabetes

Prior to September 1998, what constituted diabetes, impaired glucose tolerance (IGT), or normal blood sugar? (> means "greater than"; < means "less than.")

	Normal	**IGT**	**Diabetes**
Fasting	< 140 mg/dl (7.8)	< 140 mg/dl (7.8)	> 140 mg/dl (7.8)
2 hours after meals	< 200 mg/dl (7.8)	200 mg/dl (7.8 – < 11.1)	200 mg/dl (≥ 11.1)

Today, new guidelines stipulate the following:

	Normal	**IFG***	**Diabetes**
Fasting	<110mg/dl (6.1 mmol/L)	>110 mg/dl and <126 mg/dl (>6.1 mmol/L and < 7.0mmol/L)	>126 mg/dl (7.0)

2 hours after an oral glucose tolerance test

	Normal	**IGT†**	**Diabetes**
	< 140 mg/dl (7.8 mmol/L)	>140 mg/dl and < 200 mg/dl (>7.8 mmol/L – < 11.1mmol/L)	> 200 mg/dl (11.1 mmol/L)

*IFG stands for impaired fasting glucose.
†IGT stands for impaired glucose tolerance, referring to test results two hours after an oral glucose tolerance test.

"Side-Effect Diabetes"

This is a term I've coined to describe what's known as *secondary diabetes.* This occurs when your diabetes is a *side effect* of a particular drug or surgical procedure.

A number of prescription medications, including steroids, can raise your blood sugar levels, affecting the results of a blood sugar test. Make sure you tell your doctor about all medications you're on prior to having your blood sugar checked.

If you've had your pancreas removed (a pancreatectomy), diabetes will definitely develop. It may also develop if you've experienced one of the following:

- severe injury to your pancreas
- severe pancreatitis (see above)
- liver disease
- iron overload
- brain damage

WHEN YOUR DOCTOR SAYS "YOU HAVE DIABETES"

If you have been diagnosed with diabetes, the good news is that you are living at a time when self-managing diabetes has never been easier. There are not only brand-new treatment options available, but dozens of upgraded products to make diabetes a lot easier to monitor. The bad news is that only *you* can manage your diabetes. This is one of those diseases that can't be regulated by only your doctor. You have to take charge, while your doctor supervises. For this reason, being diagnosed with diabetes may feel like being pushed out of an airplane without a parachute. Think of this section as basic training. It will tell you what you need to know in order to plan for a safe landing.

Signs and Symptoms

By now you should have a pretty good idea of your risk profile for Type 2 diabetes, but knowing the signs of Type 2 diabetes is crucial. If you have any of the symptoms listed below, request to be screened for Type 2 diabetes.

- Weight gain. When you're not using your insulin properly, you may suffer from excess insulin, which can increase your appetite. This is a classic Type 2 symptom.
- Blurred vision or any change in sight. Often, there is a feeling that your prescription eyewear is "weak."
- Drowsiness or *extreme* fatigue at times when you shouldn't be drowsy or tired.
- Frequent infections that are slow to heal. (Women should be on alert for recurring vaginal yeast infections or vaginitis, or

vaginal inflammation, characterized by itching and/or foul-smelling discharge.)
- Tingling or numbness in the hands and feet.
- Gum disease. High blood sugar affects the blood vessels in your mouth, causing inflamed gums; the sugar content can also affect your saliva, causing cavities in your teeth.

Diabetes experts also state that the following may be signs of Type 2 diabetes:

- Irregular periods, such as changes in cycle length or flow (this could be a sign of menopause as well, discussed in chapter 5)
- Depression, which could be a symptom of either low or high blood sugar
- Headaches (from hypoglycemia)
- Insomnia and/or nightmares (from hypoglycemia)
- Spots on the shin (known as necrobiosis diabeticorum)
- Decaying toenails
- Muscle pains or aches after exercise (high blood sugar can increase lactic acid buildup, causing pain that prevents you from continuing to exercise)

You may also have diabetes if your doctor has diagnosed you with one or more of the following:

- High cholesterol
- High blood pressure
- Anemia
- Cataracts
- Salivary-gland stones

What Kind of Diabetes Do I Have?

As discussed at the beginning of this chapter, there are several types of diabetes, and even several names for the one disease we now call "Type 2 diabetes," the most common form of diabetes. Type 2 diabetes is a genetic disease that is triggered by environmental factors, such as obesity or a sedentary lifestyle. Lean, fit, healthy people who are genetically predisposed to Type 2 diabetes can still develop it, but they may also prevent the disease by modifying one or more environmental factors, discussed earlier. Type 2 diabetes is sometimes referred to as a disease of insulin resistance, which can be confusing. In fact, this is simply a description of the physiology of Type 2 diabetes.

Type 1 diabetes, explained at the beginning of this chapter, is not likely to be your diagnosis. If it is, put down this book right now and find another book on Type 1 diabetes. While some of the issues I discuss in this book will be relevant, Type 1 diabetes, once known as insulin-dependent diabetes (IDDM), is a completely different disease than Type 2 diabetes—the focus of *this* book.

There are two other kinds of diabetes, too. Diabetes can be a side effect of something else, such as pancreatic surgery (see above). Diabetes can also develop during pregnancy, known as *gestational diabetes mellitis* (GDM), which occurs between the twenty-fourth and twenty-eighth week of pregnancy (see chapter 4).

The meaning of "insulin resistance"

It wasn't until the 1960s that researchers discovered that most people with Type 2 diabetes suffered from a *resistance* to insulin, not necessarily a lack of insulin. In fact, Type 2 diabetes is usually a disease of insulin resistance rather than "no insulin." The disease causes your body to overproduce insulin. Too much insulin leads to a decrease in insulin-receptor sites, small "keyholes" on the surface of your insulin-producing cells, into which insulin (the "key") fits. Sometimes there are simply not enough receptor sites; other times, something is wrong with the connection or link between the key and keyhole.

At the beginning of this chapter, I explain the relationship between insulin and glucose, comparing insulin to a courier knocking on the cell's door with a message to "let sugar in."

Again, insulin resistance occurs when there is no answer at the door. The insulin is there; the cell isn't responding to it. The result is diabetes—too much sugar in the blood. This causes all the classic symptoms of diabetes (see above), which may have led your doctor to diagnose diabetes or screen you for the disease.

Some experts believe that insulin resistance actually causes obesity, which is why obesity is such a risk factor. When the body uses insulin properly, it not only lowers blood sugar but assists in the distribution of fat and protein. Therefore, when your body doesn't use insulin properly, obesity can be the by-product. (Refer to chapter 2 for a thorough discussion of women, obesity, and diabetes.) By the time you're diagnosed with Type 2 diabetes, it may be that you have inadequate or unreliable insulin secretion from your pancreatic beta cells.

Although Type 2 diabetes is usually a disease of insulin resistance, it is sometimes caused by a liver gone awry. In this scenario, the liver actually takes it on itself to make glucose, increasing your blood sugar levels. This is often the case in alcoholics.

Having Type 2 diabetes doesn't mean only that you have high blood sugar. This condition can cause other problems, such as hypertension (high blood pressure), high cholesterol, and insulin resistance in your muscles and liver. So even if you manage to get your blood sugar levels under control, you still may need to be treated for these other conditions, which can be greatly alleviated through diet and exercise. You don't have to have any symptoms, however, to be diagnosed with Type 2 diabetes.

When you require insulin

Insulin resistance, characterized by the body's inability to use insulin, sometimes leads to a condition in which the pancreas stops making insulin altogether. The cells' resistance to insulin causes the pancreas to work harder, resulting in too much insulin in the system (hyperinsulinemia) until it's just plumb tuckered out, as the saying goes. Your pancreas is making the insulin and knocking on the door, but the cells aren't answering. Your pancreas will eventually say, "Okay, fine! I'll shut down production since you obviously aren't using what I'm making."

But this isn't always the reason that you need insulin. Often the problem is that your body becomes increasingly more resistant to the insulin your pancreas is producing. This is sometimes exacerbated by medications or the disease over time. Controlling your blood sugar becomes harder and harder, until ultimately, you need to inject insulin.

Type 2 diabetes can also become an insulin-requiring disease if you go for long periods with high blood sugar levels. In this case, sugar toxicity occurs; the sugar poisons the cells of the body, including the insulin-producing cells in the pancreas, destroying them forever. The result is no insulin and hence, insulin-requiring Type 2 diabetes. This is not the same thing as insulin-dependent diabetes, or Type 1 diabetes, which is a completely different autoimmune disease.

If you have been told that you need insulin, and you are over age forty-five, or you were told you had impaired glucose tolerance (see page 19) and now need insulin, this is what probably happened to you.

Please remember that there is no such thing as "borderline diabetes" or a "touch of diabetes." You either have diabetes or you don't. Again, the guidelines for diagnosing diabetes are changing, and what was once clinically known as impaired glucose tolerance (IGT) may soon simply be called "diabetes."

Managing Type 2 Diabetes

Your goal in managing Type 2 diabetes is to control your blood sugar levels and weight through diet and exercise, and to prevent long-term complications of your disease. One of the most important Type 1 diabetes research projects ever undertaken is the

Diabetes Control and Complications Trial (DCCT). This trial proved beyond a doubt that when people with Type 1 diabetes kept their blood sugar levels as normal as possible, as often as possible, they could dramatically reduce the odds of developing small-blood vessel diseases related to diabetes, such as kidney disease, eye problems, and nerve disease, all discussed in chapter 9.

More recently, the results of a landmark British study, the United Kingdom Prospective Diabetes Study (UKPDS), showed that frequent blood sugar testing also helped reduce eye, kidney, and nerve damage in people with diabetes. See chapter 9 for more details.

Nevertheless, since Type 2 diabetes is associated more with cardiovascular complications, and the UKPDS did not show a direct link between frequent blood sugar testing and fewer heart attacks and strokes, two management philosophies have emerged regarding frequent self-testing of blood sugar and Type 2 diabetes.

Many physicians feel that frequent self-testing of blood sugar in Type 2 diabetes could complicate Type 2 diabetes management. In other words, it interferes with more crucial goals, such as getting your diet under control and incorporating exercise into your routine. Other physicians feel that the more involved you become in managing your blood sugar, the better off you'll be in the long run, and therefore, they support frequent self-testing of blood sugar in their Type 2 patients. The American Diabetes Association has long recommended that people with Type 2 diabetes self-test their blood sugar. In fact, in a newly diagnosed person with Type 2 diabetes, frequent daily testing will show *individual patterns* of glucose rises and dips. This information may help your health care team tailor your meal plans, exercise routines, and medication regimens. And if you do have to take insulin in the future, you will need to get into the habit of testing your own blood sugar anyway. (Of course, by getting your diet under control, you may avoid requiring insulin.)

WHEN TO TEST YOUR BLOOD SUGAR

In the days when diabetes patients went to their doctors' offices for blood sugar testing, they were usually tested first thing in the morning before eating (called a fasting blood sugar level) or immediately after eating (known as a postprandial or postmeal blood sugar level). It was believed that if either the fasting or postprandial levels were normal, the patient was stable. This is now known to be *completely false*. In fact, your blood sugar levels can bounce around all day long. Because your blood sugar is constantly changing, a blood sugar test in a doctor's office is relatively useless; it measures what your blood sugar is only for that nanosecond. In other words, what your blood sugar is at 2:15 P.M. is not what it might be at 3:05 P.M.

It makes the most sense to test yourself before each meal, so you know what your levels are before you eat anything, as well as about two hours after meals. Immediately after eating, everybody's blood sugar is high, so this is not the ideal time for testing. In a person without diabetes, blood sugar levels will drop about two hours after eating, in response to the natural insulin the body makes. Similarly, test yourself two hours after eating to make sure that you are able to "mimic" a normal blood sugar pattern. Ideally, this translates into at least four blood tests daily:

- When you wake up
- After breakfast/before lunch (two hours after breakfast)
- After lunch/before dinner (two hours after lunch)
- After dinner/at bedtime (two hours after dinner)

The most revealing information about your blood sugar control is in the answers to the following questions:

1. What is your blood sugar level as soon as you wake up? (It should be at its lowest point.)
2. What is your blood sugar level two hours *after* a meal? (It should be much lower two hours after eating than one hour after eating.)
3. What is your blood sugar level when you feel ill? (You need to avoid dipping too low or high since your routine is changing.)

Variations on the theme

- Test yourself four times a day (times indicated above) two to three times a week, and then test yourself two times a day (before breakfast and before bedtime) for the remainder of the week.

- Test yourself twice a day three to four days a week in a rotating pattern (before breakfast and dinner one day; before lunch and bedtime the next).
- Test yourself once a day every day, but rotate your pattern (day 1 before breakfast; day 2 after dinner; day 3 before bedtime, and so on).
- Test yourself four times a day (as indicated above) two days a month.

Regardless of your doctor's approach to self-testing blood sugar, the DCCT and UKPDS have caused an explosion in easy-to-use home blood sugar monitors, potentially eliminating that weekly trip to the doctor. Many people with Type 2 diabetes can now check their own blood sugar at home. And there's certainly no harm in testing your sugar frequently if you want to do so.

What about my weight?

Statistics suggest that about 80 percent of people with Type 2 diabetes weigh 20 percent more than their ideal weight, the technical definition of "obese." If you begin a meal-planning program—which means eating the right combination and amount of food—with a diabetes educator and dietitian, as well as incorporate exercise into your routine, you'll lose weight. Weight loss can greatly improve your body's ability to use insulin. There is no need to start a crash diet or panic about your weight, however. Meal planning *is* managing your diabetes. Weight loss will become a fringe benefit. As you lose weight, your blood sugar levels will drop, which may affect any diabetes medication you're on. For example, if you're taking pills that stimulate your body to make insulin, weight loss without adjusting your dosage may result in hypoglycemia (low blood sugar), discussed further on. Weight loss will also decrease the odds of developing complications from diabetes, such as heart disease. Losing weight through meal planning, however, is not as easy as it sounds, nor is exercising. See chapter 2 for a thorough discussion of women and weight issues, and chapter 6 for information on exercise.

Essentially, the point of meal planning and exercise is to eliminate your diabetes symptoms and to remain as symptom free as possible. Exercise makes insulin much more available to your cells, while your muscles use sugar as fuel.

High blood sugar (hyperglycemia)

If you can't seem to keep your fasting blood sugar levels below 126 mg/dl (7.0 mmol/L), you are probably a candidate for an antidiabetic pill or an oral hypoglycemic pill, discussed in chapter 8. Early signs of high blood sugar are extreme thirst, dry and flushed skin, mood swings, or unusual fatigue. But many people notice no symptoms at all.

Common reasons for a change in blood sugar levels include the following:

- Overeating or eating more than usual
- A change in exercise routine
- Missing a medication dose or an insulin shot (if you're taking insulin)
- An out-of-the-ordinary event (illness, stress, upset, excitement)
- A sudden mood change (extreme fright, anger, or sadness)
- Pregnancy (see chapter 4)

In response to unusual strains or stress, your body taps into its stored glucose supplies for extra energy. This will raise your blood sugar level as more glucose than usual is released into your system. Whether you're fighting off a flu or fighting with your mother, digesting the food you ate at that all-you-can-eat buffet or running away from a grizzly bear, your body will try to give you the extra boost of energy you need to get through your immediate stress.

Blood sugar levels also naturally rise when you're ill. In the event of a cold, fever, flu, or injury, you'll need to adjust your routine to accommodate high blood sugar levels, especially if vomiting or diarrhea is occurring. In some cases, you may need to go on insulin temporarily. When you're ill and you have Type 2 diabetes, it's crucial to contact your doctor.

One thing you don't need to worry about, however, is forming ketones (ketone bodies), poisonous chemicals the body manufactures in desperation as a source of energy when no glucose is available for this purpose. In people with Type 1 diabetes, high ketones along with high blood sugar cause *diabetic ketoacidosis* (DKA), which is an emergency situation. Signs of DKA include frequent urination (polyuria), excessive thirst (polydipsia), excessive hunger (polyphagia), and a fruity smell to the breath. But people with Type 2 diabetes do *not* form ketones. That's because the cells never think they are "starving" since insulin still comes to knock at the door, and the liver continues to make glucose.

Monitoring Your Performance

If you want to test your own blood sugar, discuss with your health care practitioner how frequently to do so. Use Table 1.1 as a general guideline for testing times. While there is still no conclusive proof that frequent blood sugar testing reduces cardiovascular complications for people with Type 2 diabetes, testing at home will certainly eliminate some of your trips to the doctor or lab. And that's less stress for you. The only equipment you need for self-testing blood sugar is a good glucose meter. There are several on the market; your doctor, pharmacist, or diabetes educator can recommend the right brand for you. When you get your glucose monitor, experts suggest you compare your results to one regular laboratory test, to make sure you've purchased a reliable and accurate machine.

A brief history of blood sugar testing

Twenty years ago, the only way you could test your blood sugar level yourself was by testing your urine for sugar, which meant that you had reached your renal threshold (kidney limit), where sugar spilled into your urine. The limitation of urine testing is that one can only test for *really* high blood sugar levels, over 200 mg/dl (11 mmol/L). Urine testing is also useless for checking low blood sugar. Far more accurate home blood sugar testing became available with the development of glucose meters in 1982.

Choosing and using your glucose meter

As in the computer industry, glucose meter manufacturers tend to come out with technological upgrades every year. In fact, you can now purchase systems that download the time, date, and blood sugar values for the last 125 glucose tests right onto your personal computer. This information can help you gauge whether your diet and exercise routine is working, or whether you need to adjust your medications or insulin. Of course, new upgrades cost money, but if you can't afford the "Pentium," a reliable "486" is fine. *All* glucose monitors will provide

- a battery-powered, pocket-sized device
- an LED screen (that is, a calculatorlike screen)
- accurate results in thirty to sixty seconds
- the date and time of your test result
- a recall memory of at least your last ten readings
- at least a one-year warranty
- the opportunity to upgrade
- a 1-800 customer service hotline
- mailings and giveaways every so often
- a few free lancets ("finger-pricker thingies") with your purchase; you may have to separately buy what's known as a lancing device, a sort of Pez dispenser for your lancets. (Eventually, you'll run out of lancets and have to buy those, too.)

No matter which glucose meter you choose, these instructions can serve as a general guideline:

- Wash your hands with an antibacterial soap.
- Pierce your finger on the side rather than the top, and obtain a "hanging" drop of blood (some newer devices "suck out" your blood for you).
- Smear or blot your drop of blood onto a plastic strip that looks like a strip of tape without the sticky side. (Whether you smear or wipe depends on your glucose meter.)
- Turn on your glucose meter and place the strip into the machine.
- The results will show up on the calculatorlike screen.
- Record these results in a logbook. *Hint: A good result before meals ranges from 72 to 126 mg/dl (4 to 7 mmol/L); a good result after meals ranges from 90 to 180 mg/dl (5 to 10 mmol/L).*

Factors that can taint your results

Most people are not testing their blood sugar under squeaky-clean laboratory conditions. The following outside factors may interfere with your meter's performance.

- *Other medications you're taking.* Studies show that some meters can be inaccurate if you're taking acetaminophen, salicylate, ascorbic acid, dopamine, or levodopa. As a rule, if you're taking any medications, check with your doctor, pharmacist, and glucose meter manufacturer (call the 1-800 number) about whether your medications can affect the meter's accuracy.
- *Humidity.* The worst place to keep your meter and strips is in the bathroom, where humidity can ruin your strips unless they're individually wrapped in foil. Keep your strips in a sealed container away from extreme temperatures. Don't store your meter and strips, for example, in a hot glove compartment. Don't keep them in the freezer, either.
- *Bright light.* Ever tried to use a calculator or portable computer in bright sunlight? It's not possible because the light interferes with the screen. Some meters are photometric,

which means they are affected by bright light. If you plan to test in sunlight, get a biosenser meter that is unaffected by bright light (there are several).

- *Touching the test strip.* Many glucose meters come with test strips that cannot be touched with your fingers or a second drop of blood. If you're all thumbs, purchase a meter that is unaffected by touch and/or allows a second drop of blood.
- *Wet hands.* Before you test, thoroughly dry your hands. Water can dilute your blood sample.
- *Motion.* It's always best to test yourself when you're standing still. Testing on planes, trains, automobiles, buses, and subways may affect your results, depending on the brand of glucose meter.
- *Dirt, lint, and blood.* Particles of dirt, lint, and old blood can sometimes affect the accuracy of a meter, depending on the brand. Make sure you clean the meter regularly (follow the manufacturer's cleaning directions) to remove buildup. Make sure you change your batteries, too! There are meters on the market that do not require cleaning and are unaffected by dirt, but they may cost a little more.

Glycosylated Hemoglobin

The most detailed blood sugar test cannot be done at home yet. This is a blood test that checks for glycosylated hemoglobin (glucose attached to the protein in your red blood cells), known as *glycohemoglobin* or HbA$_{1c}$ levels. This test can tell you how well your blood sugar has been controlled over a period of two to three months by showing what percentage of it is too high. I compare this test to cars with special gas tank meters that can tell you what percentage of your last quarter tank is left before you need to refuel. That information is far more telling than just "F," "½," "¼," and "E." It's recommended that you get an HbA$_{1c}$ test every three months. This test is discussed in more detail in chapter 8.

Managing Low Blood Sugar

When you're diagnosed with Type 2 diabetes, whether your treatment revolves around lifestyle modification, oral hypoglycemics, or insulin therapy, you may experience an episode of low blood sugar. This is clinically known as *hypoglycemia.* Hypoglycemia can sometimes come on suddenly, particularly overnight. If left untreated, hypoglycemia can also result in coma, brain damage, and death. Hypoglycemia is considered the official cause of death in about 5 percent of the Type 1 population. In the past, hypoglycemia was a more common problem among people with Type 1 diabetes. But since 40 to 50 percent of all people with Type 2 diabetes will eventually graduate to insulin therapy, the incidence of hypoglycemia has increased by 300 percent in this group. Moreover, hypoglycemia is a common side effect of oral hypoglycemic pills, the medication the majority of people with Type 2 diabetes take when they are first diagnosed.

Any blood sugar reading below 70 mg/dl (3.8 mmol/L) is considered too low. A hypoglycemic episode is characterized by two stages: the warning stage and what I call the *actual* hypoglycemic episode. The warning stage occurs when your blood sugar levels *begin* to drop, and can occur as early as a blood sugar reading of 108 mg/dl (6 mmol/L), in people with typically higher than normal blood sugar levels. When your blood sugar drops to below 55 mg/dl (or 3 mmol/L) you are *officially* hypoglycemic.

During the warning stage, your body responds by pumping adrenaline into your bloodstream. This causes symptoms such as trembling, irritability, hunger, and weakness, some of which mimic drunkenness. The irritability can simulate the rantings of someone who is drunk, while the weakness and shakiness can lead to the lack of coordination seen in someone who is drunk. For this reason, it's crucial that you carry a card or wear a bracelet that identifies you as having diabetes (see Table 1.2). Your liver will also release any glucose it has stored for you; but if it doesn't have enough glucose to get you back to normal, there won't be

Table 1.2 Your Diabetes ID Card

If you don't have the following information already, photocopy this section and put it in an obvious place in your wallet or on your person.

I have diabetes. If I am unconscious or if my behavior appears unusual, it may be related to my diabetes or my treatment. I am not drunk. If I can swallow, give me sugar in the form of fruit juice, a sweet soft drink, candies, or table sugar. Phone my doctor or the hospital listed below. Or phone 911 if I am unconscious.

Name _____

Address _____

Phone Number _____

Chief Contact _____ Relationship _____

My doctor's name is: _____

He or she can be reached at (phone number): _____

after hours _____ My hospital: _____

My blood type is: [ ] A [ ] B [ ] AB [ ] O [ ] Rh+ [ ] Rh–

I wear: [ ] lens implants   [ ] dentures   [ ] contact lenses

          [ ] an artificial joint   [ ] a pacemaker

I'm allergic to: _____

My Health Card/Insurance Number is: _____

My Group Insurance Number is: _____

Source: Adapted from Health Record for People with Diabetes, 1996, McNeil Consumer Products Company.

enough glucose for your brain to function properly and you will feel confused, irritable, or aggressive.

Once your blood sugar is 55 mg/dl (3 mmol/L) and falling, you'll experience a rapid heartbeat, trembling, and sweating. As the levels become lower, your pupils will begin to dilate, and you will begin to lose consciousness, and may experience a seizure. No one with diabetes is immune to hypoglycemia; it can occur in someone with long-standing diabetes or in someone newly diagnosed. The important thing is to be alert to the warning signs, be prepared, and try to avoid future episodes.

Who's at risk?

Because hypoglycemia can be the result of too high an insulin dose, it is often called insulin shock (or insulin reaction). This is a misleading term, however, because it implies that only people who take insulin can become hypoglycemic. For the record, all people with Type 1 or Type 2 diabetes can become hypoglycemic. If you are taking more than one insulin injection a day, you are at greater risk of developing hypoglycemia. But hypoglycemia can be triggered just as easily by

- delaying or missing a meal or snack (see chapter 7)
- drinking alcohol (see chapter 7)
- exercising too long or strong (without compensating with extra food) (see chapter 6)
- taking too high a dose of an oral hypoglycemic agent (this can happen if you lose weight but are not put on a lower dose of your pill)

If you're taking pills

Oral hypoglycemic agents (OHAs) can certainly cause hypoglycemia or low blood sugar. See chapter 8 for more details on the side effects of OHAs.

Recognizing the symptoms

If you can begin to recognize the warning signs of hypoglycemia, you may be able to stabilize your blood sugar before you lose consciousness. Watch out for the adrenaline symptoms; initially you will be hungry and headachy, then sweaty, nervous, and dizzy. Those who live with or spend a lot of time with you should learn to notice sudden mood changes (usually extreme irritabil-ity, "drunklike" aggression and confusion) as a warning that you are "low." Whether you notice your own mood changes or not, you will feel suddenly unwell. By simply asking yourself, "Why is this happening?" you should be able to remember that it's a warning that your blood sugar is low, and reach for your snack pack (see below). Not everyone experiences the same warning symptoms, but here are some signs to watch for:

- pounding, racing heart
- breathing fast
- skin turning white
- sweating (cold sweat in big drops)
- trembling, tremors or shaking
- goose bumps or pale, cool skin
- extreme hunger pangs
- light-headedness (feeling dizzy or that the room is spinning)
- nervousness, extreme irritability, or a sudden mood change
- confusion
- feeling weak or faint
- headache
- vision changes (seeing double or blurry vision)

Some people will experience no symptoms at all. If you've had a hypoglycemic episode without any warning symptoms, it's important for you to eat regularly, and to test your blood sugar. If you're experiencing frequent hypoglycemic episodes, diabetes educators recommend that by keeping your sugar above normal, you can prevent low blood sugar. In some cases of long-standing diabetes and repeated hypoglycemic episodes, experts note that the warning symptoms may not always occur. It's believed that in some people, the body eventually loses its ability to detect hypo-glycemia and send adrenaline. Furthermore, if you've switched from animal to human insulin, warning symptoms may not be as pronounced.

Treating low blood sugar

If you start to feel symptoms of hypoglycemia, stop what you're doing (especially if it's active) and have some sugar. Next, test your blood sugar. Regular food will usually do the trick. If your blood sugar is below 63 mg/dl (3.5 mmol/L), ingest some glucose. Real fruit juice *is* better when your blood sugar is low. The best way to get your levels back up to normal is to ingest simple sugar; that is, sugar that gets into your bloodstream fast. Half a cup of any fruit juice or one-third of a can of a sugary soft drink is a good source of simple sugar. Artificially sweetened soft drinks are useless. *It must have real sugar.* If you don't have fruit juice or soft drinks handy, here are some other sources high in simple sugar:

- two to three tablets of commercial dextrose, sold in pharmacies. If you're taking acarbose (see chapter 8) or combining it with an oral hypoglycemic agent or insulin (see chapter 8), the only sugar you can have is dextrose, due to the rate of absorption.
- three to five hard candies (that's equal to about six Life Savers)
- 2 teaspoons of white or brown sugar (or two sugar cubes)
- 1 tablespoon of honey

Once you've ingested enough simple sugar, your hypo-glycemic symptoms should disappear within ten to fifteen minutes. Test your blood sugar ten minutes after having your sugar to see if your blood sugar levels are coming back up. If your symptoms don't go away, ingest more simple sugars until they do.

If you've had a close call to the point where you experienced adrenaline symptoms, be sure to have a snack or meal as soon as possible. If your next meal or snack is more than an hour away, eat half a sandwich or some cheese and crackers. This will ensure that your blood sugar levels don't fall again. Then check your blood sugar after you eat to make sure your levels are where they should be. Try to investigate the cause of your episode by asking yourself whether your routine has varied in any way (for example, missed or delayed meals).

Glucagon

Most people will be able to treat their low blood sugar without becoming unconscious. But on rare occasions, it can happen. And if that's the case, it's too late for juice, soft drinks, or any other kind of sugar. That's where something known as a glucagon kit comes in. Ask your doctor or pharmacist about purchasing such a kit, which comes with complete instructions.

Recipes for prevention

The recipe for preventing hypoglycemia or low blood sugar is the same one for preventing high blood sugar: frequent blood sugar monitoring if your doctor feels it's necessary, following your meal plan (chapter 7), following an exercise plan (chapter 6), and taking your medication as prescribed (chapter 8). Any changes in your routine, diet, exercise habits, or medication dosages should be followed up by a period of very close blood sugar monitoring until your new routine is established.

Frequent episodes of hypoglycemia may also be a sign that your body is changing; you may be losing weight, thanks to those lifestyle changes you've made, and the dosage of pills that were prescribed to you when you weighed 190 may be too high now that you're down to 145. Or, you may be taking too high an insulin dose.

Anybody with Type 1 or Type 2 diabetes should have a snack pack with them for emergencies or for unplanned physical activity. The pack should contain

- juice (two to three boxes or cans);
- sweet soft drinks—sweetened with real sugar, not sugar substitutes (two cans);
- a bag of hard candies;
- some protein and carbohydrates (packaged cheese/crackers);
- granola bars (great for after exercise); and
- a card that says "I have diabetes" (see Table 1.2).

When you're diagnosed with Type 2 diabetes, changing your lifestyle is the optimum therapy. That means meal planning and exercising. If you can do that, you probably won't need any medication, and your body may begin to use its own insulin efficiently again. But less than 10 percent of people with Type 2 diabetes are prepared to make the necessary lifestyle changes to keep their diabetes under control. First, the older people get, the harder it is for them to change their eating habits. Second, many people may not be able to incorporate exercise or physical activity into their routines.

Third, and perhaps, most crucial, is that there are powerful social and psychological issues that affect women when it comes to food, weight, and ultimately being fat or thin. All of these complex issues are explored in the next chapter. In fact, many feminist thinkers write about fat as a *feminist* issue, not a biological one.

CHAPTER 2

Women, Weight, and Type 2 Diabetes

At least 80 percent of women with Type 2 diabetes weigh 20 percent more than they should for their height and age—the technical definition of "obese." But when women go to their doctors, diabetes educators, or dietitians, they will be given meal plans, lists of what and what not to eat, diabetes diets, and so on. The problem goes much deeper than simply eating too much food. The key to losing weight for many women is to examine *why* they got fat in the first place.

Many obese women say that they've "dieted themselves up" to their present weight. Obesity is the strongest risk factor for developing Type 2 diabetes. Basically, the longer you've been obese, the more you are at risk. Amazingly, diabetes experts have noted that when patients lose just five pounds, the body actually begins to use insulin more effectively. But the phrase "eat sensibly and exercise" just doesn't hold any weight for most women battling *theirs*.

This chapter will help you understand *why* we eat so much in North America. Part of the story is understanding the sources of the modern diet. After all, you didn't create the modern diet; you were born into it. In fact, the root word of *diet* comes from the Greek *diatta*, meaning "way of life." Since controlling your diet and weight are critical to managing Type 2 diabetes, let's start with understanding *how* diet and lifestyle became linked to Type 2 diabetes.

THE "GOOD TIMES DISEASE"

Type 2 diabetes is referred to as the "good times disease," partly because of the work of Dr. Bouchardat, a French physician in the 1870s, who noticed that his diabetic patients seemed to do rather well in war. When their food was rationed, the sugar in Dr. Bouchardat's diabetic patients' urine disappeared. It was at this point that he made a connection between food *quantity* and diabetes. This observation paved the way for low-carbohydrate diets as a treatment for diabetes; these seemed to be effective, however, only in treating "milder" diabetes, which was what Type 2 diabetes was called before the disease was better understood.

Economies and Scales

Bouchardat's discoveries were repeated throughout Europe a few decades later. The populations of many European countries experienced a significant drop, not just in "mild" diabetes, but in a number of obesity-related diseases during the first and second World Wars, when meat, dairy products, and eggs became scarce. Wartime rations forced people to survive on brown bread, oats, and barley meal and home-grown produce.

Had it not been for the Depression, we may have seen an increase in Type 2 diabetes much earlier than we did in North America. The seeds of sedentary life were already sown in the 1920s, as consumer comforts, mainly the automobile and radio, led to more driving, less walking, and more sedentary recreation. The Depression interrupted what was supposed to be prosperous times for everyone. It also stalled obesity and all related diseases, as those in most industrialized nations barely ate enough to survive.

The Depression years essentially ended when Britain declared war on Germany in 1939. While the United States did not officially enter the war until 1941, then-President Roosevelt promised Winston Churchill that the United States would help Britain fight the Germans, and he sent Americans to work to build munitions to "lend" to Britain. This, combined with four long years of war, led to an unprecedented demand for consumer goods such as cars, refrigerators, stoves, radios, and washing machines. As the boys marched home, they were welcomed with open arms into civilian bliss. There was an explosion in desk jobs and the commuter economy that exists today. The return of the veterans led to an unprecedented baby boom, driving the candy, sweets, and junk-food markets for decades to come. Moreover, a sudden influx of money from war bonds and veterans' grants meant North Americans had much more money than ever before.

Manufacturers and packaged-goods companies were looking for better ways to compete and sell their products. The answer to their prayers arrived in the late 1940s with the invention of the cathode ray tube—television. In the end, the television would become the product most responsible for dietary decline and sedentary lifestyle; it became a caretaker that mesmerized the baby boom generation for hours.

The Diet of Leisure

Naturally, after the war, people wanted to celebrate. They gave parties, drank wine, smoked, and went to restaurants. More than ever before, our diets began to include high-fat items, refined carbohydrates, sugar, alcohol, and chemical additives. As women began to manage large families, easy-to-fix meals in boxes and cans were being manufactured in abundance and sold on television to millions.

The demand for the leisure diet radically changed agriculture, too. Today, 80 percent of our grain harvest goes to feed livestock.

The rest of our arable land is used for other cash crops such as tomatoes, sugar, coffee, and bananas. Ultimately, cash crops have helped to create the modern Western diet: an obscene amount of meat, eggs, dairy products, sugar, and refined flour.

Since 1940, chemical additives and preservatives in food have risen by 995 percent. In 1959, the Flavor and Extract Manufacturers Association of the United States (FEMA) established a panel of experts to determine the safety status of food flavorings to deal with the overwhelming number of chemicals that companies wanted to add to our foods.

One of the most popular food additives is monosodium glutamate (MSG), the sodium salt of glutamic acid, an amino acid which occurs naturally in protein-containing foods such as meat, fish, milk, and many vegetables. MSG is a flavor enhancer that researchers believe contributes a "fifth taste" to savory foods such as meats, stews, tomatoes, and cheese. It was originally extracted from seaweed and other plant sources to enhance foods the same way as other spices or extracts. Today, MSG is made from starch, corn sugar, or molasses from sugar cane or sugar beets. MSG is produced by a fermentation process similar to that used for making beer, vinegar, and yogurt. While MSG is labeled Generally Recommended As Safe (GRAS) by the U.S. Food and Drug Administration (FDA), questions about its safety have been raised because of reported food sensitivities to this substance. Notwithstanding this fact, the main problem with MSG is that it arouses our appetites *even more*. MSG, widespread in our food supply, makes food taste better. And the better food tastes, the *more we eat.*

Hydrolyzed proteins are also used as flavor enhancers. These are made by using enzymes to chemically digest proteins from soy meal, wheat gluten, corn gluten, edible strains of yeast, or other food sources. This process, known as *hydrolysis,* breaks down proteins into their component amino acids. Today, there are several hundred additive substances like these used in our food, including sugar, baking soda, and vitamins (see chapters 7 and 10).

Of course, one of the key functions of food additives is to preserve foods for transport. The problem is, once we begin to eat foods that are not indigenous to our locality, the food loses many of its nutrient properties. Refrigerators make it possible for us to eat tropical foods in Canada and Texas-raised beef in Japan. As a result, few industrialized countries eat "indigenously" anymore.

Minimum wage, maximum fat

The legacy of the Western diet of leisure is that it has become cheaper to eat out of a box or can than off the land. In the developed Western world, where there's minimum wage, there is also maximum fat. At one time, fat was a sign of prosperity and wealth. Today, wealth is defined by thinness and fitness. Ironically, low-fat foods, diet programs, and fitness clubs attract the segment of our population least affected by obesity. In fact, eating disorders tend to plague women who live in higher income brackets.

In 1997, the Coalition for Excess Weight Risk Education, a Washington-based organization comprising the American Diabetes Association, the American Association of Diabetes Educators, the American Society for Clinical Nutrition, the North American Association for the Study of Obesity, and four pharmaceutical manufacturers issued statistics on obesity in the United States. The data can be used to interpret obesity patterns throughout the Western world. Based on a thirty-three-city survey, the National Weight Report found that cities with high unemployment rates and low per capita income tended to have higher rates of obesity. High annual precipitation rates and a high number of food stores also contributed to obesity. (More rainy or snowy days lead to more snacking in front of the television set!) The study also revealed the following:

- Restaurant-rich New Orleans had the United States' highest obesity rate; 37.5 percent of its adult residents were obese, while Denver, known for its outdoor living, had the lowest rate of obesity; only 22.1 percent of its residents were obese.

- Eating meals away from home and equating high-fat, fried foods to a sense of "family" was most commonly reported among obese adults. (This suggests that our commuter society increases fast-food eating, while stress and a lack of emotional support lead people to eat for comfort than in response to hunger.)

- Ethnic food (despite the fact that much of it can be lower in fat) tempted Cleveland, Ohio, residents (31.5 percent of Cleveland's adults are obese), while many people blamed their obesity on the cold climate, which made them crave meat, biscuits, and french fries to help them fuel up.

- People in hot climates, such as Phoenix, Arizona, where 24.3 percent of the adult population is obese, reported that they gained weight when the weather got too hot for outdoor exercise. (This is a case for eating *seasonably*. Heavy foods in hot climates are unnecessary. This "eating on location" concept is discussed in detail in chapter 10.)

Other statistics reveal that 35 percent of North American men and 27 percent of North American women are obese. Unfortunately, obesity, physical inactivity, and dietary fat intake are factors we must examine when trying to understand why 6 percent of North American adults (the number is much higher in aboriginal, or native populations) between the ages of eighteen and seventy-four currently have diabetes, and why 12 percent of North American adults, who were once diagnosed with *impaired glucose tolerance*, will soon be told they have diabetes under guidelines instituted in September 1998). (See chapter 1.)

Chronic Dieting

The road to obesity is paved with chronic dieting. It is estimated that at least 50 percent of all North American women are dieting at any given time, while one-third of North American dieters initiate a diet at least once a month. The very act of dieting in your teens and twenties can predispose you to obesity in your thirties, forties, and beyond. This occurs because most people "crash and burn" instead of eating sensibly. In other words, they're chronic dieters.

The crash-and-burn approach to diet is what we do when we want to lose a specific number of pounds for a particular occasion or outfit. The pattern is to starve for a few days and then eat what we normally do. Or, we eat only certain foods (such as celery and grapefruit) for a number of days and then eat normally after we've lost the weight. Most of these diets do not incorporate exercise, which means that we burn up some of our muscle as well as fat. Then, when we eat normally, we gain only fat. And over the years, that fat simply grows fatter. The bottom line is that when there is more fat in your body than muscle, you cannot burn calories efficiently. It is muscle that makes it possible to burn calories. Diet it away, and you diet away your ability to burn fat.

If starvation is involved in trying to lose weight, our bodies become more efficient at getting fat. Starvation triggers an intelligence in the metabolism; the body suddenly thinks we're living in a war zone and goes into "super-efficient nomadic mode," not realizing that we're living in modern North America. So, when we return to our normal caloric intake, or even a *lower*-than-normal caloric intake after we've starved ourselves, *we gain more weight.* Our bodies say, "Oh look—food! Better store that as fat for the next famine." Some researchers believe that starvation diets slow our metabolic rates far below normal so that weight gain becomes more rapid after each dieting episode.

This cycle of crash or starvation dieting is known as the *yo-yo diet syndrome,* the subject of thousands of articles in women's magazines throughout the last twenty years. Breaking the pattern sounds easy: Combine exercise with a sensible diet. But it's not that simple if you've been a sedentary most of your adult years. Ninety-five percent of the people who go on a diet gain back the weight they lost, as well as extra weight, within two years. As discussed further on, the failure often lies in psychological and behavioral factors. We have to understand why we need to eat before we can eat less. The best way to break the yo-yo diet pattern is to educate your children early about food habits and appropriate body weight. Experts say that unless you are significantly overweight to begin with or have a medical condition, *don't diet*. Just eat well.

But if you're gonna diet . . .

A recent study suggests that prepackaged balanced meals can help you stick to an eating program more easily if you do indeed need to lose weight. Therefore, plan your meals in advance with a nutritionist and try to prefreeze or refrigerate them. This will help curb impulse eating. If you're contemplating a diet, you should also consider the following:

- What is a reasonable weight for you, given your genetic makeup, family history, age, and culture? A smaller weight loss in some people can produce dramatic effects.
- Aim to lose weight at a slower rate. Too much too fast will probably lead to gaining it all back.
- Incorporate exercise into your routine, particularly activities that build muscle mass.
- Eat your vitamins. Make sure you're meeting your vitamin requirements. Many of the popular North American diets of the 1980s, for example, were nutritionally inadequate (the Beverly Hills Diet contained zero percent of the U.S. recommendation for vitamin B_{12}).

Eating Disorders

Imagine three steps. Chronic dieting is the bottom step; eating disorders are the middle step; obesity is the top step. Many women become obese after dieting on and off for several years.

Many other women develop eating disorders after chronic dieting, and then go on to become obese later in life.

For 2 percent of the female population in North America, starving and purging are considered a normal way to control weight. Only a small number of women are obese because of truly hereditary factors. Most women who think they are overweight are, in fact, at an *ideal* weight for their height and body size. In Western society, the fear of obesity is so crippling that 60 percent of young girls develop distorted body images between grades one and six, believing that they are "fat"; 70 percent of all women begin dieting between the ages of fourteen and twenty-one. A U.S. study of high school girls found that 53 percent were unhappy with their bodies by age thirteen; and by age eighteen, 78 percent were dissatisfied. Eating disorders are so widespread that abnormal patterns of eating are increasingly accepted in the general population. There are parents who are actually *starving* their young daughters in an effort to keep them thin.

The two most common eating disorders involve starvation. These are *anorexia nervosa* ("loss of appetite due to mental disorder"), and bingeing followed by purging, known as *bulimia nervosa* ("hunger like an ox due to mental disorder"). Women will purge after a bingeing episode by inducing vomiting and abusing laxatives, diuretics, and thyroid hormone. The most horrifying example is women with Type 1 diabetes who sometimes deliberately withhold their insulin to control their weight.

Perhaps the most accepted weight-control behavior is *overexercising*. Today, rigorous, strenuous exercise is used as a method of "purging," and has become socially accepted for women in the 1990s. A skeleton with biceps is the current ideal.

Why are we doing this?

Eating disorders are diseases of control that primarily affect women, although men have become more vulnerable in recent years. Bulimics and anorexics are usually overachievers in other aspects of their lives, and view excess weight as an announcement to the world that they are "out of control." This view becomes more distorted as time goes on, until the act of eating food in public (in bulimia) or at all (in anorexia) is equivalent to a loss of control.

In anorexia, the person's emotional and sensual desires are perceived through food. These unmet desires are so great that the anorexic fears that once she eats she'll never stop, since her appetite will know no natural boundaries; the fear of food drives the disease.

Most of us find it easier to relate to the bulimic than the anorexic; bulimics express their loss of control through bingeing in the same way that someone else may yell at her children. Bulimics then purge to regain their control. There is a feeling of comfort for bulimics in both the binge and the purge. Bulimics are sometimes referred to as "failed anorexics" because they'd starve if they could. Anorexics, however, are masters of control. They never break. I once asked a recovering anorexic the dumb question, "But didn't you get *hungry*?" Her response was that the hunger pangs made her feel powerful. The more intense the hunger, the more powerful she felt; the power actually gave her a "high."

The role of runways

Most women have a desired weight goal set at roughly ten pounds *under* their ideal weight; many women who think they are overweight are either at an ideal weight or 10 pounds underweight. Supermodels such as Kate Moss who are seriously underweight don't help much. The epidemic of eating disorders is fueled by the fashion industry, which imposes impossible standards of beauty on the average woman. Normal body fat for a healthy woman is 22 to 25 percent; most models and actresses have roughly 10 percent body fat. In order to achieve model thinness, women resort to the unhealthy habits discussed above.

To establish what is a reasonable weight for *you*, experts suggest you ask yourself four questions:

1. What is the lowest weight you have maintained as an adult for at least one year?
2. What is the largest size of clothing you feel you can "look good" in and how much do you need to weigh to wear that size?
3. Think of someone your age and height who you know (versus a model or actress) who appears to be a "normal" weight. What does that person *actually* weigh?
4. What weight can you live with?

The message is this: accepting a normal body weight in your twenties and thirties can prevent obesity in your forties and fifties.

Why we like our fat

Fat tastes good. Fat also *feels* good in our mouths. Foods that have the particular texture and taste of fat are more acceptable than foods that don't. This is why packaged-goods manufacturers describe their products as "smooth, creamy, moist, tender, and rich." All the foods that boast these qualities, from ice cream to chocolate to cheese, give us that unique feeling of satiety and satisfaction that makes us feel good.

Eating is a sensual experience. When we enjoy our food, our brains produce endorphins, "feel-good" hormones that are, ironically, also produced when we exercise. Eating fat is analogous to having a "mouth orgasm." To many of us, without the taste and texture of fat, eating is an empty experience. And when we're in emotional pain or need, the texture and taste of fat become even more important. Bingeing or falling off the diet wagon is not due to "losing control" but to regaining lost "good feelings." Food, as millions of overeaters will tell you, is our friend. It's always there; it never lets us down. (For dozens of fat-cutting tips, see chapter 10.)

The impact of "low-fat" products

Since the late 1970s, North Americans have been deluged with low-fat products. In 1990, the U.S. government launched Healthy People 2000, a campaign to urge manufacturers to double their output of low-fat products by the year 2000. Since 1990, more than a thousand new fat-free or low-fat products have been introduced into North American supermarkets annually.

Current guidelines tell us that we should consume less than 30 percent of calories from fat, while no more than one-third of fat calories should come from saturated fat (see chapter 10). According to U.S. estimates, the average person takes in between 34 to 37 percent of calories from fat and roughly 12 percent of all calories from saturated fat. Data show that in terms of "absolute fat," intake has increased from 81 grams per day in 1980 to 83 grams per day in the 1990s. Total calorie intake has also increased from 1,989 calories per day in 1980 to 2,153 calories per day. In fact, the only reason that data show a drop in the percentage of calories from fat is because of the huge increase in calories per day. The result is that we weigh more today than in 1980, despite the fact that roughly ten thousand more low-fat foods are available to us now.

Most of these low-fat products, however, actually encourage us to eat more. For example, if a bag of regular chips has 9 grams of fat per serving (one serving usually equals about five chips or one handful), you will more likely stick to that one handful. If you find a low-fat brand of chips that boasts "50 percent less fat" per serving, however, you're more likely to eat the whole bag (feeling good about eating "low-fat" chips), which can easily triple your fat intake.

Low-fat or fat-free foods trick our bodies with ingredients that mimic the functions of fat in foods. This is often achieved by using modified fats that are only partially metabolized, if at all. While some foods reduce the fat by removing it (skim milk, lean cuts of meat), most low-fat foods require a variety of "fat copy-cats" to preserve the food's taste and texture. Water, for example, is often combined with carbohydrates and protein to mimic a particular texture or taste, as is the case with a variety of baked goods or cake mixes. In general, though, the low-fat "copycats" are carbohydrate based, protein based, or fat based.

Carbohydrate-based ingredients are starches and gums that are used as thickening agents to create the texture of fat. You'll find these in abundance in low-fat salad dressings, sauces, gravies, frozen desserts, and baked goods. Compared to natural fats, which are about 9 calories per gram, carbohydrate-based ingredients are anywhere from 0 to 4 calories per gram.

Protein-based low-fat ingredients are created by modifying the proteins to make them behave differently. For example, by taking proteins such as whey or egg white, and heating or blend-ing them at high speeds, you can create the look and feel of "creamy." Soy and corn proteins are often used in these cases. You'll find these ingredients in low-fat cheese, butter, mayon-naise, salad dressings, frozen dairy desserts, sour cream, and baked goods. They are between 1 and 4 calories per gram.

Low-fat foods that use fat-based ingredients change the fat in some way so that we do not absorb or metabolize it fully. These ingredients are found in chocolate, chocolate coatings, margarine, spreads, sour cream, and cheese. You can also use these ingredi-ents as low-fat substitutes for frying foods (you do this when you fry eggs in margarine, for example). Olestra, the new fat substitute just approved by the U.S. Food and Drug Administration (FDA), is an example of a fat substitute that is not absorbed by our bodies, providing no calories (see chapter 10). Caprenin and salatrim are examples of partially absorbed fats (they contain more long-chain fatty acids; see glossary), and are more traditional fat-based low-fat ingredients. These are roughly 5 calories per gram.

There's no question that low-fat foods are designed to give you more freedom of choice with your diet, supposedly allowing you to cut your fat without compromising your taste buds. Studies show that taste outperforms "nutrition" in your brain. Yet many experts believe that low-fat products create a greater barrier to long-term weight loss.

Researchers at the University of Toronto suggest that these products essentially allow us to increase our calories even though we are reducing our overall fat intake. For example, in one study, women who consumed a low-fat breakfast food ate more during the day than women who consumed a higher-fat food at breakfast.

The good news about low-fat or fat-free products is that they are, in fact, *lower in fat,* and are created to substitute for the "bad foods" you know you shouldn't have but cannot live without. The boring phrase, "everything in moderation" applies to low-fat products, too. Balancing these products with "good stuff" is the key. A low-fat treat should still be thought of as its high-fat original. In other words, don't have double the amount because it's low fat. Instead, have the same amount as you would of the real thing.

PSYCHOLOGICAL ROLES OF FAT

There is another part of the weight story that has do with the role of food and fat in women's lives. Being fat—and/or the overeating behavior that *causes* us to be fat—is perceived by many as a very public rebellion against the role many women are asked to play in our society. So it's important to explore what being fat means to *you,* personally, and the issues surrounding food addiction.

As women, we are the ones that usually purchase and prepare the food for our families. At the same time, we are continuously being deluged with impossible standards of beauty, fitness, and thinness through media images. How do these conflicting roles affect us? For many women, the result is a feeling of powerlessness. And depending on the woman, by manipulating the body size to be bigger or smaller by eating food or refusing food, we express unconscious desires to achieve more control over our lives.

For the record, compulsive eating is more often a woman's problem, which tells us that it has much more to do with "being a woman" than we are generally told by doctors and dietitians. Psychotherapists who specialize in compulsive eating disorders stress that the only way to help women lose weight is to help them understand what conscious or unconscious needs are being met by being fat.

The Meaning of Your Fat

Therapists who work with women on weight-loss issues observe that fat both isolates a woman and makes her an object of failure. Women, of course, know this, and *sometimes* use this for psychological advantage. In other words, to the woman, the fat can "protect" her from being successful in two specific areas: sexual and financial. Many women who are striving for financial and career success find that a thin body size immediately interferes with that goal. When they are thin, they fear being perceived on sexual terms by male colleagues (or have been so perceived/noticed in the past). They may even fear their *own* sexual desires, or fear being rejected as a sexual object. But when they are fat, they can feel liberated from being perceived as a sexual or "decorative" object and enjoy the financial rewards of their success nonetheless, or simply savor being perceived as productive or competent. By being fat, women can also help to keep their families together by removing themselves from "the market" (avoiding affairs with other men).

On the flip side, many women who have never had success in their lives (sexual or financial) use their fat as a way to remain isolated. This allows them to say to themselves, "If I were thin, I'd be successful." The fatness becomes the reason for failed attempts at personal success, shielding many women from facing their own inner demons and fears, keeping them from achieving the goals they really want.

When fat means "mother"

For many women, especially women who have gained their weight after childbirth, fat has nothing to do with sexuality or personal/financial success. It has to do with their relationship with their mothers, and their own feelings of nurturing and being mothers. After all, it is a mother's breasts that initially nurture us, and it is through our mothers that we learn about food and food behaviors. Our mothers are also the source of love, comfort, and emotional support. Even when we do not receive this from our *own* mother, we still associate "mothering" with these emotions. Therapists have observed that body size and eating get tangled up in mother-daughter relationships, and can have varied meanings for the overweight woman. In other words, what your fat says to your mother can mean anything from, "I'm a big girl and can look after myself" to "I'm a mess and *can't* look after myself." Some daughters use fat to actually reject their mothers or to express anger at their mothers for inadequate nurturing.

In some cases, the "fat" is an unconscious desire to incorporate your mother into your body because she's soothing and nurturing. It's a rather brilliant way of taking your mother with you wherever you go.

When fat means "screw you"

Many women find their fat expresses anger at the beauty standard and repressive sexual role they're asked to play. The fat is not "protection" but a deliberate attempt to offend the world. Here, the fat says to the world, "Screw you! If you *really* want to get to know me, then you'll take the time to penetrate my layers. Otherwise, *I* don't want to know *you*!"

The fear that less is more

Many women fear being "seen." The belief that "the less of me there is, the more people will see" is *behind* their fat. The fat thus protects the woman from being "overexposed" emotionally and sexually.

THE ACT OF GETTING FAT: COMPULSIVE EATING

When we hear "eating disorder," we usually think about anorexia or bulimia. There are many people, however, who binge without purging. This is also known as binge eating disorder (compulsive overeating). In this case, the bingeing is still an announcement to the world: "I'm out of control." Someone who purges after bingeing is hiding her lack of control. Someone who binges and never purges is *advertising* her lack of control. The purger is passively asking for help; the binger who doesn't purge is aggressively asking for help. It's the same disease with a different result. But there is one more layer when it comes to compulsive overeating (considered to be controversial, and often rejected by the overeater): the desire to get fat is often behind the compulsion. Many people who overeat insist that fat is a consequence of eating food, not a *goal*. Many therapists who deal with overeating disagree, and believe that if a woman admits that she has an emotional interest in actually being large, she may be much closer to stopping her compulsion to eat.

Furthermore, many women who eat compulsively do not recognize that they are doing so. The following is a typical profile of a compulsive eater:

- Eating when you're not hungry;
- Feeling out of control when you're around food—either trying to resist it or gorging on it;
- Spending a lot of time thinking/worrying about food and your weight;
- Always desperate to try another diet that promises results;

Here is what women report *fat* means to them:

1. To be fat means to get into the subway and worry about whether you can fit into the allotted space.
2. To be fat means to compare yourself to every other woman, looking for the ones whose own fat can make you relax.
3. To be fat means to be outgoing and jovial to make up for what you think are your deficiencies.
4. To be fat means to refuse invitations to go to the beach or dancing.
5. To be fat means to be excluded from contemporary mass culture, from fashion, sports, and the outdoor life.
6. To be fat is to be a constant embarrassment to yourself and your friends.
7. To be fat is to worry every time a camera is in view.
8. To be fat means to feel ashamed for existing.
9. To be fat means having to wait until you are thin to live.
10. To be fat means to have no needs.
11. To be fat means to be constantly trying to lose weight.
12. To be fat means to take care of others' needs.
13. To be fat means never saying "no."
14. To be fat means to have an excuse for failure.
15. To be fat means to be a little different.
16. To be fat means to wait for the man who will love you despite the fat—the man who will fight through the layers.
17. To be fat, nowadays, means to be told by women friends that "Men aren't where it's at," even before you have had a chance to know.
18. Above all, the fat woman wants to hide. Paradoxically, her lot in life is to be perpetually noticed.

Source: Adapted from Susie Orbach, *Fat is a Feminist Issue* (New York: Berkeley Books, 1996), 32–33.

- Feelings of self-loathing and shame;
- Hating your own body;
- Obsessed with what you can or will eat, or *have* eaten;
- Eating in secret or with "eating friends";
- Appearing in public to be a professional dieter who's in control;
- Buying cakes or pies as "gifts" and having them wrapped to hide the fact that they're for you;
- Having a "pristine" kitchen with only the "right" foods;

- Feeling either out of control with food (compulsive eating), or imprisoned by it (dieting);
- Feeling temporary relief by "not eating";
- Looking forward with pleasure and anticipation to the time when you can eat alone;
- Feeling unhappy because of your eating behavior.

The Issue of Hunger

Most people eat when they're hungry. But if you're a compulsive eater, hunger cues have nothing to do with when you eat. You may eat for any of the following reasons:

1. As a social event—this includes family meals, or meeting friends at restaurants. The point is that you plan food as the "social entertainment." Most of us do this, but often we do it when we're not even hungry.
2. To satisfy "mouth hunger"—the need to have something in your mouth, even though you are not hungry.
3. Eating to prevent future hunger—"better eat now because later, I may not get a chance."
4. Eating as a reward for a bad day or bad experience; or to reward yourself for a good day or good experience.
5. Eating because "It's the only pleasure I can count on!"
6. Eating because you're nervous.
7. Eating because you're bored.
8. Eating now because you're "going on a diet" tomorrow. (Hence, the eating is done out of a real fear that you will be deprived later.)
9. Eating because food is your friend.

12 Steps to Change

Food addiction, like other addictions, can be treated successfully with a 12-step program. (For those of you who aren't familiar with this type of program, see "The 12 Steps" feature on page 62.)

THE 12 STEPS OF OVEREATERS ANONYMOUS

Step One: I admit I am powerless over food and that my life has become unmanageable.

Step Two: I've come to believe that a Power greater than myself can restore me to sanity.

Step Three: I've made a decision to turn my will and my life over to the care of a Higher Power, as I understand it.

Step Four: I've made a searching and fearless moral inventory of myself.

Step Five: I've admitted to a Higher Power, to myself, and to another human being the exact nature of my wrongs.

Step Six: I'm entirely ready to have a Higher Power remove all these defects of character.

Step Seven: I've humbly asked a Higher Power to remove my shortcomings.

Step Eight: I've made a list of all persons I have harmed and have become willing to make amends to them all.

Step Nine: I've made direct amends to such people wherever possible, except when to do so would injure them or others.

Step Ten: I've continued to take personal inventory and when I was wrong, promptly admitted it.

Step Eleven: I've sought through prayer and meditation to improve my conscious contact with a Higher Power, as I understand it, praying only for knowledge of Its will for me and the power to carry that out.

Step Twelve: Having had a spiritual awakening as the result of these steps, I've tried to carry this message to compulsive overeaters and to practice these principles in all my affairs.

Source: Overeater's Anonymous, 1997.

The 12-step program was started in the 1930s by an alcoholic, who was able to overcome his addiction by essentially saying, "God, help me!" He found other alcoholics who were in a similar position and through an organized, nonjudgmental support system, they overcame their addiction by realizing that "God" (a higher power, spirit, force, physical properties of the universe, or intelligence) *helps those who help themselves.* In other words, you have to want the help. This is the premise of

Alcoholics Anonymous—the most successful recovery program for addicts that exists.

People with other addictions have adopted the same program, using Alcoholics Anonymous and "The 12 Steps and 12 Traditions," the founding literature for Alcoholics Anonymous, as a guideline. Overeaters Anonymous substitutes the phrase "compulsive overeater" for "alcoholic" and "food" for "alcohol." The theme of all 12-step programs is best expressed through the Serenity Prayer: "God grant me the serenity to accept the things I cannot change; the courage to change the things I can, and the wisdom to know the difference." In other words, you can't take back the food you ate yesterday or last year; but you can control the food you eat today instead of feeling guilty about yesterday.

Every 12-step program also has the 12 Traditions, which, essentially, is a code of conduct. To join an OA program, you need only to take the first step. Abstinence and the next two steps are what most people are able to accomplish in a six- to twelve-month period before moving on. In an OA program, "abstinence" means three meals daily, weighed and measured, with nothing in between except sugar-free or no-calorie beverages and sugar-free gum. Your food is written down and called in. The program also advises you to get your doctor's approval before starting. Abstinence is maintained through a continuous process of one-day-at-a-time and using "sponsors"—people who call you to check in, and who you can call when the cravings hit. Sponsors are recovering overeaters who have been there and who can talk you through your cravings.

Membership is predominantly female; if you are interested in joining OA and are male, you may feel more comfortable in an all-male group. Many women overeaters overeat because they have been harmed by men, and their anger is often directed at the one male in the room; this may not be a comfortable position for a male overeater. For this reason, OA is divided into all-female and all-male groups.

BIOLOGICAL CAUSES OF OBESITY

Eating too much high-fat or high-calorie food while remaining sedentary is certainly one biological cause of obesity. Furthermore, a woman's metabolism slows down by 25 percent after menopause, which means that unless she either decreases her calories by 25 percent or increases her activity level by 25 percent to compensate, she will probably gain weight. There are also other hormonal problems that can contribute to obesity, such as an underactive thyroid gland (called *hypothyroidism*), which is very common in women over age fifty.

Because diet and lifestyle changes are so difficult, there is an interest in finding genetic causes for obesity. That would mean that obesity is *beyond our control*—and something we've inherited, which would be comforting for many people. Now that the Human Genome Project is going on that intends to map every gene in the human body, efforts are underway to find the "obesity gene" or "fat gene." But few scientists believe that obesity is *simply* genetic. In other words, there are so many environmental and social factors that can "trip" the obesity "switch," finding a specific gene for obesity is about as worthwhile as finding the "anger gene" or "crime gene."

Some Theories

An important theory about why we get fat surrounds insulin resistance. It's believed that when the body produces too much insulin, we will eat more to try to maintain a balance. This is why weight gain is often the first symptom of Type 2 diabetes. But then we have to ask what causes insulin resistance to begin with; and many researchers believe that it is triggered by obesity. So it becomes a "chicken or egg" puzzle.

There are also many theories surrounding the function of fat cells. Are some people genetically programmed to have more, or "fatter," fat cells than others? No answers have been forthcoming yet.

What about the brain and obesity? Some propose that obesity is "all in the head" and has something to do with the hypothalamus (a part of the brain that controls messages to other parts of the body) somehow malfunctioning when it comes to sending the body the message "I'm full." It's believed that the hypothalamus may control "satiation messages."

To other researchers, the problem has to do with some sort of "defect" in the body that doesn't recognize hunger cues or satiation cues; however, studies in this area are not conclusive.

What about the fat hormone?

A study reported in a 1997 issue of *Nature Medicine* showed that people with low levels of the hormone leptin may be prone to weight gain. In this study, people who gained an average of 50 pounds over three years started out with lower leptin levels than people who maintained their weight over the same period. Therefore, this study may form the basis for treating obesity with leptin. Experts speculate that 10 percent of all obesity may be due to leptin resistance. Leptin is made by fat cells and apparently sends messages to the brain about how much fat our bodies are carrying. Like other hormones, it's thought to have a stimulating action that works as a thermostat of sorts. In mice, adequate amounts of leptin somehow signaled the mouse to become more active and eat less, while too little leptin caused the mouse to eat more while becoming less active.

Interestingly, Pima Indians, who are prone to obesity and are also at highest risk for Type 2 diabetes in the United States, were shown to have roughly one-third less leptin than normal in blood analyses. Human studies involving injecting leptin to treat obesity are in the works right now, but to date have not been shown to be effective.

At present, researchers are working on using leptin as a prevention drug for Type 2 diabetes. Not only does leptin block the formation of fat in body tissues, but it apparently lowers blood sugar levels, too. It's believed that leptin somehow improves the function of insulin-producing cells in the pancreas, which helps the body to use insulin more effectively. Since you won't find leptin on your drugstore shelves just yet, you're going to have to serve as your own "fat hormone" and do the difficult work of losing some weight.

Drug Treatment for Obesity

Drug treatment for obesity has an awfully shady history. Women have been abused repeatedly by the medical system. Throughout the 1950s, 1960s, and even 1970s, women were prescribed thyroxine, which is thyroid hormone, to speed up their metabolisms. Unless a person has an underactive thyroid gland, or no thyroid gland (after surgical removal), this is a very dangerous medication; it can cause heart failure. Request a thyroid function test before you accept this medication.

Amphetamines, or "speed" were often widely peddled to women as well by doctors, but they too are dangerous, and can put your health at risk.

Antiobesity pills

The U.S. government recently approved an antiobesity pill that blocks the absorption of almost one-third of the fat people eat. One of the side effects of this new prescription drug, called orlistat (Xenical), causes rather embarrassing diarrhea each time you eat fatty foods. To avoid the drug's side effects, simply avoid fat! The pill can also decrease absorption of vitamin D and other important nutrients, however.

Orlistat is the first drug to fight obesity through the intestine instead of the brain. Taken with each meal, it binds to certain pancreatic enzymes to block the digestion of 30 percent of the fat you ingest. How it affects the pancreas in the long term is not known. Combined with a sensible diet, people on orlistat lost more weight than those not on orlistat. This drug is not intended for people who need to lose a few pounds; it is designed for medically obese people. (Orlistat was also found to lower cholesterol, blood pressure, and blood sugar levels.)

Another obesity pill, called Redux, alters brain chemicals to trick the body into feeling full. A similar competitor, sibutramine, was approved by the U.S. FDA in 1997.

One of the most controversial antiobesity therapies was the use of fenfluramine and phentermine (Fen/Phen). Both drugs were approved for use individually more than twenty years ago, but since 1992, doctors prescribed them together for long-term management of obesity. In 1996, U.S. doctors wrote a total of 18 million monthly prescriptions for Fen/Phen. Many of the prescriptions were issued to people who were not obese. (This is known as "off-label" prescribing.) In July 1997, the U.S. Food and Drug Administration, researchers at the Mayo Clinic, and the Mayo Foundation made a joint announcement warning doctors that Fen/Phen can cause heart disease. On September 15, 1997, "Fen" was taken off the market. (More bad news has surfaced about Fen/Phen wreaking havoc on serotonic levels, which only reinforces the message: In light of the safety concerns regarding current antiobesity drugs, diet and lifestyle modification are still considered the best pathways to wellness.)

Smoking and obesity

Obviously, no health care provider will "prescribe" nicotine or smoking to you as a weight-loss drug, but many women will take up the habit anyway as a tool for weight loss, or worse, revisit the habit long after they've quit.

Smoking satisfies "mouth hunger"—the need to have something in your mouth. Quitting also causes withdrawal symptoms that can drive people to eat. If you need to lose weight, also smoke, and have Type 2 diabetes, something has got to give! Smoking restricts small blood vessels, which can put you at risk for a host of complications associated with Type 2 diabetes (see chapter 9). The best way around this problem is to ask your health care team for some information on credible smoking cessation programs. There are, unfortunately, no easy answers to the dilemma of weight loss versus quitting smoking. Most health care providers will assess your current risk of heart disease and/or stroke, and help you prioritize your lifestyle changes.

TEACHING CHILDREN GOOD EATING HABITS

Type 2 diabetes is certainly a genetic disease. But, as mentioned, there are many outside factors that can "trip" the switch. The most influential factors are eating habits and lack of physical activity, which, thankfully, can be modified.

You can't change your child's genes, but you can help to offset the genetic tendency toward obesity and Type 2 diabetes by teaching your child good habits early. Because you control much of your child's diet and environment, you can make sure that you lower these odds.

For example, in young children, try to limit what I call the "Sugar Shows"—television programming for children that is basically a vehicle to sell sugar cereals and junk food. Some foods aimed at children contain as much as 22 grams of fat and 1,500 mg of sodium. And selling pies and cakes as "breakfast foods" to children raises some ethical questions as well.

Instead, play that Disney video another time or limit programs to "safe channels." Some of the worst damage is done during network Saturday-morning cartoons. You can also practice fast-food control by ordering some of the healthier foods for your kids (you know what they are) when they're begging for it. For instance, pizza, tacos, or felafel are healthier choices than greasy hamburgers, fried chicken, or fries. Try to resist fat-in-a-box meals that contain enough grease to kill your whole family, *plus* a free chocolate layer cake when you buy two!

Everything your child eats today counts in adulthood. Research shows that even infant eating patterns can lead to obesity years later. One famous baboon study found that baboons overfed early in life became obese later on. This didn't happen with baboons who were fed a normal diet in infancy.

Stop Parenting with Food

Many bad habits begin with parents forcing children to finish food when they say they're full. We all start with biological mechanisms that tell us when we're satisfied. But if we hear things such as, "Clean your plate" when we say, "But I'm full, Mom," and worse, "Good girl/boy" when we do cram that last bit of food in to please Mom, we *wreck* those biological signals designed to stop us from becoming obese. In essence, you're teaching your child not to follow natural instincts about food and eating. When your child is hungry, he will eat. If a food isn't palatable, unless your child is living in war or famine conditions, don't force the food on your child. And *never* punish a child by withholding food or, worse, *rewarding* a child with dessert. By saying, "No chocolate until you finish your carrots" you're programming your child to feel *emotional* rewards when he eats that chocolate. In other words, both these terrible parenting methods (which we learned from our parents) are recipes for eating disorders, chronic dieting, or obesity down the road.

A word about "schedules"

There are parents out there who set feeding schedules for their children. In one case, a grandmother was forbidden by the mother to feed a healthy snack to a three-year-old who was crying and begging for food out of sheer hunger (in an affluent North American suburb, I might add!). The mother apparently only allowed the child to eat at certain times. This is a recipe for disaster in later life. *Don't do this!*

Feed your children well

Why is your toddler eating toys, mud, and crayons? Because that toddler is communicating that, as a human being, she needs a *variety* of foods in her diet. And, fortunately, because we're not living under war or famine, we can give this to our children. Introduce a wide variety of normal foods (all colors of vegetables and fruits; whole grains, pastas, and so on). Without a varied diet, a child will not consume the vitamins and minerals she needs. The lack of a varied diet may also lead to childhood obesity, as the child loads up on carbohydrates, fat, and junk foods.

Babes in arms

Breastfeed your baby. And do so for as long as possible. Lots and lots of studies say breastfed children are healthier and have fewer diseases (including obesity-related diseases) than formula-fed babies. Breast-milk is perfectly balanced to satiate your baby; the "foremilk" is more watery, while the "hindmilk" is creamier and fattier—the perfect meal for someone with no teeth. (Breast milk is even more watery in hot climates for hydration, and creamier in cold climates for extra calories!)

A recent study concludes that nutrition is most important in infancy and adolescence. For example, the amount of salt in a newborn's diet could affect blood pressure later in life. The formula Similac contains 27 mg of sodium per 5-ounce serving—too high for a baby!

Today there are pills to help you manage your diabetes, if the lifestyle changes you've made aren't doing the trick. Going on diabetes medication is in no way a cure-all; but taking a pill will help you stay as healthy as possible in the event that you cannot or will not make the necessary lifestyle changes. Chapter 8 discusses all these medications in detail.

CHAPTER 3

The Estrogen Connection

E strogen definitely influences your blood sugar levels and insulin requirements. There is also evidence that estrogen-containing products can even trigger insulin resistance in women who have a family history, or genetic predisposition to Type 2 diabetes. Estrogen usually *raises* blood sugar levels, which interferes with medication or insulin doses. This is why estrogen-containing medications, such as oral contraceptives or hormone replacement therapy after menopause, were once considered "no-no's" for women with diabetes. It is also why diabetes is still considered a *contraindication* (meaning a condition that is not compatible with a given therapy or medication) for many estrogen-containing products. In recent years, however, the thinking surrounding estrogen and diabetes has been changing, and guidelines for women with diabetes are being revised to reflect, in part, more knowledge about the health benefits of various therapies, as well as the lower doses of estrogen contained in newer generations of medications.

As this chapter outlines, there are certain benefits for women with diabetes who opt for hormonal contraception, or hormone replacement therapy. There are also health risks that need to be carefully weighed by each individual woman with Type 2 diabetes.

Some of the material in this chapter previously appeared in M. Sara Rosenthal, *The Gynecological Sourcebook*, 3d ed. (Los Angeles: Lowell House, 1999).

Unfortunately, there is no surefire mathematical equation you can use to calculate just how severely your own blood sugar levels will be affected by the estrogen your ovaries naturally produce, or by the external estrogen that may be prescribed for you. Much of the risk has to do with how well controlled your blood sugar already is. Therefore, the message of this chapter is a simple one: You may need to adjust your diabetes medication, insulin, or blood sugar monitoring habits to accommodate the estrogen that is affecting your system. That estrogen, as mentioned, can be from your own ovaries (some women find that they need to adjust their blood sugar monitoring habits or medication at certain times in their monthly cycles), or synthetic sources, in the form of pills, patches, and so on. If taking estrogen from external sources is too high a risk for you (something you must determine in consultation with your health care practitioner), this chapter outlines alternative forms of birth control and postmenopausal therapy.

THE ESTROGEN REFRESHER COURSE

Okay—back to health class or gym class for you. Let's review where estrogen comes from in Mother Nature's world. Low levels of sex hormones are continuously produced during a woman's reproductive years. It is the continuous *fluctuation* of hormones, however, that establishes the menstrual cycle, which can affect your blood sugar levels.

The main organs involved in the menstrual cycle are the hypothalamus (a part of the brain), the pituitary gland, and the ovaries. The hypothalamus is the omniscient figure, watching over the cycle and controlling the symphony of hormones from above. It tells the pituitary gland to start the hormonal process, which signals the ovaries to "do their thing." The hypothalamus is sensitive to the fluctuating levels of hormones produced by the ovaries. When the level of estrogen drops below a certain level, the hypothalamus turns on *gonadotropin releasing hormone*

(GnRH). This stimulates the pituitary gland to release *FSH, follicle stimulating hormone*. FSH triggers the growth of ten to twenty ovarian follicles, but only one of them will mature fully; the others will start to degenerate sometime before ovulation. As the follicles grow, they secrete estrogen in increasing amounts. The estrogen affects the lining of the uterus, signaling it to grow, or proliferate (*proliferatory phase*). When the egg approaches maturity inside the follicle, the follicle secretes a burst of progesterone in addition to the estrogen. This progesterone/estrogen "combo" triggers the hypothalamus to secrete more GnRH, which signals the pituitary gland to secrete FSH and *LH* (*luteinizing hormone*) simultaneously. The FSH/LH levels peak and signal the follicle to release the egg. This is ovulation.

To simplify this process, think of it as a thunderstorm. The lightning that precedes the storm is the hypothalamus, sending out GnRH. The thunder that follows is the pituitary gland, answering with FSH. Then the rain starts—lightly at first. The ovaries are the rain, which are beginning to grow follicles and trickle estrogen and progesterone into the bloodstream. This light rain goes on for a few minutes until suddenly, *two* bright bursts of lightning ignite the sky: the hypothalamus again with GnRH. Then, BANG, BANG. The pituitary gland answers the lightning, sending out FSH and LH simultaneously. The intensity of the rain increases and it starts *pouring*; the follicles burst and estrogen and progesterone pour out into the bloodstream, which is when you ovulate. Slowly the rain dies down, as hormonal levels taper off until the storm stops. It is at this point that you menstruate.

Under the influence of LH, the follicle changes its function and is now called a *corpus luteum,* secreting decreasing amounts of estrogen and increasing amounts of progesterone. The progesterone influences the estrogen-primed uterine lining to secrete fluids that nourish the egg (the secretory phase). Immediately after ovulation, FSH returns to normal, or base levels, and LH decreases gradually, as the progesterone increases. If the egg is fertilized, the corpus luteum continues to secrete estrogen and progesterone to maintain the pregnancy. In this case, the corpus luteum is stimulated by human chorionic gonadotropin (HCG), a hormone secreted by the developing placenta. If the egg isn't fertilized, the corpus luteum degenerates until it becomes nonfunctioning, (at this point called a *corpus albicans*). As the degeneration progresses, the progesterone levels decrease. The decreased progesterone fails to maintain the uterine lining, which causes it to shed. Then, the whole thing starts again.

Menstrual cycles range anywhere from twenty to forty days, and the bleeding lasts from two to eight days, four to six days being the average. It's important to count *the first day of bleeding as day one of your cycle.*

Periods with Diabetes

When estrogen levels are naturally high in the cycle, your body may be more resistant to its own insulin or to the insulin you inject. Most women find that their blood sugar levels will be high for about three to five days before, during, or after their periods. Every woman is different, so the only way to manage your blood sugar levels at this time is to test your levels and chart them along with your cycle. Many experts advise that you check your blood sugar levels two to four times a day the week before, during, and after your period for two to three months. (See chapter 1 for details on blood sugar monitoring.) This will help you establish an accurate chart, and find your own individual pattern.

PMS and High Blood Sugar

Most women will experience premenstrual symptoms seven to ten days before their periods. (You know the ones—feeling tender, bloaty, and bitchy!) Some evidence points to the fact that high blood sugar can exacerbate these symptoms, meaning that instead of feeling "blue" or "sad" or "moody," you would feel *intensely* blue, sad, or moody. This creates a vicious cycle (no pun intended) because these feelings of anxiety and moodiness can raise your blood sugar even higher, making blood sugar control more difficult. The only way to prevent severe PMS is to keep your blood sugar as controlled as possible around this time in your cycle. Charting your cycles and keeping track of when in the cycle your PMS strikes will help to pinpoint when you need to more frequently monitor your blood sugar.

Many of you may also be approaching menopause, and experiencing changes in your cycles as a result of your station in life, rather than high blood sugar. You may wish to ask your doctor to test your levels of follicle stimulating hormone (FSH) to see if they are high, which is an indication that you're approaching menopause. This will help sort out whether severe PMS is related to sugar or your age. In many cases, it is, unfortunately, related to both.

Food cravings, PMS, and diabetes

Food cravings are a classic symptom of PMS, but can be especially problematic for women trying to manage diabetes. The cravings are caused by an increase in progesterone at this time in your cycle, and affect all women equally—regardless of whether they have diabetes. These cravings, like all PMS symptoms, will diminish after menopause. Most often, these desires point women in the direction of chocolate or sweet foods. The advice from many experts is to simply allow yourself the food you are craving in perhaps a sugar-free or fat-free format, such as fat-free chocolate pudding, or "lite" chocolate desserts (see chapter 7). If you deprive yourself of the particular food you're longing for, you may wind up bingeing, which can be far more destructive, and which can set off a pattern of bingeing and purging, or bingeing and guilt. (See chapter 2.)

Bear in mind, however, that the food you eat during this craving period may, alone, be responsible for a rise in your blood sugar. Charting the foods you eat during your cycle may help to pinpoint when to anticipate a change in blood sugar levels. It's also important to note that many women have less energy as a result of PMS or because of the period itself. This can interfere with daily activities or exercise routines, also causing your blood sugar levels to rise.

BIRTH CONTROL AND DIABETES

There is a widely circulated myth that diabetes causes infertility, and that women with poorly controlled diabetes cannot get pregnant. This is completely false; it's important to understand how various birth control options affect you if you have diabetes.

When oral contraceptives (OCs)—"the pill"—were first introduced in the 1960s, contraceptive technology evolved around refining OCs. Now there are probably as many estrogen/progesterone combination OCs as there are cough medicines. (In the late 1980s, the "mini-pill" came out, which is a progesterone-only OC. It was developed because many women suffer side effects from estrogen, discussed below.) Until the late 1980s, unless women were taking OCs, they had to rely on fairly ancient but reliable barrier methods, such as the diaphragm and IUDs (intra-uterine devices). North American women had relatively few contraceptive choices: oral contraception, condoms and foam, diaphragm and foam, or IUDs. By the early to mid-1980s, more barrier methods became available to North American women— methods that had been popular in Europe for decades. They included the cervical cap and the vaginal sponge. Then in the late 1980s, there was an *explosion* in new contraceptive products that are now FDA approved and readily available. These include sub-dermal implants (Norplant), contraceptive injections, the abortion pill (not yet available in North America), and the female condom. There are also several male oral contraceptive products being developed that may be ready by the early 2000s.

Many women in their late thirties and forties find hormonal contraceptives the best method of preventing unwanted pregnancy. This is particularly the case with the advent of new studies showing that women who stay on hormonal contraception beyond age thirty-five, right up until menopause, have greater protection from ovarian cancer, ovarian cysts, and endometrial cancer (discussed further on). Since Type 2 diabetes often strikes women prior to menopause, women need to know how diabetes will affect their contraceptive options.

Oral Contraception

Any hormonal contraceptive can affect women who have diabetes or high cholesterol (also called lipid, or blood fat disorders). The synthetic progesterone that is used in many hormonal contraceptives (called progestin) can decrease your glucose tolerance by *increasing* insulin resistance, while estrogen has the exact opposite effect; you may need to adjust your meal/exercise routine, insulin dosage, or diabetes medication while taking an estrogen-containing contraceptive. Women who go on low-dose oral contraceptives have fewer problems with balancing blood sugar than women on high-dose pills. In the general population, low-dose oral contraceptives have fewer side effects, too. There are only a small number of situations where a high-dose oral contraceptive may be clinically necessary (this may be the case where heavy bleeding needs to be controlled).

When it comes to cholesterol, progestin (the synthetic progesterone) can exacerbate high cholesterol because it reduces high-density lipoprotein (HDL) or "good" cholesterol and raises low-density lipoprotein (LDL) or "bad" cholesterol. If your cholesterol levels are normal, progestin can put you at risk for a cholesterol problem, which aggravates Type 2 diabetes. Therefore, a progestin-only contraceptive, such as the mini-pill (see below) or Norplant would not be as good a choice as a combination hormonal contraceptive, which contains estrogen; estrogen can help to *counteract* the lipid effect of the progestin. The amount of estrogen in your combination oral contraceptive will influence how severely your cholesterol is affected.

There have also been conflicting results in studies that looked at how Norplant or Depo Provera affects blood sugar levels and insulin. Right now, doctors recommend that women with Type 2 diabetes be cautious about either form of contraception. If you do opt for Norplant or Depo Provera, you should be monitoring your blood sugar levels frequently. (See chapter 1.)

Oral contraception is about 4,000 years old. There is a long history of women consuming a wide compendium of potions and toxins to prevent pregnancy. Women in China drank mercury to prevent conception. Women in India swallowed carrot seeds as a "morning after" contraceptive in the 1500s. Dried beaver testicle was brewed in a strong alcoholic solution and drunk by women in the backwoods of northern New Brunswick. Today's modern oral contraceptive pills were developed in the 1930s from the Mexican plant *Barbasco Roota,* which led to the discovery of steroids.

In 1960, when the pill first came on the market, it seemed like the answer to our prayers. It soon became evident, however, that the pill had not been properly tested and evaluated before its release, and that serious risks were linked to it. Most of the problems with the early pills had to do with their high estrogen content. To counteract the problem, combination pills were developed with lower amounts of estrogen; triphasic pills were introduced, which were combination pills that released different *amounts* of hormones throughout the cycle; and the mini-pill, or progesterone-only pill was marketed, which works the same way as Norplant (see further on) by blocking ovulation, causing cervical mucus to thicken, and preventing the endometrium from thickening.

Over 56 million women worldwide are using OCs, which have a success rate of 98 percent. The 2 percent failure rate is due to human error; for example, forgetting to take the pill. Even though the estrogen content of the pill has been reduced by at least half, it is still a very potent contraceptive that carries risks. The pill affects every system in the body, and some of its side effects can persist even when it is stopped. For women over age thirty-five who smoke, the risks are substantial.

How OCs work

OCs work by preventing ovulation and causing the cervical mucus to thicken, making it difficult for the sperm to reach the egg. With combination OCs, the estrogen causes the uterine lining to thicken, which means that it *needs* to shed. The difference between combination OCs and the new "time-release" hormonal contraceptives is that your periods are induced on OCs. All OCs come in a packet or case containing either a twenty-one-day or a twenty-eight-day supply of pills. For the twenty-eight pack, the last week of your supply contains only sugar pills; the twenty-one-day package requires a little more thought. You'll need to remember to start your next package seven days later. Because you're off the synthetic hormones for seven days, you will get a period, known in "clinicalspeak" as "withdrawal bleeding." These periods are incredibly punctual and usually come on exactly the same day at the same time, every month. You'll have less cramping, and a shorter, lighter flow. You'll need to take the pills at exactly the same time every day. This is to keep the hormonal levels in your body consistent.

This induced period is what makes OCs so popular. Anyone who suffers from irregular cycles, painful periods, PMS, or heavy flows will benefit from the pill—so long as they want to prevent pregnancy.

The progesterone-only pill, or mini-pill has *exactly* the same advantages and disadvantages as Norplant (see further on) because it is the same drug, except taken orally. Mini-pill users will therefore experience irregular menstrual cycles, but more women can take the "mini-pill" than the traditional combination pill (for example, smokers, older women, and women who are breast-feeding).

Who can be on combination OCs

If you don't smoke and are healthy, you can be on a combination OC from the time of your first period (called *menarche*) right up until menopause. That's because there are a number of fringe health benefits to taking OCs, known by clinicians as "noncontraceptive benefits." Because OCs prevent ovulation, they also help prevent diseases associated with the ovaries, such as ovarian cancer, ovarian cysts, and endometrial cancer. In fact, if you have no children, or have no plans to get pregnant and breast-feed, staying on an OC will have the same therapeutic effect on your ovaries as pregnancy and breast-feeding because it will "give your ovaries a break." The following are considered clear, undisputed benefits of OCs:

1. OCs reduce the incidence of endometrial cancer and ovarian cancer.
2. OCs reduce the likelihood of developing fibrocystic breast conditions.
3. OCs reduce the likelihood of developing ovarian cysts.
4. OC users have less menstrual blood loss and have more regular cycles, which reduces the chance of developing iron deficiency anemia.
5. The severity of cramps and PMS are reduced.
6. You'll see an improvement in what's called "androgen-related side effects," such as acne, or unwanted facial hair. (Androgen is to the male body what estrogen is to the female body; it is the sex hormone that makes his body "go.") Progestin, which is synthetic progesterone, can cause these kinds of side effects, which include weight gain, acne, and unwanted

facial hair. See Table 3.1 for a complete list of androgenic side effects.

7. Some brands may improve your cholesterol levels, as discussed above.

Will I get a blood clot?

Women with Type 2 diabetes should be alert to the risk of blood clots, because their risks when taking an OC increase. The rule for the general population is that if you're healthy and don't smoke, serious cardiovascular problems linked to OCs are rare in women taking *low-dose* pills. Nevertheless, it's important to make sure that you're not *already* at risk for blood clots. If you have a history of thrombophlebitis, pulmonary emboli, and other cardiovascular diseases, you should not be encouraged to take OCs. Your risk of blood clots also increases if you

- smoke;
- don't exercise;
- are overweight;
- are over age fifty;
- are hypertensive; or
- have high cholesterol.

Unfortunately, many women with Type 2 diabetes will check off all the risk factors above. So if you decide, despite warnings to the contrary, to opt for an oral contraceptive anyway, you must have your cholesterol and blood pressure checked regularly. If you currently have high blood pressure, you should also note that OCs can aggravate eye or kidney disease (see chapter 9).

Estrogen versus progestin side effects

Many of the side effects of OCs are dose related. In other words, if you switch to a lower-dose OC, your side effects will likely disappear. In some cases, you may even require a slightly higher-dose OC—

Table 3.1 Progestin-Related Side Effects of Oral Contraceptives

Caused by too much	Caused by too little
appetite increase	bleeding/spotting days 10–21
depression	delayed withdrawal bleeding
fatigue	dysmenorrhea
hypoglycemia symptoms	heavy flow and clots
weight gain	bloating
hypertension	dizziness*
dilated leg veins	edema*
cervicitis	headache*
flow length decrease	irritability*
yeast infections	leg cramps*
acne†	nausea/vomiting*
jaundice†	visual changes*
hirsutism†	weight gain*
libido increase†	amennorrhea
libido decrease	
oily skin and scalp†	
rash and pruritis†	
edema†	

*PMS-related symptoms.
†Due to excess androgen.
Source: R. P. Dickey, *Managing Contraceptive Pill Patients,* 7th ed. (Ontario: EMIS Canada, 1993).

particularly if you have a history of heavy uterine bleeding. Tables 3.1 and 3.2 will help you sort out whether your side effects are caused by too high a dose of estrogen or too high a dose of progestin, the synthetic progesterone that's found in combination OCs. Too much progestin is what creates those androgenic side effects, which are basically appearance related (sometimes referred to as "nuisance side effects"): weight gain, acne, and facial hair (*hirsutism*), discussed earlier. The older progestins can cause a complex chemical reaction in the body that basically makes more testosterone available, which is what causes these side effects. In fact, most women who discontinue OCs will do so because of androgenic side effects (and that's understandable!). The good news is that if you're experiencing androgenic side

Table 3.2 Estrogen-Related Side Effects of Oral Contraceptives

Caused by too much	Caused by too little
Splotchy face	bleeding/spotting days 1–9
chronic nasal congestion	continuous bleeding/spotting
flu symptoms	flow decrease
hay fever and allergic rhinitis	pelvic relaxation symptoms
urinary tract infections	atrophic vaginitis
bloating*	
dizziness*	
edema (water retention)*	
headaches*	
irritability*	
leg cramps*	
nausea/vomiting*	
visual changes*	
weight gain*	
cervical changes	
breast cysts	
dysmenorrhea (painful periods)	
heavy flow and clotting	
increase in breast size	
excessive vaginal discharge	
uterine enlargement	
uterine fibroid growth	
capillary fragility	
blood clots and related disorders	
spidery veins on the chest area	

*PMS-related symptoms.

Source: R. P. Dickey, *Managing Contraceptive Pill Patients,* 7th ed. (Ontario; EMIS Canada, 1993).

effects, it's *very* easy to fix! Simply request a low-dose, *triphasic* OC with a low-activity selective progestin. Studies show these do make a difference in reducing side effects.

The "new generation" OC

When you compare the chemical recipes of today's OC brands with those of thirty years ago, it's like comparing a Commodore 64 (the very first home computer, circa 1980) with a Pentium note-book computer. In short, the OC you take now is a very different product from the OC you (or your mother) may have taken in the 1960s or 1970s.

Not only has estrogen content been substantially reduced, but so has the amount of progestin. The OCs of yesteryear were also all *monophasic,* meaning that the dose did not change over the course of the cycle. In other words, monophasic OCs release estrogen and progestin in constant doses. *Triphased* OCs deliver different doses of hormone over the course of the cycle. Most recently, there are OCs available with triphased estrogen *and* progestin, designed to minimize side effects. When the pro-gestin is triphased, it delivers less hormone, but is equally effec-tive. In essence, you get more "bang for your buck." Studies comparing women on monophasic OCs and triphasic estrogen and progestin OCs show that a reduced progestin dose slightly improves cholesterol levels, raising HDL (high-density lipids or "good cholesterol").

When your doctor is prescribing an OC, there are three things you should ask:

1. What is the estrogen dose? Anything above 30–35µg is con-sidered high.
2. Is the OC monophasic or triphasic? Triphasic OCs may not contain a triphased progestin.
3. Which progestin "recipe" is in the OC? The newer progestins, norgestimate or desogestrel, are considered to be far gentler on your body in terms of side effects. Gestodene is a third new progestin that has not yet been approved in North America, but is expected to be very soon.

There is also another wrinkle to the progestin story. The new ones are now "selective"; this means they are closer in appear-ance and behavior to natural progesterone, which in theory, spells less side effects.

The bottom line is that you should walk out of your doctor's office with the lowest-dose OC possible to prevent pregnancy or, as I like to say: ALAP—as low as possible. In fact, ask your doctor to show you all the OC samples and play a role in selecting the one you want.

A Word About the Mini-Pill

You'll need to follow the same instructions as outlined above. You will not be getting regular periods, however. So just keep track of when you do get them. If you go for more than forty-five days without a period, take a pregnancy test, just in case. You'll also need to religiously take your pill at the same time each day. *If you're even three hours off, you'll need a backup method of birth control for the next forty-eight hours.*

Norplant

Norplant is a *subdermal* implant, which means that it's inserted underneath the skin. The Norplant contraceptive was approved by the FDA in December 1990, and has been on the market since February 1991. To use Norplant, your doctor inserts six silicone rubber matchstick-sized capsules that contain a synthetic progestin hormone, long used in oral contraceptives, under the skin of your upper arm. Once in place, they steadily release a low dose of hormone into the bloodstream to prevent pregnancy.

The hormone prevents ovulation, and also causes the cervical mucus to thicken, making it more difficult for sperm to reach the egg. In addition, the lining of the uterus becomes thinner, making it less receptive to an egg implanting in it. Norplant should be inserted either during your period or no later than the seventh day of your menstrual cycle. This is to prevent inserting it during a possible pregnancy. It absolutely *should not be inserted if you either are or suspect you're pregnant.* Norplant can also be inserted immediately after an abortion or miscarriage, and six weeks after delivery; it does not interfere with breast-feeding. Norplant is effective within twenty-four hours after insertion, and one insertion keeps working for five years.

The insertion process is fairly simple. Before the procedure, you'll be given a local anesthetic. Your doctor will then make a tiny incision. Using a special instrument called a *torcar,* your doctor will place six capsules, one at a time, in a fan shape just under your skin. The incision is then covered with protective gauze and a small adhesive bandage. Stitches are not required. The bandage should be left on for three days, and kept dry. When the anesthetic wears off, there will be some tenderness or itching, and even some discoloration, bruising, and swelling. This is all normal. If this doesn't clear up, it means that you have developed an infection, and you'll need to see your doctor again to get the infection treated or the capsules removed. (Infection is pretty rare with insertion and removal of Norplant, however.) You can't see the capsules once they're in place, unless you're very thin or muscular, and even then, they look like protruding veins. The inserts have also been known to come out, which happens only if they're not inserted properly. (Again, this is rare.) The insertion process takes between fifteen and twenty minutes. The upper arm was selected as the insertion site because it's not a noticeable part of your body. These inserts do not move around, unlike breast implants. They stay exactly where they're inserted until they're removed. In fact, they're made from the same material as heart valves and other surgical devices—material used in surgery since the 1950s. The implants can be taken out *at any time,* also under a local anesthetic; the removal process is exactly the same as the insertion process. Or, every five years, you can get another set of capsules and resume using Norplant.

Each Norplant capsule is about one-tenth of an inch in diameter, and just under one and a half inches long. It holds 36 milligrams of the synthetic progestin *levonorgestrel,* in the form of powdered crystals. The tubes are made of Silastic, a silicone material. The hormone seeps through the permeable tubes into the bloodstream, initially at a rate of about 85 micrograms a day. The amount declines gradually to about 50 micrograms by nine months, 35 by eighteen months, and about 30 micrograms at the end of five years. In comparison, oral contraceptives that contain progestin release about 50 to 150 micrograms of progestin a day, *plus* estrogen. The progestin-only pill, or mini-pill releases about 75 micrograms of levonorgestrel a day. When the capsules are removed, fertility is restored five to fourteen days later. Twenty percent of Norplant users got pregnant within the first month of removal; 49 percent got pregnant within four months of removal; 73 percent got pregnant within six months of removal, and 86 percent got pregnant within one year of removal. No side effects have been reported in children conceived after Norplant removal (although the product is still too new for this data to be compiled).

Interestingly, Norplant has been marketed in other countries for quite a few years. More than half a million women in forty-six countries have used Norplant since it was first approved in Finland in 1983. It now has regulatory approval in seventeen other countries as well, including Sweden, Indonesia, the Dominican Republic, Thailand, China, and Peru. In fact, the first subdermal implants were tested in 1968, and what was to be called Norplant was developed in 1974.

How effective is Norplant?

Norplant is very effective. With the exception of male sterilization, *Norplant is the most effective contraceptive there is.* Pregnancy rates, however, were slightly higher in women weighing over 153 pounds (who probably needed a higher dose). Even then, Norplant was effective. For example, among 100 women of all weights using the implant for five years, 4 will become pregnant on Norplant. That compares to 15 out of 100 women becoming pregnant on oral contraceptives. The main reason why Norplant is so effective is that it doesn't depend on patient compliance; there are no pills to forget, no human error involved. It's also important to remember that Norplant does not protect women against STDs. Used with a latex condom, however, it is an excellent contraceptive/prophylactic system.

What are the side effects?

The most common side effect is menstrual cycle irregularity, and irregular bleeding. The bleeding irregularities result from the *continuous* hormone release, and the thinning of the endometrium. Basically, when there's no thickened lining to be shed, it just doesn't. With OCs, estrogen and progestin are taken for three weeks, and withdrawn for one week, causing *regular* bleeding. Over a five-year period of use, about 45 percent of Norplant users will have irregular periods, and another 45 percent will have normal periods. The remaining 10 percent will have long periods of time (three to four months) with no bleeding. Usually, the number of days of menstruation increase, while the flow decreases. In the first year, about 70 percent of users will experience changes in their menstrual cycles. Studies so far show that Norplant causes irregular periods in the first year, with regular periods developing over the next four years. Twenty-five percent of users will have no periods at all for the first ninety days. If you decide to use Norplant (or already are), chart your periods. If you go longer than six months without any bleeding, see your doctor or gynecologist and find out whether you should continue to use Norplant. Often, you need to wait out the first year before your cycle gets more regular.

Other side effects reported are headaches, nervousness, depression, nausea, dizziness, skin rash, acne, change of appetite, breast tenderness, weight gain, ovarian cysts, and excessive growth of body or facial hair. Breast discharge, vaginal discharge, inflammation of the cervix, abdominal discomfort, and muscle and skeletal pain are also reported. It's important to note, however, that many of these latter side effects are also common complaints in *general,* and have not yet been linked specifically to Norplant, as the irregular bleeding has. If you suffer side effects other than irregular bleeding, they will probably be weight gain, headaches, acne, depression, excessive hair growth, occasional itching at the site of the implants, and possibly a benign ovarian cyst.

The statistical breakdown of why women stop using Norplant is as follows: 9 percent stop because of irregular bleeding; 5 percent stop because of other symptoms, such as dizziness or headaches; and 5 percent stop because they want to conceive. Most countries report a very high continuation rate after one year (80 to 98 percent) and more than 40 percent continuation after five years (meaning they've had it reinserted.) *In contrast, 50 percent of the women who stop using OCs do so after one year.*

Who shouldn't use Norplant?

You should definitely avoid Norplant if you're pregnant or have acute liver disease or liver tumors (benign or malignant), unexplained vaginal bleeding, breast cancer, or blood clots in the legs, lungs, or eyes. If you become pregnant while Norplant is in, have it removed right away. You should also avoid Norplant if you

- are happy with your current form of contraception;
- cannot afford the upfront cost of Norplant (see below);
- cannot tolerate irregular menstrual bleeding; or
- don't want to visit a doctor to control your own contraception.

IUDs

After reading the section above, you may well decide that hormonal contraception and Type 2 diabetes don't mix. Therefore, another option may be the IUD, or intrauterine device.

The IUD actually dates back 3,000 years. Smooth pebbles were apparently inserted into the uteruses of camels to prevent pregnancy during long trips through the desert. IUDs are tiny devices with thin silky threads attached to them that are fitted inside the uterus. The thread hangs down through the cervix, just barely into the vagina, in a tamponlike fashion, to indicate that the device is in place correctly. Some IUDs are shaped like rings, with a thread attached; some are shaped like tiny sewing scissors with a thread extending from the base; some are shaped liked capital Ts with a thread extended from the base; and the earlier IUDs were loopshaped, like a tiny "Crazy Straw." The amazing thing about IUDs is that no one really knows *why* they prevent pregnancy. The main theory is that as a foreign object in the uterus, they interfere with the sperm reaching the egg and the egg implanting itself in the uterus. At any rate, the IUD has a failure rate ranging between from 3 to 6 percent.

The first IUD was developed in 1909, by a German gynecologist and sex researcher, Ernst Grafenberg. It was a ring-shaped device that wasn't used widely until the 1920s. In 1934, Tenrei Ota, a Japanese physician, came up with another design. Both designs had no strings, and both physicians ran into resistance to using the device because of the fear of uterine infection. Once antibiotics were discovered, however, physicians felt comfortable prescribing the IUD. The most extensive IUD study was done in Israel between 1930 and 1957; a doctor there reported his success with the 1909 model. The Israeli results were promising, and IUDs began to be engineered in the United States by the 1960s. One of the key figures in American IUD engineering was Jack Lippes, a gynecologist from Buffalo, New York. He tried both the Grafenberg and Ota rings, but found they were difficult to remove. He ingeniously attached a simple blue string, and changed the ring to a loop instead. The string would allow women to check to see if the device was still in place, as well as assist the doctor in removal. This string has been the springboard for IUD engineering ever since. The Lippes Loop became the best-known and most widely used IUD in developing countries outside of China. Currently 85 million women use IUDs, and 59 million of them are in China (where the stringless IUD is still used).

After the Lippes Loop came out, several IUD series were soon developed, including the Saf-T-Coil series and copper-bearing IUDs in the late 1960s. In the 1970s, a second generation of IUDs arose, and the shift was toward copper IUDs, which yielded fewer complications, and hormone-impregnated IUDs, which released progestin into the bloodstream. (Today, Progestasert, a hormone-releasing IUD, is the only one widely available in the United States) By the mid-1970s, everyone wanted to get in on the IUD market. Untested devices were marketed, and IUDs have been dogged by lawsuits and controversy ever since.

The IUD Disaster

The most controversial IUD was the Dalkon Shield, which was banned in 1975 and recalled in 1980. This was a badly designed, untested IUD that was rushed onto the market by the pharmaceutical firm A.H. Robins Company. At this time, IUDs did not require FDA approval. By 1986, several pharmaceutical companies in the United States discontinued their IUD lines. To date, the Progestasert system is the only IUD widely marketed in the United States, although some clinics have some Lippes Loops, Cu-7s, and Cu-T 200s (from the copper series) still around.

IUDs in the post-Dalkon Shield era were—and still are—alive and well in Canada and the rest of the world, however. The reason why they were virtually banned in the United States had more to do with liability insurance, because U.S. health care is all private. Since the "Dalkon Disaster," IUDs must now receive FDA approval before they're marketed, and several are about to be approved.

IUD side effects

IUDs increase your risk of pelvic inflammatory disease (PID), an infection in the upper genital tract that can cause infertility. Since many of you reading this may be finished having your families, this may not be of as much concern to you as to younger women. Recent studies show that the risk is highest in the first four months after insertion. Basically, the infection results because your uterus is "rejecting" the IUD, just as transplant patients suffer infections. You're also at a higher risk of getting PID with IUDs if you have been exposed to an STD. In other words: *STD + IUD = PID!* Another potential risk with IUDs is an ectopic pregnancy, or tubal pregnancy. Since IUDs prevent the egg from implanting in the uterus, the egg decides to stay in the fallopian tube, which is very dangerous. Periods may also be much heavier with IUDs, and you'll either get more severe cramps, or *develop* cramps. Because of this, anemia is common in IUD users. IUDs have also been linked to uterine and cervical cancers, but this area is still murky. About 15 percent of IUD users have them removed because of bleeding, spotting, hemorrhaging, or anemia.

Other complications arise when the IUD partially expels (comes out), which means lots of cramping, painful intercourse, unusual discharge, and spotting. Lost strings are another problem, making removal difficult. Full-term pregnancies have been reported with an IUD in place, but if you do get pregnant with one in, there's a 50 percent chance you'll miscarry for obvious reasons. Punctures in the uterus or cervix that lead to pelvic infections are another drawback.

Don't go anywhere *near* an IUD if you

- have PID, an active pelvic or vaginal infection, or an STD;
- suspect you're pregnant;
- have multiple sexual partners;
- have no access to an emergency clinic (for example, you live on a farm);

- ever had an abortion or an ectopic pregnancy;
- have hemophilia or a blood coagulation disorder; or
- have an allergy to copper (many IUDs are copper).

In the past, women with diabetes were cautioned against IUDs, but this view is changing. Many doctors feel that the IUD has advantages for women with diabetes because it does not affect blood sugar and insulin. It's wise to have a checkup prior to IUD insertion to make sure that you have no sexually transmitted diseases, review your diabetes control history with your doctor, and be checked out for other gynecological problems. If you have diabetes, smoke, are finished with having children, have high blood pressure, or have any of the diabetes complications discussed in chapter 9, an IUD may be a good contraceptive option.

Women who are at high risk for developing Type 2 diabetes (see chapter 1), as well as women who developed gestational diabetes with a prior pregnancy, may also be good IUD candidates.

Barrier Methods

Barrier methods are the oldest contraceptive methods there are, and simply refer to placing some kind of obstacle inside the vagina that prevents the sperm from entering the uterus. Many women are returning to barrier methods, weary of the risks associated with hormonal contraception, not to mention IUD risks. Not much has really changed in barrier method design, other than the materials. In Sumatra, for example, women molded opium into a cuplike shape and inserted it into the vagina to cover the cervix; Chinese and Japanese women covered the cervix with oiled silky paper; Hungarian women used beeswax melted into 5 to 10 centimeter disks. Some barrier devices recorded were particularly ingenious: Casanova recommended women squeeze half a lemon and then insert the lemon rind into their vaginas, fitting it over the cervix. The citric acid from the lemon acted as a spermicide, while the rind served as a diaphragm, covering the cervix.

Natural sea sponges have been used since antiquity for contraception, and did much the same thing as a contraceptive sponge does today. Barrier methods are also very safe, and pose few risks to the user. Unless they're combined with spermicide and a condom, however, they offer no protection against STDs. The only risk that is considered significant with barrier contraceptives is toxic shock syndrome (TSS), which occurs in 10 out of every 100,000 barrier users (a very low occurrence rate). TSS can occur for the same reasons it occurs with tampon use. So, whatever barrier method you decide on, here are some rules to follow that will greatly reduce your risk of TSS, however rare it may be:

1. Wash your hands with soap and water before inserting or removing a barrier (diaphragm or cervical cap).
2. Do not leave your barrier in place longer than twenty-four hours (cervical caps can be left in up to forty-eight hours).
3. Don't use your barrier during your period, when you're bleeding for any other reason, or if you have any abnormal vaginal discharge. (The menstrual flow may also break the suction.)
4. After a full-term pregnancy, wait six to twelve weeks before using your barrier again. (The cervix may still be dilated.)
5. If you think you may have TSS, remove your barrier immediately, and see your doctor.
6. If you have a history of TSS, choose another method of birth control.

The Diaphragm

A diaphragm is a dome-shaped cup with a flexible rim that fits over your cervix and rests behind your pubic bone. It looks like a tiny rubber flying saucer. It's inserted before intercourse, and blocks the sperm from entering the uterus through the cervix. Rubber diaphragms have been around since the early 1880s, and were introduced into the United States by Margaret Sanger. Not much happened to diaphragm technology until the 1950s, when spermicides were introduced and used in conjunction with the diaphragm. Typically, you place spermicidal jelly inside the diaphragm before you put it in. The jelly helps to hold the diaphragm in place. The most recent development in the history of the diaphragm was the introduction of a new model in 1983. This product incorporates a soft latex flange, attached to the rim, intended to create a seal with the vaginal wall. Along with the new model, the same manufacturer introduced a spermicide packaged in foil, in premeasured amounts, for convenient, one-time use and portability. Disposable spermicidal diaphragms are also being developed, which haven't yet received FDA approval.

The failure rate ranges from 10 to 20 percent. This is considerably higher than hormonal methods, but much of the failure has to do with improper use and insertion. Diaphragms come in different sizes and styles. You'll need to be fitted for one by either your family doctor (who probably does it all the time) or your gynecologist. Once you're fitted, you'll be given a prescription to purchase the diaphragm at any drugstore. Then you'll need to go back to your doctor to be shown how to use it. Sometimes you'll need a plastic inserter, sometimes you won't. Go home and practice and see your doctor one more time before you use it, so she can make sure you're putting it in correctly. (See below for instructions.)

Fitting

There are three basic types of diaphragms on the market: *The Arcing Spring* has a double spring in the rim, which produces strong pressure against the vaginal walls. It's most suitable for women with poor vaginal muscle tone, or those who have a mild uterine prolapse. This style tends to flip in place by itself and is almost impossible *not* to fit correctly. In fact, many physicians recommend this one to new users because it's so easy to fit. *Coil Spring Rim* is the most common style in North America. It's suitable for women who have strong vaginal muscles, no displacement of the uterus, and a normal size and contour of the vagina. It can be inserted by hand without an inserter. *The Flat Spring Rim* has a thin, delicate rim with gentle springs. It's most useful for women who haven't had children.

Before your doctor recommends a diaphragm, he should perform a pelvic exam to make sure you don't have any physical abnormalities that would prevent you from using one in the first place. It's important to get a diaphragm that fits well; if it's too small, it will expose the cervix, if it's too big, it will buckle. You should also be refitted if you've gained or lost more than fifteen pounds, had pelvic surgery, had a child or an abortion, or if you found the first fitting uncomfortable. If you just can't get the hang of a diaphragm, it's probably not for you.

Side Effects

Aside from the minimal risk of TSS, there is evidence suggesting a link between urinary tract infections and diaphragm use. If you have a history of urinary tract infections, don't use a diaphragm, just to be safe. Some women are also allergic to rubber or the spermicide. Again, don't use a diaphragm if you have these allergies. Other side effects include irritation caused by the spermicide, foul-smelling discharge associated with prolonged wearing of the diaphragm, pelvic discomfort, cramps, or pressure on the rectum or bladder (usually caused by poor fit).

There *is* a benefit to diaphragm use, however. Women who use them have lower rates of STDs and PID. This may be because the diaphragm helps block bacteria from entering the cervix and the spermicide helps to kill them.

How to Use a Diaphragm

Hold the diaphragm as if it were a cup and apply one teaspoon of spermicide in the center, making a circle about the size of a quarter. Spermicide may be applied to the rim of the diaphragm to ease insertion. Then squeeze the diaphragm firmly between your thumb and forefinger into an even fold. This should make it narrow enough to fit inside the vagina. Assume a comfortable position—stand with one foot on a chair, the bed, or the toilet seat, squat on the floor, or lie back on the bed with your knees up. Then insert the folded diaphragm into the vagina and push it up as far as it will go. When you release the diaphragm, the rim will regain its shape and fit around the cervix. When it's in place comfortably, you shouldn't be able to feel it. If you do, take it out and reinsert it. You might also want to incorporate the diaphragm insertion into foreplay. Partners can insert and check the diaphragm as well.

To remove it, hook your finger or thumb over the rim toward the front, and pull the diaphragm down and out. Use the same position to remove it as you did to insert it. You may also try breaking the suction by slipping a finger between the diaphragm and the sides of the vaginal wall, and then pulling the diaphragm out. Don't panic if you can't get it out at first. It just means you're tensing up. Wait a while and try again. There's no way it can "get lost" inside the body. You'll need to take it out after twenty-four hours, however, or you may get a foul smell as bacteria grow on it. These bacteria can also cause irritations and discharge.

Things to keep in mind

1. Be sure to use the diaphragm with spermicidal cream or jelly *every time you have intercourse.*
2. After intercourse, leave your diaphragm in place for at least six to eight hours. Don't douche during that time (or ever, in fact!). Then remove the diaphragm when it's convenient.
3. If you are going to have intercourse again, *after* eight hours, wash the diaphragm with mild soap and water, dry it with a clean towel, apply new spermicidal jelly or cream, and reinsert it. Try to remove your diaphragm at least once every twenty-four hours.

4. If you have intercourse more than once within the six to eight hour "leave the diaphragm in place" period, insert more spermicide with an applicator into your vagina each time you have intercourse. Don't remove the diaphragm, however. Just leave it alone.

5. Make sure you always have your diaphragm supply kit on hand—either at home or when you travel: a diaphragm in a plastic case, one or two tubes of spermicidal jelly or cream, and a plastic applicator for inserting extra spermicide.

6. *Each time you use your diaphragm, check for holes!* Diaphragms wear out after about two years. Hold your diaphragm up to the light first, to see if there are any defects, and stretch it a little bit. Then pour water into it and see if any water leaks out. If it does have holes, *don't use it.* You'll need a new one.

7. Your diaphragm shouldn't interfere with normal activities. Urination or bowel movements shouldn't be affected, and you should be able to bathe and shower as usual. If it is interfering with these activities, it may not be in properly or might be the wrong size.

8. Keep your diaphragm away from Vaseline or petroleum jelly. It can erode the rubber.

9. Although this may sound like a broken record, diaphragms do not offer any protection against STDs. You'll need to use a latex condom along with it if you're not in a monogamous relationship.

The Cervical Cap

The cervical cap is a small thimble-shaped cap that blocks only the cervix and *not* the entire upper part of the vaginal canal, the way a diaphragm does. In essence, the cervical cap is a "mini-diaphragm" with a tall dome. It was actually invented forty-four years before the diaphragm. Dr. Adolphe Wilde in Germany (contraceptive devices seem to always come from there!) took an individual impression of a woman's cervix and then made a custom-fitted cap out of rubber to wear over it. At about the same time, a New York physician, Dr. E. B. Foote, invented his own version of the cap. The cervical cap has always been widely available in Europe. The caps that were popular in North America thirty to forty years ago were actually made out of silver or copper (more recently, plastic) and were left in place for up to four weeks. The caps currently available in North America are manufactured in England. They are now made of soft rubber and the *exact same instructions apply to the cap as to the diaphragm.* The only differences between the cervical cap and the diaphragm are that it doesn't need to be squeezed or folded to fit in—you simply insert the cap with your forefinger and place it over the cervix yourself; that you can leave the cervical cap on for a longer time frame—thirty-six to forty-eight hours instead of twenty-four hours; and that because it is smaller, you need far less spermicide inside it.

The cervical cap was not available in North America until 1988. Although it was popular at the beginning of the century, it became less so because it is a little more difficult to fit than a diaphragm (although many women do report that it is easier to use, and less messy than a diaphragm). The main problem with the cap was that it required women to be very comfortable with their bodies. It eventually drifted out of North American bedrooms. In the early 1970s, feminist health organizations in the United States lobbied for its return to the U.S. market. By 1976, all contraceptive manufacturers had to provide the FDA with data on the safety and failure rates of their products; Lamberts Ltd., the British manufacturer of the cap, for some reason failed to provide the necessary data to the FDA. As a result, the FDA put the cervical cap on its Class III list, banning its use. Finally, after much protest, tests were done, data was provided, and the ban was lifted in 1988. The FDA approved one type of cap, the Prentif cavity-rim cervical cap, for general use. Like the diaphragm, it must be fitted (cervices come in different sizes). It has a failure rate of about 17 percent, very similar to the diaphragm. The cap also has the same side effects and advantages as the diaphragm except for this: there's no risk of bladder infections with the cap, but there can be some irritation to the cervical lining—mainly because of improper use. About 6 percent of cervical cap candidates will not be able to find one that fits (shorter or longer cervices are apparently a problem). Obviously, as with a diaphragm, until you're using it correctly, use a backup method of birth control.

The only women who shouldn't use the cervical cap are these:

- women who have a history of abnormal Pap tests, cervical or vaginal infections, or PID
- women who have had a cervical biopsy or cryosurgery within the past six to twelve weeks
- women allergic to rubber (plastic caps are also available)
- women who can't seem to use it properly

Cervical cap users will need to follow both the general barrier rules outlined at the beginning of this section, and the diaphragm instructions above.

Tubal Ligation

Tubal ligation is having your "tubes tied," a once-permanent procedure that can now be successfully reversed. This surgical procedure is actually a good option for women who are finished having babies, although it is much more invasive than a vasectomy. Before deciding to undergo tubal ligation, you should first have some thoughtful discussions with your partner and gynecologist.

HORMONE REPLACEMENT THERAPY AND DIABETES

The average North American woman will live until age seventy-eight, meaning that she will live one-third of her life after menopause. In a survey of the general North American population,

11 percent of those between ages sixty-five and seventy-four reported having diabetes. Heart disease is a major complication of Type 2 diabetes, and postmenopausal women are more prone to heart disease as a result of estrogen loss; therefore, the current recommendation is for women with Type 2 diabetes to seriously consider hormone replacement therapy. Right now, the Women's Health Initiative (WHI) is studying 25,000 postmenopausal women, many of whom have diabetes. The results of this study (expected by 2003) should present more concrete facts regarding the perceived benefits of HRT on postmenopausal women with Type 2 diabetes.

Many women, of course, are also concerned about their risk of breast cancer. Taking estrogen can stimulate or trigger the growth of an estrogen-dependent breast cancer cell (that is, a breast cancer cell that "feeds," or thrives on the hormone estrogen). Current studies show that these types of cancers are far more treatable than other kinds of breast cancers. And, as I'll discuss further on, since many more women die of heart attacks than breast cancer—particularly if they have Type 2 diabetes—preventing heart disease, as well as fractures from osteoporosis (see chapter 5) is a benefit. Nevertheless, you have some thinking to do if you're considering hormone replacement therapy. So here are the facts you need to make an informed choice.

What Is HRT?

Hormone replacement therapy (HRT) refers to estrogen *and* progesterone; the progesterone is given to women after menopause who still have a uterus to prevent its lining from overgrowing and becoming cancerous. Estrogen replacement therapy (ERT) refers to estrogen only, which is given to women after surgical menopause who no longer have a uterus. Both HRT and ERT are prophylactic therapy and a cure for the menopausal symptoms discussed in chapter 5. They are designed to replace the estrogen lost after menopause; they:

1. prevent or even reverse the long-term consequences of estrogen loss (osteoporosis, skin changes, vaginal thinning, and a list of other ailments discussed in chapter 5); and
2. treat the short-term symptoms of menopause, such as hot flashes and vaginal dryness.

You have the choice of taking HRT or ERT as either a *short-term therapy* or a *long-term therapy*. There are also some risks involved with HRT and ERT that you'll need to weigh against the benefits.

The Benefits

What exactly is estrogen responsible for in our bodies? In addition to protecting our bones, and maintaining our reproductive organs, estrogen also helps to maintain appropriate levels of high-density lipoprotein (HDL), which keeps our arteries clear of

---

THE BENEFITS OF HRT (PROGESTERONE AND ESTROGEN)

- Reduces bone loss during and after menopause
- Reduces menopausal symptoms
- Reduces the risk for heart disease by 40 to 50 percent*
- Reduces thinning of vaginal tissue and associated discomforts

THE RISKS OF HRT (PROGESTERONE AND ESTROGEN)

- HRT is not effective for every woman
- It can raise cholesterol levels
- Side effects of depression and anxiety have been reported
- In women with a high risk of breast cancer, or a history of severe blood clotting disorders, HRT is not recommended

*Benefits are less clear when progesterone is added to the estrogen. Some studies suggest that progestin added to the estrogen may even cancel out the protection against heart disease.

Source: Laurinda M. Poirier and Katharine M. Coburn, *Women & Diabetes: Life Planning for Health and Wellness* (American Diabetes Association and Bantam Books, 1998), 133.

plaque, preventing them from clogging and causing heart attacks and strokes. By raising HDL, known as the "good cholesterol," the "bad" cholesterol (the low-density lipoproteins that cause fatty substances to *collect* in the arteries, causing arteriosclerosis) drops. Estrogen also helps protect us from rheumatoid arthritis. It's our ovaries, of course, that make estrogen, but other sources of estrogen come from androstenedione (a hormone) and testosterone, which are converted by our tissues into a form of estrogen called *estrone,* a weaker type of estrogen than the kind our ovaries produce. Obese women have estrone in greater amounts. Although this may prevent severe menopausal symptoms, estrone is *not* considered a potent enough form of estrogen to protect against osteoporosis or heart disease.

Thirty years ago, all women, regardless of whether they still had a uterus, were placed on pure estrogen hormone without any progesterone. This is known as "unopposed estrogen therapy" because in a natural cycle the progesterone "opposes" the estrogen and counterbalances high estrogen levels, preventing you from becoming "estrogen toxic." This created several problems. First, women experienced side effects, similar to the early oral contraceptives: nausea, dizziness, bloating, and so on. Second, women who went into menopause naturally tended to develop endometrial hyperplasia (overgrowth of the uterine lining) which often became uterine cancer. Finally, both surgical and natural menopause recipients of this estrogen therapy were at higher risk of developing estrogen-dependent cancers, such as breast cancer and ovarian cancer.

Today, all women who have gone through menopause naturally and decide to go on HRT will be given estrogen *and* progesterone. The progesterone, of course, triggers the uterine lining to shed regularly, *which prevents endometrial hyperplasia,* which is what predisposed women on unopposed estrogen to uterine cancer. Estrogen and progesterone *together* also mimic the normal menstrual cycle, and help prevent the side effects normally felt with estrogen alone. The estrogen levels prescribed now are much lower than those of the past; current HRT doses are about ten times lower than the average combination oral contraceptive.

If you're in surgical menopause, you won't *need* progesterone because you're no longer at *risk* for endometrial hyperplasia. Because your menopausal symptoms will be more severe (discussed in chapter 5), however, your need for estrogen may be greater. Again, since estrogen doses are so much lower now, you'll likely not experience any short-term side effects from the estrogen.

What to expect in the short term

Generally, HRT/ERT will begin to relieve your estrogen-loss menopausal symptoms within days of starting the therapy. Your hot flashes will disappear, your vagina will become moist again and will lubricate on its own during sex, and your vagina's acidic environment will be restored, preventing yeast and other vaginal infections from plaguing you. If you change your mind and go *off* the therapy, however, your symptoms will return in a far more severe form!

What to expect in the long term

Your HDL levels will be maintained, and you won't experience any severe bone loss, which can put you at risk for fractures and breakages. Research shows that HRT is more effective than ERT, however, in preventing osteoporosis.

As for heart disease, roughly half a million North American women die of heart disease every year. Heart attacks are much less frequent in premenopausal women than in postmenopausal women. In the premenopause age group, men are much more vulnerable. After menopause, however, women equal men in numbers of heart attacks. To date, most of the research shows that estrogen *protects* women from heart disease.

But it's also important to review these studies in the proper context. First, the women selected for these studies are generally upper middle class, and educated: two major factors that appear to decrease the risk of heart disease *anyway*! Second, women who take estrogen are usually healthier, and are more willing to make *other* lifestyle changes that will lower their risk—such as improving their diet or not smoking.

Finally, some animal research has revealed that the progesterone added to HRT *may* have the *opposite* influence on HDL as estrogen. If you decide to go on HRT strictly for the heart benefit, have your cholesterol levels checked before you start, as a "baseline"; then get your levels checked after you're on HRT for about three months. If there's no improvement in your cholesterol levels, you may want to review your decision with your doctor.

The heart benefits from estrogen only if the estrogen is taken orally, not in patches or vaginal creams. In order for the estrogen to work its magic with HDL, it needs to be metabolized in the liver.

Finally, estrogen will not counteract a poor diet and lifestyle. If you smoke, drink excessively, are under tremendous stress, eat copius amounts of the wrong foods (you know the ones), or have a family history of heart attack, don't expect estrogen alone to shield you from heart disease.

Don't expect miracles

If your decision for going on ERT or HRT is based on cosmetic reasons ("Gee, I won't get any wrinkles with hormone therapy!") you're in for a big surprise: hormone/estrogen replacement therapy *does not prevent wrinkles*. Estrogen can cause you to retain water, making your skin puffier, and your wrinkles less noticeable. The majority of women, however, have wrinkles because of heredity, excessive or accumulative sun exposure, smoking, and drinking too much alcohol. Estrogen can also cause skin dryness, rashes, and permanent brown blotches on your skin (harmless skin discoloration known as hyperpigmentation).

Estrogen therapy will not prevent weight gain, another myth that has been passed down through the estrogen folklore. Weight gain has to do with our metabolism slowing down as we age, something estrogen cannot prevent or reverse.

Some women want to take estrogen to keep their breasts full and shapely; this is not a good reason to go on HRT. Although estrogen promotes cell growth in the breasts, and the retention of body fluid can make breasts swollen and fuller, your breasts can also become tender and painful. Taking HRT to keep your breasts full is not recommended, because of the health risks.

The Risks

The risk that we hear about most regarding the estrogen issue is uterine cancer. Today, this is no longer a risk! Here's why: In the past, as discussed earlier, unopposed estrogen was given to both women who still *had* a uterus and women without one. Of course, if you don't have a uterus, there is no risk of uterine cancer. But what about the women who had one? Well, a funny thing happened; doctors *forgot* about the uterus, ignoring the fact that the female body is very smart. When it detects estrogen in the body, it says, "Oh, look—estrogen again! Better start preparing the endometrium for a baby!" And guess what? There's no progesterone to trigger the lining to shed, and certainly no baby—so the lining just keeps growing until you wind up with endometrial hyperplasia, overgrowth of the uterine lining, and eventually, uterine cancer. When the uterine cancer rate began to increase in uterus "owners" on unopposed estrogen, the medical community realized its mistake and remembered the uterus and the importance of progesterone. *Today, unopposed estrogen is not given to any woman with a uterus.*

Just for the record, women in natural menopause have a 1 in 1,000 risk of uterine cancer; women with a uterus on unopposed estrogen increase their risk to anywhere from 4 to 8 in 1,000. What if you were on unopposed estrogen in the past and have your uterus? This is still in debate. It seems that once you go off the estrogen, your uterine cancer risk drops. A Boston University School of Medicine study, using 1,217 women, revealed that the risk of cancer may not drop until you've been off the estrogen for as long as ten years, however.

With HRT and progesterone added to the estrogen therapy, the risk of uterine cancer decreases: it's lower in women on HRT than in women on nothing. As for the risk of breast cancer and HRT, refer to chapter 5, page 163.

The risks you don't read about . . .

It might interest you to know that you *triple* your chances of developing gallbladder disease on ERT or HRT. Gallbladder disease is easily treated, however, by removing the gallbladder, which is one of the most common surgeries performed.

If you have fibroids, they may grow larger on HRT. Estrogen also causes fluid retention, which can exacerbate *existing* conditions such as asthma, epilepsy, preexisting heart disease, kidney disease, and migraine headaches.

The Forms of HRT and ERT

You can take estrogen in a number of ways. The most common estrogen product is *Premarin*. Premarin uses a synthesis of various estrogens derived from the urine of pregnant horses. That way the estrogen mimics nature more accurately. Premarin literally means "pregnant mare's urine" from "pre" (pregnant) "mar" (mare's) and "in" (urine). Premarin is a trade name for this type of replacement estrogen, and comes in either pills, patches (transdermal), or vaginal creams. Other common, synthetic forms of estrogen include micronized estradiol, ethinyl estradiol, esterified estrogen, and quinestrol.

As a short-term therapy, you may only need the vaginal cream to help with vaginal dryness or bladder problems. As a long-term therapy, you'll need the pill form if you want to protect yourself from heart disease. This drug is available under a variety of brand names, each just as good as the other. Estrogen can also be "worn." In this case, it's placed in a small plastic patch about the size of a silver dollar, placed on the abdomen, thighs, or buttocks, and changed twice weekly.

When estrogen is in patch or cream form, it goes directly to the bloodstream, bypassing the liver, and hence does not affect HDL or protect against heart disease. Some women also have an allergic reaction to the skin patch and get a rash. If you're one of them, you can investigate taking estrogen in other forms.

Finally, you can also have estrogen injected. Each shot lasts from three to six weeks, but this is expensive and inconvenient because the dosages aren't as flexible as with pills.

Women react differently to Premarin or other synthetic forms of estrogen; some do better than others on different chemical recipes. So if you don't do well on Premarin, for example, see if estradiol is better for you, or vice versa. Don't just give up and go off the HRT or ERT altogether; explore all the estrogen possibilities. Dosages are discussed below.

Progesterone

Synthetic progestins (a family of progesterone drugs that includes natural progesterone) are norethridone or norethindrone acetate. Natural progestin is medroxyprogesterone.

Progestins are taken in separate tablets along with estrogen. Together, the estrogen and progestin you take is called HRT. HRT can be administered two ways: *cyclically* or *continuously.* Taking HRT cyclically is very similar to taking an oral contraceptive because the hormones closely mirror a natural cycle. The first day you start is considered day "1" of your mock "cycle." You take estrogen from day 1 to 25; you then add the progesterone from day 14 to 25. Then you stop all pills and bleed for two or three days—just as you would on a combination OC. This vaginal bleeding is called "withdrawal bleeding," and is lighter and shorter than a normal menstrual period. In fact, if the bleeding is heavy or prolonged, this is a warning that something's not right, and you should be checked.

In addition, you may experience "breakthrough bleeding"—spotting during the first three weeks after you begin HRT. This kind of bleeding is also similar to what happens on a combination OC. This bleeding usually goes away after a few months, but report it anyway. You may need to switch to a lower dose of estrogen or take a higher dose of progestin. Once your mini-period of withdrawal bleeding is finished, you simply start the cycle again. Many women can't tolerate cyclical HRT because they feel they should be *rid* of their periods by now, and not have to deal with pads and tampons ever again. It is believed, however, that cyclical HRT offers slightly better heart protection.

When HRT is taken continuously, you simply take one estrogen pill and one progestin pill each day. When you do it this way, the progesterone *counteracts* the estrogen; no uterine lining is built up, so no withdrawal bleeding needs to happen.

The appropriate dosages

Every woman requires a different dosage of estrogen and progestin. You will always be placed on the *lowest* possible dosage of either one, and the dosage increased gradually if necessary. If your estrogen dosage is too high, you'll experience side effects similar to those seen with estrogen OCs: headaches, bloating, and so on. Before you determine how much estrogen you'll need, it's crucial to first determine how much your body is *still* producing; this depends on your weight, menopausal symptoms, and a hundred other things.

Estrogen

Estrogen tablets come in dosages of 0.3 mg, 0.625 mg, 0.9 mg, or 1.25 mg. Dosages also depend on why you're taking estrogen. For women who are at high risk for osteoporosis, the most common starting dosage is 0.625 mg. But for women who just want short-term relief from their menopausal symptoms, such as hot flashes, starting at 0.3 mg is more usual. If you forget to take your estrogen tablet one day, don't worry about it. You will not need to double up the way you would with birth control pills. (The reason you double up then is to avoid pregnancy. Obviously, pregnancy, in this case, is not a concern anymore.) It's important, however, that once you begin the estrogen, you continue to take it daily without a substantial break (like more than two days). Studies show that when you stop your estrogen, you can suffer from far more severe hot flashes and insomnia than you did before you started it.

If you're not taking estrogen orally, and are on the vaginal estrogen cream, you can use the cream for about three weeks on, and one week off. Women who opt for the vaginal cream have decided on estrogen for short-term relief of vaginal dryness and thinning, as well as relief from urinary incontinence, another post-menopausal problem, discussed below. But vaginal cream does not relieve hot flashes or offer any protection from osteoporosis or heart disease. Using the vaginal cream occasionally, the way you would lubricant, for example, will do you no good. Again, every woman is different, as are brands and dosage measurements in each brand. Make sure you discuss how much estrogen you're getting per application with either your doctor or pharmacist.

As for skin patches, they contain either 4 or 8 mg of estrogen. The 4-mg patch releases 0.05 mg of estrogen daily; the 8-mg patch releases twice that amount. You'll need to change the patch twice a week. Some doctors recommend that you wear the patch for three weeks, then take a one-week break before you start again. You'll need to discuss this with your doctor and decide what's right for you. Women who use the patch will not derive any HDL benefits, but they will be protected from bone loss and menopausal symptoms. In fact, the patch delivers a more continuous flow of estrogen than pills because there is no fluctuation in terms of dosage. With pills, it's impossible to be perfectly consistent about when you take your pill; there is more human error involved.

The androgen strain

ERT or HRT sometimes contain androgens, male hormones. Doctors will prescribe androgens to improve your libido, if you're experiencing problems. This may indeed be appropriate, but it's important to *know what you're getting*! If your androgen dosage is too high, you can develop male features, such as increased body hair, a deeper voice, and shrinking breasts. These symptoms do not magically vanish once you go off the androgens. Some studies also show that added androgens may have a negative effect on blood cholesterol, actually *increasing* heart disease risk. This may explain why men on estrogen derive no HDL benefits!

Common side effects

If you're taking *cyclical* progestins with your estrogen because you still have your uterus, bleeding is *not* a side effect! The whole point of adding progestin to your estrogen is to trigger withdrawal bleeding, and get your uterine lining routinely shed. If you're taking continuous progestins with your estrogen, however, bleeding is not the norm, and should be reported to your doctor.

A common side effect of estrogen is fluid retention, because estrogen will decrease the amount of salt and water excreted by the kidneys. Legs, breasts, and feet can swell. Because of the fluid retention, you may weigh more.

Nausea is another common side effect, also seen with OCs. This occurs during the first two or three months of therapy, and should disappear on its own. Some women find that taking their pills at night may remedy this. Decreasing the dosage is also an option.

Some other side effects reported include headaches, facial skin color changes called *melasma,* more cervical mucous secretion, liquid secretion from breasts, change in curvature of the cornea, jaundice, loss of scalp hair, and itchiness. Again, these side effects vary and depend on the brand you're taking, the dosage, your medical history, and so on. Many women suffer no side effects at all.

Finally, a minor side effect estrogen causes is vitamin B_6 deficiency, also seen with OCs. Symptoms are vague and include fatigue, depression, loss of concentration, loss of libido, or insomnia. This is easily remedied by taking a vitamin B_6 supplement.

Are You a Candidate for HRT or ERT?

Again, HRT or ERT is not for everyone. Some women make better candidates than others. Here's a guide that may help you make the decision:

- Do you suffer from severe hot flashes that don't respond to natural remedies, outlined below?
- Are your vaginal changes causing painful intercourse, urinary tract infections, or vaginitis, which does not respond to natural remedies, such as more stimulation of the clitoris during sex or sexual lubricants?
- Are you in a high-risk category for endometrial cancer? If so, taking progestin to trigger withdrawal bleeding will lower your risk.
- Are you in a high-risk group for heart attacks or strokes? If so, ERT or HRT will lower your risk.
- Are you in a high-risk group for developing osteoporosis? Again, ERT or HRT will lower your risk.

Women who shouldn't be on ERT or HRT

- Women with a history of endometrial cancer should not be on unopposed estrogen ERT. Again, if you still have a uterus, you'll be placed on HRT (estrogen and progesterone), which lowers your cancer risk anyway.
- Women with breast cancer. You shouldn't be on either ERT or HRT if you have a history of breast cancer.
- Women who have had a stroke. Neither ERT or HRT is recommended.
- Women who have a blood clotting disorder. Neither ERT nor HRT is recommended.
- Women with undiagnosed vaginal bleeding. Neither therapy is recommended.
- Women with liver dysfunction. You can be on the estrogen patch or vaginal cream to relieve your menopausal symptoms but you shouldn't take any pills.

Women who should think twice about HRT or ERT

Women with Type 2 diabetes are encouraged to discuss whether they are candidates for HRT, given its protective effects against heart disease. You may need to think twice, however, if you have the following *other* conditions:

- sickle cell disease
- high blood pressure
- migraines
- uterine fibroids
- a history of benign breast conditions such as cysts or fibroadenomas
- endometriosis
- seizures
- gallbladder disease
- a family history of breast cancer
- a past or current history of smoking

Common HRT Questions

Q. What if I begin my estrogen therapy while I'm still peri-menopausal, and am still getting my period? Will estrogen delay or reverse menopause?
A. *Estrogen won't interfere with your natural menopause because your ovaries will run out of eggs with or without hormone treatment.*

Q. What if I just take progesterone?
A. *Progestin alone can relieve up to 80 percent of your menopausal symptoms—especially hot flashes—but it won't affect your vaginal changes.*

Q. So I can't go on and off hormone therapy the way I could with oral contraceptives?
A. *You shouldn't go on and off estrogen because it may cause either irregular uterine bleeding or hyperplasia. Moreover, any protection from bone loss or heart disease is negated by going on and off.*

Phytoestrogens: The HRT Alternative

If you are uncomfortable with the idea of taking hormone replacement therapy, you may wish to consider the therapeutic benefits of phytoestrogens, or plant estrogens. Women are treating their symptoms with capsules of powdered herbs, such as licorice, burdock, wild yam, motherwort, and dong quai (*Angelica sinensis*).

These herbs contain a multitude of chemicals, including estrogenic substances. Although phytoestrogens have been used in Asian cultures for centuries to treat hot flashes, they're just beginning to catch on in the West. The first controlled trial began in 1996 at Columbia-Presbyterian Medical Center in New York.

Many food sources, such as tofu and soy, contain high concentrations of phytoestrogens. Scientists believe this may account for the incredible lack of menopausal symptoms in

Japan, which has a soy-heavy diet. Blood levels of phytoestrogens are ten to forty times higher in Japanese women than in their Western counterparts, and Japanese women report hot flashes about one-sixth as often as Western women. Even the average vegetarian would not consume nearly as much soy as does the average Japanese woman.

More interesting, plant hormones not only help prevent menopausal symptoms, but may protect you from breast cancer; breast cancer rates are dramatically lower in Japan than in the United States (but there may be other factors involved, such as childbearing habits and low-fat diets). After menopause, high-fat diets can increase your risk of heart attack and stroke, no matter how much estrogen you take. Meanwhile, bad habits, such as coffee, alcohol, and smoking, can increase your risk of osteoporosis. Right now, most doctors will tell you to go ahead and add as much soy as you want to your diet. It may well help; and it certainly can't hurt!

What are the drawbacks?

Licorice root increases your blood pressure if you already have hypertension, while wild yam occasionally causes gastrointestinal cramps. Moreover, many people have allergic reactions to a variety of herbs. Finally, because herbal products are not regulated, there is a danger of misuse, overuse, or using poor-quality products.

Phytoestrogens can be taken orally or even in creams, which can be applied to your body parts. Creams are "quasi-natural," however, because the plant hormones they contain are modified in a lab. One good question many women are asking is whether phytoestrogens carry the same risks as HRT.

Because plant-based hormones contain chemicals that are similar but not identical to natural estrogen, questions remain about their use.

This chapter has focused on the estrogen connection in women who are not pregnant. The rules of the game change when pregnancy is in the cards. The next chapter is the one to read if you are planning a pregnancy and already have diabetes, or you are concerned about gestational diabetes (diabetes developing in pregnancy).

CHAPTER 4

Type 2 Diabetes, Fertility, and Pregnancy

There is such a "splintered" market when it comes to pregnancy and diabetes that reliable information is difficult to find. This chapter is designed for two specific groups of women: The first group has already been diagnosed with Type 2 diabetes and has delayed having children (probably for social reasons) but is nevertheless planning a pregnancy or is already pregnant. Many of the women in this group also have been dealing with infertility, or are undergoing assisted reproductive technology. Women in their mid- to late forties, for example, have more options regarding pregnancy as a result of egg donation. Therefore, the old thinking that "women with Type 2 diabetes are too old to have babies and don't need this information" is being radically revised. In fact, there has been an upsurge in what is called "postmenopausal pregnancy" as a direct result of new fertility treatments. Fertility treatments and diabetes are therefore discussed, as well as how Type 2 diabetes often affects fertility. Everything you need to know about managing Type 2 diabetes *during* pregnancy is discussed as well in the section Being Pregnant on page 126.

Some of the material in this chapter previously appeared in M. Sara Rosenthal, *The Pregnancy Sourcebook*, 2d ed. (Los Angeles: Lowell House, 1997).

The second group of women reading this chapter have not been diagnosed at all with Type 2 diabetes, but instead, have been diagnosed with *gestational diabetes,* which means "diabetes during pregnancy." Gestational diabetes is not the same disease as Type 2 diabetes, even though it usually *behaves* the same way. It is a condition during pregnancy in which the body becomes resistant to the insulin it makes; it can often be managed through dietary changes and meal planning. It often disappears after pregnancy. Gestational diabetes, however, is often a "warning" that unless lifestyle and dietary habits change between pregnancies or *after* childbirth, Type 2 diabetes may be "in the cards" in the long run. If this describes you, go directly to the section Gestational Diabetes on page 129. Finally, if you have Type 1 diabetes, this is *not* the book for you, although you may indeed find certain sections of this chapter helpful.

GETTING PREGNANT

Okay. You have Type 2 diabetes. But you still want to get pregnant. What do you need to do in order to have a healthy baby, while staying healthy yourself?

The first step is to *plan ahead*! Get yourself under tight control through diet, exercise, and frequent blood sugar monitoring. If you are taking oral diabetes medication, you must stop; these drugs cannot be taken during pregnancy. You must either manage your diabetes through diet and exercise alone, or go on insulin during your conception phase and pregnancy. If you have to go on temporary insulin, consult Chapter 8 for "getting started" information, as well as useful tables that explain what kinds of insulin are available. Be forewarned: you must be able to *handle* taking insulin and going through a fairly radical change in your lifestyle habits, as well as being able to deal with another huge lifestyle change—having a baby! Have a frank discussion with your partner and doctor prior to making this decision.

Experts recommend that, ideally, you should plan your pregnancy three to six months in advance, so that you can make sure that your glycosylated hemoglobin levels (known as HbA_{1c} levels—see chapters 1 and 8) are within normal ranges during this period. A normal level means that your diabetes is well managed; therefore, the risk of birth defects is low. (This is a risk if you have high blood sugar in the early stages of pregnancy.) The following tests are also recommended prior to getting pregnant:

- Eye exam (to rule out diabetic eye disease)
- Blood pressure and urine tests to check your kidney function
- A gynecological exam (this should include a pelvic exam, breast exam, Pap test, and screening for vaginal infections or sexually transmitted diseases)
- A general checkup to rule out heart disease or other circulatory problems

Obesity

Regardless of your diabetes, obesity is a warning that your pregnancy may become high risk. For the record, the definition of *obese* means that you weigh at least 20 percent more than you should for your height and age. In the United States, roughly 32 million women (one-sixth of the population) fit this definition. And 40 percent of these women are young. There is some additional bad news. A recent study showed that women who are obese prior to conceiving are 60 percent more likely to have a cesarean delivery than women of average weight. If you are obese with your first pregnancy, the news is even worse: you're 64 percent more likely to require a cesarean section. The heavier you are, the more likely you are to have that C-section.

This is not a conspiracy. It just so happens that when you're obese *prior* to pregnancy, the odds of a number of complications *during* pregnancy increase, including gestational diabetes, discussed below.

Experts strongly suggest that the only way to combat this problem is to help women achieve a normal weight prior to conceiving, which would lead to a marked decrease in C-section deliveries. In fact, the current first-time cesarean delivery rate of 20 to 25 percent is blamed on this obesity issue. If all women were of normal weight for their ages and heights, experts muse that the C-section rate in the United States would drop to roughly 12 percent for first-time cesareans and 3 percent for repeat C-sections.

Having Sex

Getting pregnant means having sex (usually!). For women with diabetes, the act of having sex can interfere with blood sugar levels; it is, afterall, an *activity.* Therefore, many experts recommend that you treat sexual activity as any other physical exercise and plan for it accordingly. The risk of developing low blood sugar, or hypoglycemia, is not uncommon with sexual activity and diabetes. You may need to eat after sex, or eat something beforehand to ward off low blood sugar.

Another problem can arise: *no desire* for sex. This can occur because of vaginal infections (see chapter 9), or due to changing hormones if you are approaching menopause. Studies that looked specifically at the effect diabetes has on women and sexuality found that loss of libido was often caused by high blood sugar; vaginal infections and resulting pain or itching during intercourse; the sheer fear of pain or itching during intercourse; and nerve damage, which affects blood flow to the female genitalia, and hence, can interfere with pleasure, sensation, and orgasm.

Many women with diabetes also report that they feel unattractive as a result of their diabetes. They are concerned with not just their own performance, but their ability to please their partners. Fears of a "low blood sugar attack in the sack" are particularly common. The only way around feelings of unattractiveness or fears is openness with your partner. Discussing these issues with a sex therapist or counselor may also be of value.

Who should not get pregnant?

If your diabetes has affected your kidneys (see chapter 9), then pregnancy is not in your best interests. You will need to weigh your desire to procreate against the risks of dying from kidney failure. By controlling your diabetes during pregnancy, it is possible to give birth to a healthy child even when *you* have kidney disease, but it is unlikely that you will live to see that child's fifth birthday. Since people with diabetic kidney disease do not do well on dialysis, unless you have a kidney transplant, pregnancy will put your life in danger. I recommend that any woman with diabetic kidney disease contemplating pregnancy rent the film *Steel Magnolias*. It may give you a different perspective.

Infertility and Diabetes

Of course, there are those of you who want to get pregnant, but cannot. This section will shed some light on a common problem affecting many women with Type 2 diabetes. It is a condition known as Polycystic Ovarian Syndrome (PCO), a classic female infertility problem in the general population.

What happens in PCO is that your body secretes far too much androgen, the male hormone, which counteracts your ovaries' ability to make enough progesterone necessary for a normal cycle. (Review the first part of chapter 3 before reading on.) Here, your estrogen levels are fine, and in fact, your luteinzing hormone (LH) levels are higher than usual, working overtime to try to kick-start the cycle. But the androgen levels interfere with your FSH (follicle stimulating hormone), which you need to trigger progesterone. So your follicles never develop, and instead turn into small, pea-sized cysts on your ovaries. Your ovaries can then enlarge. Because your androgen levels are out of whack, you may develop facial hair, or hair on other parts of your body (this happens in 70 percent of the cases and is called *hirsutism*), or even a balding problem. Acne is another typical symptom because of an increase in androgen, as well as obesity (although women who are normal weight or are thin can also have this syndrome). Your periods will be irregular, and as a result, you might be at greater risk for developing *endometrial hyperplasia,* where your uterine lining thickens to the point of becoming precancerous. (If you have endometrial hyperplasia, you will be given progesterone supplements to induce a period, or a D&C may be required to get rid of the lining.) Because of your high levels of androgens, you may also be at increased risk for cardiovascular disease. Diet can help reduce the onset of heart problems.

If PCO was caught earlier in your menstrual history, you would have been put on a combination oral contraceptive to induce normal withdrawal bleeding and pump your system with normal levels of estrogen and progesterone. Or you would have been put on progestin, a synthetic progesterone supplement, and been instructed to take it about midcycle.

If you were treated earlier with progestin, you won't experience problems with your cycle unless you go off it for some reason. Women, however, who were treated with oral contraceptives for irregular cycles at a very young age may not know *why* they suffered from irregular periods in the first place. When these women go off contraception to conceive, they'll be plagued by the same symptoms that warranted oral contraception initially.

Sometimes, women who had normal cycles for many years develop PCO later in life. In this case, they will suddenly develop irregular cycles (called *secondary amenorrhea*) out of the blue.

It's recently been discovered that insulin resistance and polycystic ovary syndrome go hand in hand. Women with insulin resistance are either at risk for, or have been diagnosed with, Type 2 diabetes. Women who are obese (many of whom are also insulin resistant) are predisposed to PCO because their fatty tissues produce estrogen, which can confuse the pituitary gland.

Lowering insulin in women with polycystic ovary syndrome seems to help restore menstrual cycles, and lower male hormone levels. Oral hypoglycemic agents used to treat Type 2 diabetes are now being used to treat PCO, although these drugs must be stopped once you become pregnant. Only about half of women diagnosed with PCO have insulin resistance, however. Before you take an insulin-lowering drug, ask your doctor about how diet and exercise can help your body use insulin more efficiently.

In general, PCO is hereditary; it is more common among women of Mediterranean descent. It's also uncommon to develop PCO later in life, although it can happen, as stated above. Generally, a woman with PCO will begin to experience menstrual irregularities within three to four years after her menarche (first period). About 4 percent of the general female population suffer from PCO, which accounts for half of all hormonal disorders affecting female fertility.

Why are estrogen levels normal in women with PCO?

Normal estrogen levels come as a surprise to women with PCO. In normally fertile women, estrogen is made from the follicles. In this case, however, your body converts the *androgens* into estrogen. If you're obese, estrogen will also be stored in fat cells. This constant estrogen level really confuses the hypothalamus, which assumes that high estrogen levels are present because of a developing egg inside the follicle. The hypothalamus will then tell the pituitary to slow down the release of FSH. Without FSH, your follicles won't mature and won't burst, and hence, you won't ovulate.

Reversing PCO

To reverse infertility in women with PCO, doctors use the fertility drug, clomiphene citrate, in tablet form. You'll start clomiphene citrate around day five of your cycle, and then go off the tablet at about day ten. If you've had long bouts of amenorrhea, before starting on clomiphene citrate, your period will first be induced via a progesterone supplement. An average dosage of clomiphene citrate in this case ranges from 25 to 50 milligrams. In some cases, an anti-estrogen drug, called tamoxifen (also used as treatment in certain kinds of breast and gynecological cancers) will be given along with clomiphene citrate. Roughly 70 to 90 percent of all women with PCO on clomiphene will ovulate, but pregnancy rates really vary; 30 to 70 percent of women with PCO on clomiphene will conceive.

If you're still not ovulating after taking clomiphene citrate, human chorionic gonadotropin (HCG) may be added to your hormonal "diet" during the luteal phase of your cycle, roughly one week after your last dose of clomiphene citrate.

If this regimen fails, you'll graduate to a very potent fertility drug, human menopausal gonadotropin (HMG—Pergonal or Metrodin). This drug is *pure* FSH, made from the urine of menopausal women. (During menopause, FSH levels naturally soar to compensate for tired ovaries.)

Prior to starting HMG, you'll need to have a hysterosalpingogram (a procedure that checks whether your fallopian tubes are clear). You may also need a pelvic ultrasound to rule out other structural abnormalities. Women with PCO don't do as well on HMG as they do on clomiphene citrate. While 70 to 80 percent will ovulate with HMG, only 20 to 40 percent will conceive. While taking HMG, you'll also need to be monitored through blood tests (to check estrogen levels) and ultrasound (to check follicle growth).

For more information on the side effects, costs, and risks associated with fertility drugs and other fertility treatments, consult *The Fertility Sourcebook*, 2d edition (1998).

I caution any woman with diabetes, however, to consult her diabetes specialist prior to going on *any* fertility drugs. Estrogen can raise blood sugar levels, and you need to know how these drugs will affect your blood sugar, not just your ovaries.

Other treatments for PCO

In many women with PCO, weight loss is considered the "cure"—
just as it often is for insulin resistance. When infertility is a concern, and your birthdays are coming "fast and furious," weight
loss may not be a realistic short-term treatment; it's a slow, time-
consuming process. If you have PCO, and are being treated with
fertility drugs, you may be able to improve your fertility through
natural weight loss for future pregnancies. Your diabetes educator or a dietitian can help you with meal planning, which will not
only help control your diabetes, but may help you get pregnant.

If the ovaries have large cysts on them, some fertility specialists may want to attempt cauterizing the ovary (in about eight to
ten small spots) through laparoscopic surgery. This procedure is
still considered experimental, but roughly 62 percent of women
with PCO go on to conceive after this surgery, and when the
surgery is combined with fertility drug therapy, pregnancy rates
are as high as 80 percent.

In some women with PCO, androgens are also produced in the
adrenal glands. Under these circumstances, your doctor may want to
put you on a corticosteroid to suppress the adrenal gland, lowering
the production of androgens. This will help induce ovulation as well.

Bromocriptine, which suppresses prolactin, will be given to
15 to 20 percent of all women with PCO. The high levels of estrogen associated with PCO commonly cause hyperprolactenemia,
meaning "too much prolactin," which can interfere with fertility.

A hairy situation

Women who have had diabetes for a long period of time may
notice hirsutism, or overgrowth of hair. Some studies show that
prolonged use of insulin can trigger higher levels of testosterone,
which can cause facial hair growth. This is also one of the
unpleasant symptoms of PCO. Typically, this hair appears on the
face, navel, or breasts; many women will want to treat this. An

anti-androgen drug, which is available in pill or cream form, will take care of the hair growth problem. You'll need to discuss your exact dosage of this drug with your doctor, and specifically how this drug will affect your blood sugar. You'll begin to see hair growth slow down after about five months on the drug.

In the interim, electrolysis is the most effective treatment for hair growth on the face, navel, or breasts. Make sure you go to a reputable clinic, and ask for referrals to past clients. Sloppy electrolysis can result in burning and other skin problems.

Other causes of infertility

There are many other causes of female-factor and male-factor infertility that are completely unrelated to blood sugar. For the record, roughly 80 percent of all female-factor infertility is caused by structural problems, where the fallopian tubes become blocked. This may be due to pelvic inflammatory disease, a condition that results when bacterial infections (from a sexually transmitted disease or bacteria entering during pelvic surgery or previous childbirth) travel up the reproductive tract, causing tubal scarring and inflammation. Endometriosis is another cause of tubal blockage. For more information on other causes of infertility, please refer to *The Fertility Sourcebook,* 2d edition (1998).

BEING PREGNANT

If you've been diagnosed with either Type 1 or Type 2 diabetes *prior* to becoming pregnant, this section is for you. This means you have what's known as *pregestational diabetes* (diabetes before pregnancy). If you have developed diabetes *during* pregnancy, see the separate section on page 129 about gestational diabetes (diabetes during pregnancy).

So long as your blood glucose levels are normal throughout your pregnancy and you have normal blood pressure, you are "allowed" to be pregnant and you and your baby should be fine. Nevertheless, there are some concerns unique to women with Type 2 diabetes.

For example, if you have Type 2 diabetes, statistics indicate that you're probably in worse shape than your Type 1 counterparts. First, you don't have the years of practice Type 1 women do at monitoring your blood sugar levels. Second, if you were taking oral hypoglycemic agents prior to your pregnancy, you may not have learned to be as strict with your diet as you should be—something you *must* do during pregnancy. Since these pills cannot be taken during pregnancy (they cause birth defects), your doctor will switch you to insulin before you conceive, which puts you in the difficult predicament of "learning" a whole new disease. The danger of taking oral hypoglycemic agents during pregnancy is that the drug crosses the placenta and gets into the baby's bloodstream, causing very low blood sugar in the fetus. Insulin, however, does not cross the placenta, and is safe during pregnancy.

Unfortunately, unless you became an expert on your diabetes *prior* to conceiving, you're in for a bumpy ride. In fact, the early weeks of pregnancy are so critical that if your blood sugar levels were not under control *three to six months prior to your pregnancy,* you should seriously consider asking your practitioners whether they advise continuing the pregnancy.

It is during the first three months of pregnancy that the fetus develops its brain, nervous system, and other body organs. It is also during this time when your blood sugar levels are most vulnerable as a result of hormonal changes, vomiting due to morning sickness, and fatigue.

Staying in Control

No matter what type of diabetes you have, every diabetes book will tell you that a healthy pregnancy depends on how well *you* manage your disease. If you can keep your blood sugar levels as close to normal as possible throughout your pregnancy, then, as most books will also tell you, your chances of a healthy baby are as good as a nondiabetic woman's. The only way to do this is to carefully plan out your meals, exercise, and insulin requirements (if needed) with your doctor. And if you do need insulin, your requirement will continue to increase as your pregnancy progresses. Keep in mind that the state of pregnancy means that blood sugar levels are usually lower than those of nonpregnant women. Therefore, what's considered to be in the normal range for nonpregnant women will be different than what is considered normal for pregnant women. Consult your doctor about what the normal range should be for you.

When you lose control

If you lose control of your blood sugar levels in the first eight weeks of pregnancy, your baby is at risk for birth defects. High blood sugar levels may interfere with the formation of your baby's organs, causing heart defects or spina bifida (open spine). Once your baby's organs are formed, the risk of birth defects from high blood sugar levels disappears, but new problems surface.

High blood sugar levels will cross the placenta and feed the baby too much glucose, causing the baby to make extra fat, and therefore, to grow too big and fat for its gestational age. This condition is called *macrosomia,* defined as birth weight greater than 4,000 grams, or greater than the ninetieth-percentile babies.

In addition, the baby is at risk for becoming lethargic and developing a malfunctioning metabolism in utero, which can lead to stillbirth. This problem is solved when you regain control of your blood sugar levels. Babies with macrosomia are usually not able to fit through the birth canal; they often sustain damage to their shoulders (the shoulders get stuck) during a vaginal birth. So if your baby is too big, you will need a cesarean section.

The extra glucose that gets into the baby also causes the baby's pancreas to make extra insulin. Then, after birth, the baby's body needs time to adjust to normal glucose levels (since the placenta is gone); this can cause the baby to suffer from hypoglycemia, or low blood glucose levels. These babies are at higher risk for breathing problems, and are at a higher risk for developing obesity and Type 2 diabetes later in life.

Your baby may also develop jaundice after birth. This is very common for all newborns, but tends to happen more frequently in babies born to mothers with diabetes. Newborn jaundice is caused by a buildup of old, "leftover" red blood cells that aren't clearing out of the body fast enough. Breastfeeding is the best cure for newborn jaundice. Consult the book *The Breastfeeding Sourcebook*, 2d edition (1998) for more information.

GESTATIONAL DIABETES

Gestational diabetes (GDM) refers to diabetes that is first diagnosed during the twenty-fourth to twenty-eighth week of pregnancy. If you had diabetes prior to your pregnancy (Type 1 or Type 2), it is known as *pregestational diabetes,* which is a completely different story, in that the risks to the fetus exist throughout pregnancy.

Technically, gestational diabetes means "high blood sugar (hyperglycemia) first recognized during pregnancy." Three to 12 percent of all pregnant women will develop gestational diabetes between weeks twenty-four and twenty-eight of their pregnancies. The symptoms of gestational diabetes are extreme thirst, hunger, or fatigue, but many women do not notice these symptoms.

What is GDM?

During pregnancy, hormones made by the placenta can block the insulin the pancreas normally makes. This forces the pancreas to work harder and manufacture three times as much insulin as usual. In many cases, the pancreas isn't able to keep up and blood

FOUR STEPS TO GOOD GLUCOSE LEVELS

1. Use a home blood glucose monitor to test your blood sugar levels. Pregnancy can mask the symptoms of low blood glucose so you cannot rely on how well you "feel." The goal is to get your blood glucose levels to match those of a non-diabetic pregnant woman, *which are lower than in a nondiabetic, nonpregnant woman.*

2. Ask your doctor *when* you should test your blood glucose levels. During pregnancy, it's common to test up to *eight times per day,* especially after eating.

3. Record your results in a journal you keep handy. Take the journal with you when you go out—especially to restaurants.

4. In a *separate* journal, keep track of when you're exercising and what you're eating.

5. Check with your doctor or diabetes educator before you make any changes to your diet/insulin plan whatsoever. And, no, midwives and doulas are *not* the appropriate practitioners to rely on for this information!

YOUR DIABETES PRENATAL TEAM

A healthy pregnancy depends on a good prenatal team who can help you stay in control. In the same way that you would handpick various skill sets for a baseball team, you must do the same for this team. Here are the specialists to look for:

1. An endocrinologist or internist who specializes in diabetes—and diabetic pregnancies.

2. An obstetrician who specializes in high-risk pregnancies, particularly diabetic pregnancies. You may wish to use a *perinatologist,* a doctor who exclusively specializes in high-risk pregnancies.

3. A neonatologist (a specialist for newborns) "waiting in the wings" or a good pediatrician who is trained to manage babies of diabetic moms.

4. A nutritionist or registered dietitian who can help you work out a realistic diet/insulin plan during your pregnancy.

5. A diabetes educator who is available to answer questions throughout your pregnancy.

6. For additional support, a midwife or doula.

sugar levels rise. Gestational diabetes is therefore a common pregnancy-related health problem, and is in the same league as other pregnancy-related conditions that develop during the second or third trimesters, such as high blood pressure.

Since pregnancy is a time when you're gaining weight, some experts believe that it is the sheer weight gain which contributes to insulin resistance, as the pancreas cannot keep up with the new weight, and hence new "demand" for insulin. It's akin to the situation when a small restaurant with only ten tables suddenly is presented with triple the amount of customers. It will be understaffed, and unable to accommodate the new demand for "tables."

GDM usually takes the form of Type 2 diabetes in that it can be managed through diet and blood sugar monitoring. Recent research on California women with gestational diabetes, however, showed that only one-third were able to control their condition through diet and blood sugar monitoring. Therefore, insulin may be necessary if your GDM cannot be controlled. GDM will usually disappear once you deliver, but it recurs in future pregnancies two out of three times. In some cases, GDM is really the unveiling of Type 2 or even Type 1 diabetes *during* pregnancy.

If you are genetically predisposed to Type 2 diabetes, you are more likely to develop Type 2 in the future after a bout of gestational diabetes.

Moreover, if you have GDM, you're more at risk for other pregnancy-related conditions, such as hypertension (high blood pressure), preeclampsia, and polyhydramnios (too much amniotic fluid). If you're carrying more than one fetus, your pregnancy is even more risky. Therefore, it's wise to seek out an experienced obstetrician if you have GDM. In very high-risk situations, a perinatologist (an obstetrician who specializes in high-risk pregnancies) may have to be consulted.

Diagnosing GDM

GDM is diagnosed through a test known as *glucose screening.* Obviously, if you've already been diagnosed with Type 2 diabetes, you will not need to be screened for diabetes during pregnancy. Candidates for glucose screening are women who are worried about developing diabetes during pregnancy because they believe they have risk factors (see chapter 1), have a family history of gestational diabetes, or have a personal history of gestational diabetes from a previous pregnancy.

There is debate in the medical community over the issue of universal glucose screening during pregnancy. Many practitioners feel that *all* women should be given a glucose tolerance test between their twenty-fourth and twenty-eighth weeks, regardless of risk factors (see chapter 1). U.S. studies show that by screening only women with risk factors, almost half of all gestational diabetes is missed.

Since blood sugar levels rise steadily throughout pregnancy, it's entirely possible to have normal blood sugar levels at week twenty-four and high levels at week twenty-eight, which is why many physicians feel that universal screening produces more problems than it catches. Many feel that the anxiety it creates in women who have high blood sugar levels is an issue worth considering. And some doctors wonder if even selective screening (meaning screening only those women with risk factors) reduces the problem of macrosomic babies (fat, glucose-gorged babies).

Jelly beans versus cola

If your doctor decides on testing, the good news is that a new jelly bean glucose test is available in some areas instead of the test with a colalike beverage now used, which causes nausea, vomiting, abdominal pain, bloating, and profuse sweating. Apparently by eating just eighteen jelly beans, and having blood glucose tested an hour later, gestational diabetes is as accurately rooted out as it was with the old, horrid cola test. Furthermore, the jelly beans do not cause any side effects other than a mild headache or nausea in a tiny percentage of women. If you are going to have your blood glucose tested, show your doctor this passage of the book and ask for the jelly beans! Many women are worried that a history of gestational diabetes means they will eventually develop Type 2 diabetes. If you developed (or will develop) gestational diabetes during pregnancy, consider yourself put on alert. Approximately 20 percent of all women with gestational diabetes develop Type 2, presuming no other risk factors. Gestational diabetes develops more often in women who were overweight prior to pregnancy and women who are over age thirty-five.

Who should be screened?

The symptoms of gestational diabetes are extreme thirst, hunger, or fatigue, all of which can be masked by the normal discomforts of pregnancy. Therefore, all women should be screened for GDM during weeks twenty-four to twenty-eight of their pregnancies (see the glucose screening section above). This is particularly crucial if

- you are of aboriginal, African, or Hispanic descent;
- your mother had GDM;
- you previously gave birth to a baby with a birth weight of more than nine pounds;
- you've miscarried or had a stillbirth;
- you're over twenty-five years of age;
- you're overweight or obese (20 percent above your ideal weight); or
- you have high blood pressure.

Some doctors believe it isn't necessary to screen a woman for GDM if she has no symptoms or any of the risk factors above; their attitude is that universal screening can create unnecessary anxiety. U.S. studies show, as mentioned, that by screening only women with risk factors, almost half of all gestational diabetes is missed.

Risks to the Fetus

Fortunately, because gestational diabetes occurs well after the baby's body has been formed, birth defects are not a risk with GDM as they are with pregestational diabetes. Gestational diabetes is only linked to heart defects when the condition is severe enough to necessitate insulin treatment in the last trimester.

The main risk to the fetus with GDM is that the high blood sugar levels cross the placenta and feed the fetus too much glucose, causing it to grow too fat and large for its gestational age. This condition, as described earlier, is called *macrosomia,* technically defined by a birth weight greater than 4,000 grams.

Babies with macrosomia are usually not able to fit through the birth canal because their shoulders get stuck (known as *shoulder dystocia*). Therefore, most women with macrosomic babies will need to deliver by cesarean section.

The extra glucose that gets into the baby can also cause its pancreas to work harder, which can cause hypoglycemia after birth.

Treating GDM

The treatment for GDM is controlling blood sugar levels through diet, exercise, insulin, if necessary, and blood sugar monitoring. To do this, you must be under the care of a pregnancy practitioner (obstetrician or midwife), a diabetes specialist, and a dietitian. Guidelines for nutrition and weight gain during a diabetic pregnancy depend on your current health, the fetal size, and *your* weight.

At least 80 percent of the time, gestational diabetes disappears after delivery. Unfortunately, it is destined to return in subsequent pregnancies 80 to 90 percent of the time, unless you get yourself in good physical shape between pregnancies. Experts report that each subsequent bout of gestational diabetes is more severe than the previous one.

Treating low blood sugar in pregnancy

Many women with gestational diabetes will have episodes of low blood sugar, which are not harmful to the fetus, but very unpleasant for the mother. The thinking is that it's better to risk low blood sugar (hypoglycemia) in pregnancy to avoid high blood sugar (hyperglycemia), which is damaging to the fetus. Treating low blood sugar is the same in pregnancy as any other time. Review chapter 1, pages 38–39 for details.

SPECIAL DELIVERY

About one in four babies is delivered by cesarean section. A cesarean section, or C-section is a surgical procedure that is essentially "abdominal delivery." The procedure, as the name suggests, dates back to Julius Caesar, who, as legend tells us, was born in this manner. Whether Caesar's truly was a cesarean birth is hotly debated among historians, but what historians *do* know is that the abdominal delivery dates back to ancient Rome. In fact, Roman law made it legal to perform a cesarean section *only* if the mother died in the last four weeks of pregnancy. The procedure therefore originated *only as a means to save the child.* Using the procedure to save the *mother* was not even *considered* until the nineteenth century, under the influence of two prominent obstetricians, Max Sanger and Eduardo Porro.

Women who have diabetes during pregnancy (pregestational or gestational) are at a higher risk of requiring a cesarean section than the general pregnant population. That's because they may give birth to very large babies, who may not be able to fit through the birth canal. Prior to your due date you need to have a frank discussion with your pregnancy health care provider about what situations would warrant a cesarean section.

This is major pelvic surgery, and usually involves either a spinal or epidural (a type of local anesthetic). A vertical or horizontal incision is made just above your pubic hairline. Then the surgeon cuts (usually) horizontally through the uterine muscle and eases the baby out. Sometimes, this second cut is vertical, known as the "classic incision." It is this *second cut*, into the uterine muscle, that determines the possibility of a VBAC (vaginal birth after cesarean). With a horizontal cut, women have gone on to have normal second vaginal births; with the classic cut, the scar is less stable, and will mean that for *you*, "once a C-section, always a C-section" is a reality.

In some instances, you'll know in advance whether you need to have a cesarean section. Your pelvis may be clearly too small, or you may have irreparable scarring on your cervix from previous pelvic surgery that will prevent dilation. Or, an emergency situation may be detected that requires the fetus to be taken out immediately.

A Dozen Good Reasons to Have a C-Section

Below are twelve legitimate reasons why a cesarean section may be performed.

1. When a vaginal delivery, even with intervention, is risky. *Note: You may fall into this category if your baby is large.*
2. A prolonged labor (caused by failure to dilate, failure of the labor to progress, too large a head, and several other reasons).
3. A failed induction attempt (labor induction sometimes fails, and when the baby is overdue, a cesarean is the next alternative).
4. When the baby is in a breech position.
5. Placental problems.
6. Fetal distress.
7. Health problems in the mother that prevent normal vaginal delivery.

8. A history of difficult deliveries or stillbirth.
9. When the baby is in a transverse lie (horizontal position).
10. When the mother has primary genital herpes or other sexually transmitted diseases, such as genital warts, chlamydia, or gonorrhea, which may be passed on to the newborn via vaginal delivery.
11. When the mother is HIV positive.
12. A multiple birth.

Unnecessary Versus Necessary Cesareans

There are, of course, many *unnecessary* cesarean sections performed. Most *second* cesareans are not necessary, for instance, if the uterine cut *was* horizontal. Another common practice is to perform a C-section when a woman fails to go into labor after being induced. Inducing labor is often because of the pregnancy progressing past the due date. In this case, if the fetus isn't in distress, you may want to wait, or get a second opinion regarding a C-section. In a U.S. study, situations where a C-section was performed depended more on the *doctor* than on any other single factor; the rate of C-sections varied from 19 to 42 percent according to the individual doctor's preference. This is a huge discrepancy. What it boils down to is the *doctor's* definition of "emergency," which may arise in the event of any of the problems listed above. No competent doctor will delay a C-section if he or she thinks that the labor is endangering the baby's or mother's health.

Again, to avoid an unnecessary procedure, consult with your practitioner and midwife *before* the third trimester. Find out what situations truly warrant a C-section, and whether you're a VBAC (pronounced vee-back) candidate. If you're experiencing a difficult or high-risk pregnancy or will be having a multiple birth, you *may* be more likely to have the procedure than a woman with a low-risk pregnancy.

AFTER THE BABY IS BORN

The first question you may have after you give birth is whether your diabetes is "gone." This is only a valid question for women who have had gestational diabetes. In this case, the only way to tell is to have another glucose tolerance test when you get your first postpartum menstrual period (if you're breast-feeding), or alternatively, six weeks after childbirth. If the test results are normal, then your diabetes is, indeed, gone—but should not be forgotten. It's a warning to you that you better "shape up" between pregnancies, or forever after. Otherwise future bouts of gestational diabetes or Type 2 diabetes in later years could come back to haunt you. Of course, there are some other issues that will surface for mothers who have (or had) diabetes.

If your test results show continuing high blood sugar, it's probably safe to assume that you have Type 2 diabetes that simply revealed itself during your pregnancy. In this case, your diabetes is a permanent health condition that was diagnosed during pregnancy, or even, perhaps, triggered by it.

Should I Breastfeed?

Yes. Next question.

Why Was I Told Not to Breastfeed?

Ignorant practitioners may tell you that you can't breastfeed if you've had diabetes. *This is completely false!* If your diabetes is well controlled, and you've given birth to a healthy baby, than breastfeeding is the normal way to feed your baby, and does not place your baby at risk for the numerous, undisputed, and well-documented health problems associated with babies fed artificial milk. Stick to your "pregnancy rules" and keep self-monitoring your blood sugar levels so that you can adjust your diet and exercise routine to your new hormone levels. As stated in chapter 3, estrogen levels affect blood sugar levels; when they rise, your blood sugar rises; when they drop—which is what happens during breast-feeding as a result of the hormone prolactin—blood sugar levels may drop. This could mean you may need to eat more while breastfeeding to keep your levels up.

If you had gestational diabetes, this natural drop in blood sugar levels is nature's way of helping you bounce back to health faster if you breastfeed. If you need to take insulin to control high blood sugar after childbirth, your baby doesn't care! Insulin cannot be ingested, so even if it "crosses" into the breast-milk, it will have zero effect on the baby. Remember, if insulin could be ingested, *you* wouldn't need to inject it in the first place!

Furthermore, several studies show that breastfed babies have lower incidences of both Type 1 and Type 2 diabetes later in life.

If you have high blood sugar in the days and/or weeks following childbirth, then your milk will be much sweeter than usual. That's not dangerous *per se* to the baby; the baby has his or her own functioning pancreas, which can produce the insulin she needs to handle the sweetness. But the baby could put on too much weight and get fat as a result of the sweet milk. There may be cases when the sweetness is a "turnoff" to the baby, and he may not nurse as vigorously, which may cause problems with your milk supply. This can also cause engorgement, which is painful and can put you at risk for mastitis (inflammation in the breast, usually due to bacterial infection). In general, the main danger of high blood sugar during breastfeeding is to *you*; you'll want to control your diabetes so that you can be as healthy and fit as possible. This is the case, however, for every woman—whether she has children or not, and whether she's breastfeeding or not. For more information about breastfeeding, consult *The Breastfeeding Sourcebook*, 2d edition (1998).

Postpartum "Blues" and Diabetes

Many women find the enormous lifestyle adjustment after child-birth tiring. They may feel fatigued, stressed, overwhelmed, and many other normal emotions that accompany giving birth. Unfortunately, some women may also suffer from postpartum depression, characterized by a loss of interest in formerly plea-surable activities, changes in appetite and sleep patterns (which happen anyway after childbirth), sadness, and a host of other emotional and physical symptoms.

Just because you have diabetes does not mean that you can't develop another condition on top of it, such as postpartum depression. But keeping your blood sugar in check after child-birth will help to avoid the common problem of high or low blood sugar levels—and their associated mood swings—masking post-partum depression, or vice versa. It's also recommended that you have your thyroid checked after childbirth to make sure that you are not also suffering from postpartum thyroid disease, which affects about 18 percent of the postpartum population. This can be misdiagnosed as postpartum depression as well.

For more information on postpartum depression, consult *The Pregnancy Sourcebook,* 2d edition (1997).

Diabetes never ceases to affect women in unique ways at dif-ferent stages of their lives. The next chapter is the one to read after your baby-making days are over.

CHAPTER 5

Type 2 Diabetes and the Menopausal Woman

Menopause is a recent phenomenon in our society. Previous to one hundred years ago, many women died before the age of menopause. Only in this century have women outlived their ovaries.

Menopause is a Greek term taken from the words *menos,* meaning "month," and *pause,* meaning "arrest"—the arrest of the menstrual cycle. It is a time in every woman's life when her ovaries slow down, run out of eggs, and get ready to retire. The process involves a complex shutting down of the hormones that have sustained the menstrual cycle until this point. As a result, the normal hormonal fluctuations women are accustomed to throughout their menstrual cycles become far more erratic, causing the infamous "menopausal mood swings" that have created much of the negative mythology surrounding menopause in our culture.

Nevertheless, natural menopause and *menarche* (the first menstrual period) have a lot in common; they are both processes that women ease into gradually. A woman doesn't suddenly wake up to find herself in menopause any more than a young girl wakes up to find herself in puberty. When menopause, however,

---

Some of the material in this chapter previously appeared in M. Sara Rosenthal, *The Gynecological Sourcebook,* 3d ed. (Los Angeles: Lowell House, 1999).

occurs *surgically*—the by-product of an oopherectomy, ovarian failure following a hysterectomy, or certain cancer therapies—it can be an extremely jarring process. *One out of every three women in North America will not make it to the age of sixty with the uterus intact.* These women may indeed wake up one morning to find themselves in menopause, and as a result, will suffer far more noticeable and severe menopausal symptoms than those who experience natural menopause. It is because of *surgical* menopause that hormonal replacement therapy (HRT) and estrogen replacement therapy (ERT or "unopposed estrogen") have become such hotly debated issues in women's health. The loss of estrogen, in particular, leads to drastic changes in the body's chemistry that trigger a more aggressive aging process (discussed below).

Women with Type 2 diabetes have a little more to be concerned about than women without Type 2 diabetes. Estrogen loss increases *all* women's risk of heart disease, which is the major cause of death for postmenopausal women. In postmenopausal women with diabetes, however, the risk of heart disease is two to three times higher than in the general female population. Furthermore, as estrogen and progesterone levels drop, women with diabetes can expect fluctuations in their blood sugar levels, and possibly more episodes of low blood sugar (see chapter 1). After menopause, women taking insulin may find that their insulin requirements have dropped by 20 percent.

The purpose of this chapter is to discuss both the natural and surgical menopausal facts of life for women with diabetes, which include myths about menopause, the symptoms of menopause, the osteoporosis issue, and the variety of health problems that women with diabetes face as they age. The benefits and risks of HRT and ERT are discussed in chapter 3. Remember that your age, medical history, and menopausal symptoms all need to be factored into the HRT or ERT decision, and weighed against the health risks your diabetes poses.

NATURAL MENOPAUSE

When menopause occurs naturally, it usually takes place between the ages of forty-eight and fifty-two, but it can occur as early as your late thirties, or as late as your midfifties. When menopause occurs *before* age forty-five, it is technically considered early menopause; just as menarche is genetically predetermined, however, so is menopause. What the average woman with an unremarkable medical history eats or does in terms of activity will *not* influence the timing of menopause. Women who have had chemotherapy or who have been exposed to high levels of radiation (such as radiation therapy in the pelvic area for cancer treatment), however, may experience earlier menopause than normal. In any event, the average age of menopause is fifty to fifty-one.

Other causes of early menopause include mumps (in a few women, the infection causing mumps spreads to the ovaries, prematurely shutting them down) and specific autoimmune diseases, such as lupus or rheumatoid arthritis (some women develop antibodies to their own ovaries, which attack the ovaries).

The Stages of Natural Menopause

Socially, the word *menopause* refers to a process, not a precise moment in the life of your menstrual cycle. But medically, *menopause* does indeed refer to one precise moment: the date of your last period. The events preceding and following menopause amount to a huge change for women, both physically and socially, however. Physically, this process is divided into four stages:

1. *Premenopause*—Although some doctors may refer to a thirty-two year-old woman in her childbearing years as "premenopausal," this is not really an appropriate label. The term *premenopause* refers to women on the cusp of menopause. Their periods have just *started* to get irregular, but they do not yet experience any classic menopausal symptoms such

as hot flashes or vaginal dryness. A woman in premenopause is usually in her mid- to late forties. If your doctor tells you that you're premenopausal, you might want to ask her how she is using this term.

2. *Perimenopause*—This term refers to women who are in the thick of menopause—their cycles are wildly erratic, and they are experiencing hot flashes and vaginal dryness. This label is applicable for about four years, from the first two years prior to the official "last" period through the two years following the last menstrual period. Women who are perimenopausal are aged between the midforties to about fifty-one.

3. *Menopause*—This refers to your final menstrual period. You will not be able to pinpoint your final period until you've been completely free from periods for one year. Then you count back to the last period you charted, and *that* date is the date of your menopause. *Important: After more than one year of no menstrual periods, any vaginal bleeding should be considered abnormal.*

4. *Postmenopause*—This term refers to the last third of most women's lives, ranging from women who have been free of menstrual periods for at least four years to women celebrating their one-hundredth birthdays. In other words, once you're past menopause, you'll be referred to as postmenopausal for the rest of your life. Sometimes, the terms *postmenopausal* and *perimenopausal* are used interchangeably, but this is technically inaccurate.

In a *social* context, however, nobody really bothers to break down menopause this precisely. When you see the word *menopausal* in a magazine article, you are noting what's become acceptable medical slang, referring to women who are premenopausal and perimenopausal—a time frame that includes the actual menopause. When you see the word *postmenopausal*, you are seeing more accepted medical slang, which includes women who are in perimenopause and "official" postmenopause.

"Diagnosing" premenopause or perimenopause

When you begin to notice the signs of menopause, discussed next, either you'll suspect the approach of menopause on your own, or your doctor will put two and two together when you report your "bizarre" symptoms. There are two very simple tests that will accurately determine what's going on, and what stage of menopause you're in. Your FSH levels will dramatically rise as your ovaries begin to shut down; these levels are easily checked from one blood test. In addition, your vaginal walls will thin, and the cells lining the vagina will not contain as much estrogen. Your doctor will take a Paplike smear from your vaginal walls—simple and painless—and then analyze the smear to check for vaginal atrophy—the thinning and drying out of your vagina. In addition, as discussed below, you need to keep track of your periods and chart them as they become irregular. Your menstrual pattern will be an additional clue to your doctor about what stage of menopause you are in.

Signs of Natural Menopause

In the past, a long list of hysterical symptoms have been attributed to the "change of life," but medically, there are really just three classic *short-term* symptoms of menopause: erratic periods, hot flashes, and vaginal dryness. All three of these symptoms are caused by a decrease in estrogen. The emotional symptoms of menopause, such as irritability, mood swings, melancholy, and so on, are actually caused by a *rise in FSH*. As the cycle changes and the ovaries' egg supply dwindles, FSH is secreted in very high amounts and reaches a lifetime peak (as much as fifteen times higher than usual); it's the body's way of trying to "jump-start" the ovarian engine. This is why the urine of menopausal women is used to produce Human Menopausal Gonadotropin (HMG), the potent fertility drug which consists of pure FSH.

Women make the understandable mistake of assuming that mood swings are caused by estrogen deficiency. But during the childbearing years, premenstrual symptoms are caused by *peak* levels of estrogen and progesterone; the symptoms are relieved when the flow starts, and the estrogen and progesterone levels *drop*. So, it's not possible for low levels of estrogen to cause *premenstrual* symptoms during menopause. Ironically, the only other time in a woman's life when her FSH levels are as high as they are in menopause is during puberty. (This may be why the classic mother/daughter "hormone clash" tends to occur when a daughter is entering puberty while the mother is entering menopause. At this stage, both mother and daughter are more "sex hormone matched," in terms of hormonal levels, than at other times in their relationship.) The erratic "up and down" moods of puberty mirror the mood swings that can characterize menopause for the same reasons. Decreased levels of estrogen can, however, make you *more vulnerable* to stress, depression, and anxiety because estrogen loss affects REM sleep. When we're less rested, we're less able to cope with stresses that would normally not affect us.

Every woman entering menopause will experience a change in her menstrual cycle, discussed below. Not all women, however, will experience hot flashes or even notice vaginal changes. This is particularly true if a woman is overweight. Estrogen is stored in fat cells, which is why overweight women tend to be more at risk for estrogen-dependent cancers. The fat cells convert fat into estrogen, creating a type of estrogen reserve that the body uses during menopause, reducing the severity of estrogen loss symptoms.

Erratic periods

Every woman will experience irregular cycles before her last period. Cycles may become longer or shorter, with long bouts of amenorrhea. There will also be flow changes; periods may suddenly become light and scanty, or very heavy and crampy. The impact of suddenly irregular, wild cycles can be disturbing, however, because menstrual cycle changes may also signify other problems, discussed throughout previous chapters. It's imperative to chart your periods and try to sort out your own pattern of "normal" irregular cycles. It's also crucial to bring your chart to your gynecologist and confirm your suspicions that you are indeed entering menopause. As mentioned, this involves a few simple diagnostic procedures, using blood tests to check your FSH levels (high FSH levels indicate that your estrogen levels are dropping and you are entering menopause) or vaginal smears that analyze whether the vaginal walls are thinning out (another indication that your estrogen levels are dropping.) If you're not entering menopause, you'll need to isolate the cause of your cycle changes.

Of course, since you can go into menopause earlier than you might have anticipated, irregular cycles may not make you suspect menopause. Is there any way you can predict more accurately when your own menopause might occur? Yes. If you can, try to find out how old your *mother* was when *she* went into menopause. If she's no longer living, you might ask other women still alive who were close to her, or your father if he's still living. Although most women can expect menopause in their fifties, women who experience earlier menopause usually have a family history of earlier menopause. Periods will generally become erratic approximately two years before the final period. Some women, however, experience a longer premenopausal process than others.

Hot flashes

Roughly 85 percent of all pre- and perimenopausal women experience what are known as "hot flashes." These can begin when periods are still regular, or have just started to become irregular. Hot flashes usually end from one to two years after your final menstrual period. A hot flash feels different for each woman. Some women notice a feeling of warmth in the face and upper body; others experience hot flashes as simultaneous sweating with chills. Some women feel anxious, tense, dizzy, or nauseous just before the hot flash; some feel tingling in their fingers or heart palpitations at this time. Some women have hot flashes during the day; others will experience them at night, and may wake up so wet from perspiration that they need to change their bedsheets and/or nightclothes.

Nobody really understands what causes a hot flash, but researchers believe that it has to do with mixed signals from the hypothalamus, which controls both body temperature and sex hormones. Normally, when the body is too warm, the hypothalamus sends a chemical message to the heart to cool off the body by pumping more blood, causing the blood vessels under the skin to dilate, which makes you perspire. During menopause, however, it's believed that the hypothalamus gets confused and sends this "cooling off" signal at the wrong times. A hot flash is not the same as being overheated. Although the skin temperature often rises from 4 to 8 degrees Fahrenheit, the internal body temperature drops, creating this odd sensation. Why does the hypothalamus get so confused? Decreasing levels of estrogen. We know this because when synthetic estrogen is given to replace natural estrogen in the body, hot flashes disappear. Some researchers believe that a decrease in LH is also a key factor, and a variety of other hormones that influence body temperature are being examined as well. Although hot flashes are harmless in terms of health risks, they are disquieting and stressful. Certain groups of women will experience more severe hot flashes than others:

- *Women who are in surgical menopause* (discussed further on page 152).
- *Women who are thin.* When there's less fat on the body to store estrogen reserves, estrogen loss symptoms are more severe.
- *Women who don't sweat easily.* An ability to sweat makes extreme temperatures easier to tolerate. Women who have trouble sweating may experience more severe hot flashes.

Just as you must chart your periods when your cycles become irregular, it's also important to chart your hot flashes. Keep track of when the flashes occur and how long they last, and number their intensity from 1 to 10. This will help you determine a pattern for the flashes, and allow you to prepare for them in advance—this will reduce the stress involved in the flashes. It's also crucial to report your hot flashes to your doctor, just as you would any changes in your cycle. Hot flashes can also indicate other health problems, such as circulatory difficulties.

What can I do about my hot flashes?

Short of taking ERT or HRT, discussed in chapter 3, the only thing you can do about hot flashes is to lessen your discomfort by adjusting your lifestyle to cope with the flashes. The more comfortable you are, the less intense your flashes will feel. Once you establish a pattern by charting the flashes, you can take a few preventive actions around the time of day your flashes occur. Some suggestions:

- Avoid synthetic clothing, such as polyester, because it traps perspiration.
- Use only 100 percent cotton bedding if you have night sweats.
- Avoid clothing with high necks and long sleeves.
- Dress in layers.
- Keep cold drinks handy.
- If you smoke, cut down, or quit. Smoking constricts blood vessels and can intensify and prolong a hot flash. It also leads to severe complications from diabetes, discussed in chapter 9.
- Avoid "trigger" foods such as caffeine, alcohol, spicy foods, sugar, and large meals. Substitute herbal teas for coffee or regular tea.
- Discuss the benefits of taking vitamin E supplements with your doctor. Evidence suggests that it's essential for proper circulation and the production of sex hormones.

- Exercise to improve your circulation.
- Reduce your exposure to the sun; sunburn will aggravate your hot flashes because burnt skin cannot regulate heat effectively.

Vaginal changes

Estrogen loss will also cause vaginal changes. Since it is estrogen that causes the vagina to continuously stay moist and elastic through its natural secretions, the loss of estrogen will cause the vagina to become drier, thinner, and less elastic. The vagina may also shrink slightly in terms of width and length. In addition, the reduction in vaginal secretions causes the vagina to be less acidic. This can put you at risk for more vaginal infections, particularly if you have high blood sugar. As a result of these vaginal changes, you'll notice a change in your sexual response. Your vagina may take longer to become lubricated, or you may have to depend on artificial lubricants to have comfortable intercourse.

Estrogen loss can affect other components of your sex life as well. Your sexual libido may actually increase, because testosterone levels can rise when estrogen levels drop. (Your testosterone levels will generally either stay the same or increase.) Women who *do* experience an increase in sexual desire, however, will also be frustrated with their vaginal changes. First, there is the lubrication problem: more stimulation is required to lubricate the vagina naturally. Second, a decrease in estrogen means that less blood flows to the vagina and clitoris, so orgasm may be more difficult to achieve or may not last as long as it has in the past. Other changes involve the breasts. Estrogen causes blood to flow into the breasts during arousal, which makes the nipples more erect, sensitive, and responsive. Estrogen loss causes less blood to flow to the breasts, which makes them less sensitive. Finally, since the vagina shrinks as estrogen decreases, it doesn't expand as much during intercourse, which may make intercourse less comfortable, particularly with less lubrication.

Menopause and Blood Sugar

As you approach menopause, you'll want to revisit your blood sugar monitoring habits. That's because menopause often masks the symptoms of low or high blood sugar, and vice versa. For example, hot flashes (or sweating), moodiness, and short-term memory loss are also associated with low blood sugar. Experts recommend that before you decide that "you're low" and bite into that chocolate bar, you may want to test your blood sugar first to see if your symptoms are caused by sugar or hormones. Otherwise, ingesting more sugar than you need could unnecessarily cause high blood sugar.

That said, many women find that because estrogen and progesterone levels drop, they experience more frequent and severe episodes of low blood sugar. As mentioned, estrogen can trigger insulin resistance; the loss of estrogen will therefore have the opposite effect, causing insulin to be taken up more quickly by the body, resulting in low blood sugar. An easy way to remember how estrogen levels affect blood sugar is to note that when estrogen is up, so is blood sugar; when estrogen is down, so is blood sugar. Therefore, high estrogen levels = high blood sugar; low estrogen levels = low blood sugar.

The only way to cope with these fluctuations is to try to eliminate other causes for blood sugar fluctuations, such as stress, deviating from meal and exercise plans, and so on. If you're on oral hypoglycemic agents, you may need to adjust your dosages around menopause to compensate for less resistance to insulin as your hormone levels drop. (If you go on hormone replacement therapy, however, you may need to readjust your dosages again.)

Women who have persistent high blood sugar levels may find the normal menopausal symptoms, such as vaginal dryness, exacerbated. In this case, by gaining more control over blood sugar levels, they may find their menopausal symptoms are less severe.

Mood swings

Mood swings can be an especially tricky symptom of both meno-pause and varying blood sugar levels. Many women with diabetes struggle with severe mood swings, which can make controlling blood sugar more difficult. While anger and depression can be symptoms of low blood sugar, anxiety and irritability can be symp-toms of high blood sugar. Factor in hormonal changes during menopause, and moods can be severely affected. Unfortunately, depression and irritability can lead women to poor control of their diabetes. Frequent monitoring of your blood sugar levels and stick-ing to your meal plan can help to prevent drastic mood swings.

SURGICAL MENOPAUSE

Surgical menopause is the result of a bilateral oophorectomy— the removal of both ovaries before natural menopause. Surgical menopause can also be the result of ovarian failure following a hysterectomy or following cancer therapy, such as chemotherapy or radiation treatments. A bilateral oopherectomy is often done in conjunction with a hysterectomy, or sometimes as a single procedure (when ovarian cancer is suspected, for example).

Bilateral Oopherectomy Symptoms

If you've had your ovaries removed after menopause, you won't be in surgical menopause. You won't feel any hormonal differences in your body, although you may experience some structural prob-lems. If you've had your ovaries removed before you've reached natural menopause, you'll wake up from your surgery in *post-*

menopause. Once the ovaries are removed, your body immediately stops producing estrogen and progesterone. Your FSH level will skyrocket in an attempt to "make contact" with ovaries that no longer exist. Unlike women who go through menopause naturally, women wake up after a bilateral oopherectomy in immediate estrogen "withdrawal." It's that sudden: One day you have a normal menstrual cycle, the next, you have none whatsoever. This can cause you to become understandably depressed, but you'll also *feel* more the physical symptoms of estrogen loss far more intensely than a woman in natural menopause. That means that your vagina will be *extremely* dry, your hot flashes will feel like sudden violent heat waves that will be very disturbing to your system, and of course, your periods will cease altogether, instead of tapering off naturally. The period that you had prior to your surgery will have been your last, so you won't even experience premenopause or perimenopause, just postmenopause. That means you'll need to begin estrogen replacement therapy (ERT) *immediately* following surgery to prevent these sudden menopausal symptoms. As discussed below, if you no longer have your uterus, you'll be on estrogen only, or unopposed estrogen. If you still have your uterus, you'll be placed on estrogen and progesterone hormone replacement therapy (HRT), for the reasons explained in the HRT/ERT section below. Any short-term menopausal symptoms will be alleviated by HRT/ERT. Prior to going on HRT/ERT, your doctor will perform a vaginal smear and a blood test to determine your FSH levels, which will tell him how much estrogen you need. Dosages will vary from woman to woman, so don't compare notes with your friends and wonder why "she's taking only X amount" when you're taking Y amount. ERT and HRT is discussed later in the chapter.

If you've just had one ovary removed . . .

If the blood supply leading to your ovary was not damaged during your surgery, you should still be able to produce enough estrogen for your body. If you begin to go into ovarian failure, the symptoms will depend on how fast the ovary is failing; you may have symptoms more akin to natural menopause, or you may have sudden symptoms, mirroring the surgical menopause experience.

Ovarian Failure Resulting from Cancer Therapy

Chemotherapy and radiation treatments that involve the pelvic area may throw your ovaries into menopause. You may experience a gradual menopausal process, or you may be overwhelmed by sudden symptoms of menopause. This depends on what kind of therapy you've received, and the speed at which your ovaries are failing. Before you undergo your cancer treatment, discuss how the treatments will affect your ovaries, and what menopausal symptoms you can expect.

LONG-TERM EFFECTS OF ESTROGEN LOSS: POSTMENOPAUSAL SYMPTOMS

The long-term effects of estrogen loss are the traditional symptoms of aging. One of the key reasons why women will choose HRT or ERT (discussed in chapter 3) is to slow down or even reverse these symptoms. It's important to keep in mind that the long-term effects of estrogen loss will not set in immediately after menopause. These changes are subtle, and happen over several years. Even women who experience severe menopausal symptoms will not wake up to find that they've suddenly aged overnight; these changes occur gradually whether you experience surgical or natural menopause.

Blood Sugar Levels

As stated above, decreasing levels of estrogen and progesterone in your bloodstream lead to decreased blood sugar levels as your body's responsiveness to insulin improves. As a result, you may need to adjust your diabetes medication or insulin regimen if you require insulin.

You may also need to adjust your meal and exercise plan, because menopause slows down your metabolism. That means it will be easier to gain weight on fewer calories. The only way around this is to increase activity or decrease your calorie intake.

Skin Changes

As estrogen decreases, skin, like the vagina, tends to lose its elasticity; it too becomes thinner because it is no longer able to retain as much water. Sweat and oil glands also produce less moisture, which is what causes the skin to gradually dry, wrinkle, and sag.

Good moisturizers and skin care will certainly help to keep your skin elastic, but there is one known factor that aggravates and speeds up your skin's natural aging process, damaging the skin even more: *the sun.* If you cut down your sun exposure, you can dramatically reduce visible aging of your skin. Period. The bad news is that much of the sun's damage to our skin is cumulative, from many years of exposure. In fact, many researchers believe that when it comes to visible signs of aging, *estrogen loss is only a small factor.* For example, it's known that ultraviolet rays break down collagen and elastin fibers in the skin, causing it to sag. This also puts us at risk for skin cancer, the most notorious of which is melanoma, one of the most aggressive and malignant of all cancers.

Other sun-related problems traditionally linked to estrogen loss are what we call "liver spots"—light brown or tan splotches that develop on the face, neck, and hands as we age. These spots have *nothing* to do with the liver; they are sun spots and are caused by sun exposure. In fact, they are sometimes the result of HRT, known in this case as *hyperpigmentation.*

Currently, dermatologists recommend sunblocks with a minimum of SPF 15. In fact, sun damage is so widespread in our population that sunblock should be part of all North American women's daily cosmetic routine; women often put it on as regularly as a daily moisturizer.

Women who have high blood sugar levels may find that their skin is drier and more scaly, while vaginal dryness may be more severe. They may also notice that their nails are deteriorating more rapidly. Controlling blood sugar can reverse this.

The Osteoporosis Issue

Osteoporosis literally means "porous bones" and is perhaps the most feared condition in postmenopausal women. Unfortunately, osteoporosis is not always preventable, and is a classic symptom of aging. Normally, for a healthy, unremarkable woman, by her late thirties and forties her bones become less dense. By the time she reaches her fifties, she may begin to experience bone loss in her teeth, and become more susceptible to wrist fractures. Gradually, the bones in her spine weaken, fracture, and compress, causing upper back curvature and loss of height, known as a "dowager's hump." Osteoporosis is more common in women because when skeletal growth is completed, they typically have 15 percent lower bone mineral density and 30 percent less bone mass than a man of the same age. Studies also show that women lose trabecular bone (the inner, spongy part making up the internal support of the bone) at a higher rate than men.

Women are prone to three types of osteoporosis: *postmenopausal, senile,* and *secondary. Postmenopausal osteoporosis* usually develops roughly ten to fifteen years after the onset of menopause. In this case, estrogen loss interferes with calcium absorption, and you begin to lose your trabecular bone three times faster than the normal rate of trabecular bone loss. You will also begin to lose parts of your *cortical* bone (the outer shell of the bone) but not as quickly as the trabecular bone.

Senile osteoporosis affects men and women. Here, you lose cortical and trabecular bone because of a decrease in bone cell activity that results from aging. Hip fractures are seen most often with this kind of osteoporosis. The decreased bone cell activity affects your capacity to rebuild bone in the first place. It is also aggravated by low calcium intake.

Secondary osteoporosis means that there is an underlying condition that has caused bone loss. These conditions include chronic renal disease, hypogonadism (overstimulation of the sex glands, or gonads), hyperthyroidism (an overactive thyroid gland), some forms of cancer, gastrectomy (removal of parts of the intestine, which interferes with calcium absorption), and the use of anticonvulsants.

Fractured statistics

At least 30 million North American women over the age of forty-five are affected by osteoporosis; more than 500,000 postmenopausal women in the United States alone will have an osteoporosis-related fracture each year. These fractures usually involve the spine, hip, or distal radius (forearm). In North America, the number of hip fractures linked to osteoporosis will have increased by 73.7 percent between 1987 and 2006.

Fractures lead to death 12 to 20 percent of the time as a result of pneumonia. As the rib cage moves forward toward the pelvis, gastrointestinal and respiratory problems increase. Meanwhile, at least 23 percent of all fractures lead to permanent disability after one year. Osteoporosis-related fractures of the wrist, usually the result of a fall on the outstretched hand, are painful and can require a cast for four to six weeks.

Women with diabetes who are suffering from other complications (see chapter 9), such as nerve damage, poor vision, or foot problems, are also more likely to fall and suffer a fracture.

What causes bone loss anyway?

Our bones are always regenerating (known as "remodeling"). This process helps to maintain a constant level of calcium in the blood, essential for healthy heart functioning, blood circulation, and blood clotting. About 99 percent of all the body's calcium is in the bones and teeth; when blood calcium drops below a certain level, the body will *take* calcium from the bones to replenish it. But by the time we reach our late thirties, our bones lose calcium faster than it can be replaced. Bone calcium loss speeds up for "freshly postmenopausal" women, who are three to seven years beyond menopause. The pace then slows once again, but as we age, the body is less able to absorb calcium from food. One of the most influential factors on bone loss is estrogen; it slows or even halts the loss of bone mass by improving our absorption of calcium from the intestinal tract, allowing us to maintain a higher level of calcium in our blood. The higher the calcium levels in the blood, the less you lose calcium from your bones. In men, testosterone serves the same function regarding calcium absorption, but men never reach a particular age when their testes completely *stop* producing testosterone. If they did, they would be just as prone to osteoporosis as women are.

Estrogen alone cannot prevent osteoporosis. There is a long list of other factors that affect bone loss. One of the most obvious is calcium in the diet. Calcium is regularly lost to urine, feces, and dead skin. We need to continuously replace this loss in our diet. The less calcium we ingest, the more we force our body to take it out of our bones. Exercise also greatly affects bone density; the more we exercise, the stronger we make our bones. In fact, the bone mass we have in our late twenties and early thirties will affect our bone mass at menopause.

Finally, there are several physical conditions and external factors that may weaken our bones, contributing to bone loss later in life. These include:

- *heavy caffeine and alcohol intake*—because these are diuretics, they cause you to lose more calcium in your urine;
- *smoking*—research shows that smokers tend to go into earlier menopause, while older smokers have 20 to 30 percent less bone mass than nonsmokers;
- *women in surgical menopause who are not on ERT*—losing estrogen earlier than you normally would have naturally increases your bone loss;
- *corticosteriods;*
- *diseases of the small intestine, liver, and pancreas*—which prevent the body from absorbing adequate amounts of calcium from the intestine;
- *lymphoma, leukemia, and multiple myeloma;*
- *chronic diarrhea from ulcerative colitis or Crohn's disease*—this causes calcium loss through feces;
- *surgical removal of part of the stomach or small intestine*—this affects absorption;
- *hypercalciuria*—a condition where one loses too much calcium in the urine;
- *early menopause (before age forty-five)*—the earlier you stop producing estrogen, the more likely you are to lose calcium;
- *lighter complexions*—women with darker pigments have roughly 10 percent more bone mass than fairer women because they produce more *calcitonin,* the hormone that strengthens bones;
- *low weight*—women with less body fat store less estrogen, which makes the bones less dense to begin with and more vulnerable to calcium loss;
- *women with eating disorders (yo-yo dieting, starvation diets, binge/purge eaters)*—when there isn't enough calcium in the bloodstream gained through diet, the body will go to the bones to get what it needs. These women also have lower weight;
- *a family history of osteoporosis*—studies show that women born to mothers with spinal fractures have lower bone mineral density in the spine, neck, and midshaft;

- *high-protein diet*—this contributes to a loss of calcium in urine;
- *women who have never been pregnant*—they haven't experienced the same bursts of estrogen in their bodies as women who have been pregnant;
- *antacids with aluminum*—they interfere with calcium absorption;
- *lactose intolerance*—since so much calcium is in dairy foods, this allergy is a significant risk factor;
- *teenage pregnancy*—when a woman is pregnant in her teens, her bones are not yet fully developed and she can lose as much as 10 percent of her bone mass unless she has an adequate calcium intake of roughly 2,000 mg during the pregnancy and 2,200 while breast-feeding; and
- *scoliosis.*

Osteoporosis and diabetes

If you are overweight, as at least 80 percent of women with Type 2 diabetes are, then you're less at risk for osteoporosis, but at greater risk of developing other health problems. If you have a history of chronic dieting, however, or eating disorders, your risk of osteoporosis increases because you may have deprived yourself of vital nutrients in the past, necessary for healthy bone density.

Regardless of your weight, however, high blood sugar levels can also increase your risk of osteoporosis, although high insulin levels—the nature of Type 2 diabetes—are conversely associated with a lower risk of osteoporosis.

Preventing osteoporosis

As boring and repetitive as it may sound, the best way to prevent osteoporosis is to ingest more calcium, and increase your bone mass. This boils down to eating right and exercising. It's not enough to just take calcium supplements or eat high-calcium foods; you need to cut down on foods that are diuretics: caffeine and alcohol. How much is "enough" calcium? According to the National Institutes of Health Consensus Panel on Osteoporosis, premenopausal women require roughly 1,000 mg of calcium a day; for perimenopausal or postmenopausal women already on HRT or ERT, 1,000 mg; and for perimenopausal and postmenopausal women not taking estrogen, roughly 1,500 mg per day. For women who have already been diagnosed with osteoporosis, the panel recommends 2,500 mg of calcium a day. Foods that are rich in calcium include all dairy products (an 8 oz glass of milk contains 300 mg of calcium), fish, shellfish, oysters, shrimp, sardines, salmon, soybeans, tofu, broccoli, and dark green vegetables (except spinach, which contains oxalic acid, preventing calcium absorption). It's crucial to determine how much calcium you're getting in your diet *before* you start any calcium supplements; too much calcium can cause kidney stones in people who are at risk for them. In addition, not all supplements have been tested for absorbency. Dr. Robert Heaney, in his book *Calcium and Common Sense,* suggests that you test absorbency yourself by dropping your supplement into a glass of warm water, and stirring occasionally. If the supplement doesn't dissolve completely, chances are it won't be efficiently absorbed by your body. It's crucial to remember that a calcium supplement is, in fact, a *supplement*; it should not replace a high-calcium diet. The dosage of your supplement should only need to be roughly the usual 400 to 600 mg per day; your diet should account for the remainder of your 1,000 to 1,500 mg daily intake of calcium. Calcium is examined more thoroughly in chapter 10, which discusses nutrition.

As for exercise, the best kinds of activity are walking, running, biking, aerobic dance, or cross-country skiing. These are considered good ways to put more stress on the bones, increasing their mass. Lifting weights is also a good way to increase bone mass.

The most accurate way to measure your risk of osteoporosis is through a bone densitometry (or "DEXA") test, which measures bone mass and provides you with a "fracture risk estimate." This test involves low-dose X-rays and takes about thirty minutes. For more information about osteoporosis, contact the National Osteoporosis Foundation at 1-800-223-9994.

OTHER POSTMENOPAUSAL CONCERNS

As you age, there are several health problems that might plague you as a result of estrogen loss. Here is a brief overview.

Concerns About Heart Disease

If you have Type 2 diabetes, you must educate yourself about the signs and symptoms of heart disease. Again, heart disease kills more postmenopausal women than lung cancer or breast cancer because estrogen loss increases the risk of coronary artery disease. If you have Type 2 diabetes, your risk increases two to three times. Other factors, such as smoking, high blood pressure, high cholesterol, obesity, and an inactive lifestyle will further increase your risk. In fact, the Nurses' Health Study, a study that looked at 120,000 middle-aged women, found that women who were obese had a two- to threefold increase in heart disease, particularly women with "apple-shaped" figures (having abdominal or upper-body fat).

Studies show that hormone replacement therapy, cholesterol-lowering drugs, and lifestyle changes can significantly reduce your risk of heart disease. Women who are physically active have a 60 to 75 percent lower risk of heart disease that inactive women. For more information on women and heart disease, see chapter 9, page 262–263.

Concerns About Breast Cancer

As you probably know, breast cancer is considered to be epidemic among women over age fifty. There are many reasons for this, all of which are discussed in *The Breast Sourcebook*. Women with Type 2 diabetes will probably be told that they should consider hormone replacement therapy to reduce their risk of heart disease. Therefore, you may be concerned about breast cancer risk and HRT.

It's still not clear whether hormone replacement therapy (HRT) increases your risk of breast cancer, but there's actually more consensus in the medical research community over this issue than many others. That's because the incidence of breast cancer in Western nations dramatically rises *anyway* after menopause—whether you're on HRT or not. So it's not clear whether HRT really contributes to this increase. The current thinking seems to be that if you're on HRT, there's a slight increased risk of developing breast cancer. If you do develop it, however, it's apparently a very treatable type of cancer that's estrogen-receptor positive, which means that your risk of dying from breast cancer is *decreased*. If you add up all the data, you may want to rethink HRT if your risk of breast cancer is significant (due to other factors such as family history, for example), or if the risk of breast cancer significantly outweighs your risk of heart disease. For the record, heart disease kills more women than breast cancer, and HRT can definitely lower your cholesterol levels, lower your risk of heart disease, and reduce your risk of dying from heart disease. Furthermore, if you are at greater risk for osteoporosis (we're all somewhat at risk, but women who exercise or have heavier bones will not develop it as quickly), HRT stops bone loss. In fact, if started in the first few years after menopause, HRT will even increase bone mass. Remember—hip and spinal fractures can be very debilitating (often life threatening) and can truly affect quality of life. What if you're on HRT and are diagnosed with breast cancer? A 1995 study in Ottawa, Ontario, found that women on HRT had more difficulty battling breast cancer once it was diagnosed. This led to an unnecessary scare in Canada. Doctors will simply take you *off* hormone replacement therapy if a breast cancer is diagnosed, which completely eliminates the problem, and restores your survival rate to that of the general population. That being said, many medical papers suggest that women undergoing breast cancer treatment can still be on HRT; it is not necessarily a conflict.

Your menstrual and pregnancy history

Your menstrual history can apparently affect your risk of breast cancer, but many experts are in conflict as to how significant a role it truly plays in the big picture. For example, one factor is what experts call "early menarche." Menarche refers to your first period; early menarche means that you got your first period prior to age 12. This somewhat trivial detail also means that you've been making estrogen longer than the average woman, which is why this is examined. Menarche ages can vary enormously. The average age of menarche is 12.8 in the United States and 17 in China. Some researchers say this is why breast cancer in China occurs one-third as often as in the United States. And even within China, provinces with later menarche tend to have lower rates of breast cancer.

Another factor is cycle length. If your cycles are either longer (big maybe, here!) or shorter (more evidence for this) than average, your breast cancer risk increases by some estimates as much as 50 percent. (An average cycle is anywhere from twenty-six to twenty-nine days.) It's believed that shorter or longer cycles indicate a hormonal imbalance at work, which *may* contribute to an increased breast cancer risk. Shorter cycles also indicate that you're making more estrogen than women with longer cycles.

Pregnancy history is a *huge* factor in determining your overall risk of breast cancer. In fact, according to a 1751 edition of the *Chambers Encyclopedia*, breast cancer is described as "a most dread disease, particularly of the celibate and barren." To a large extent, this is still true today. For example, according to the National Cancer Institute, lesbians are two to three times more likely to develop breast cancer than heterosexual women, while childless women are 50 percent more likely to develop breast cancer than women who had children before the age of thirty-five. Curiously, if you bear your first child after age thirty-five, your pregnancy no longer offers you the same protection against breast cancer—*unless you decide to breast-feed.*

Urinary Incontinence

Urinary incontinence means "involuntary urination." This tends to plague women with diabetes, as well as women who do a lot of sitting; who have had several children; who have repeated urinary tract infections; who have diseases that affect the spinal cord or the brain such as Parkinson's disease, multiple sclerosis, or Alzheimer's disease; who have (a history of) bladder cancer; or who have had major pelvic surgery, such as a hysterectomy.

The muscles of your pelvic floor and abdomen weaken and your urinary apparatus drops down. On top of this, less estrogen causes the urethra to thin and change, similar to the vaginal changes you experience.

When we're younger, we have tremendous control over one particular muscle: the *pubococcygeal (levator ani) muscle.* This muscle controls the vaginal opening as well as the urinary opening. Normally, we feel the urge to urinate, but we hold it in until we get to the right place! When we get to the toilet, urine doesn't come out immediately. First we relax slightly, and then urinate. This "relaxing" prior to urination is the relaxing of the pubococcygeal muscle. We can also stop and start the stream. Anyone who's had to have a urinalysis has probably mastered this technique. Again, this ability is controlled by the same muscle. Sometimes after an orgasm, this muscle takes longer to kick in. We may sit on the toilet and try to urinate, but find we are unable to do so. But after the postorgasmic phase passes, we are once again in control of this muscle.

Urinary incontinence is categorized into one of four groups: *stress incontinence, urge incontinence, overflow incontinence,* or *irritable bladder.* Stress incontinence is when urine leaks out during a sudden movement, such as a sneeze, cough, or even uncontrollable laughing. This can happen to women of all ages, and is the most common form of incontinence. It also results when the urethra becomes stretched out from overuse. You may be in the habit of "holding it in" or simply have aged.

Urge incontinence refers to a sudden, sometimes painful urge to urinate that is so unexpected and powerful you may not always be able to make it to the toilet. This is almost exclusively a postmenopausal problem in women over age sixty.

Overflow incontinence occurs in only a small percentage of overall incontinence problems. Here, with no warning, urine suddenly overflows after you change your position (from sitting to standing or vice versa, for example). You may lose just a few drops of urine, or enough to require a maxipad. Sometimes these episodes are followed by the urge to urinate a few minutes later, but when you try, nothing comes out. This is a condition that often precedes or accompanies a urinary tract infection (UTI). Causes of this type of incontinence are similar to the causes of UTIs.

Finally, an irritable bladder is a mishmash of all three incontinence symptoms and UTIs. You'll need to see a urologist to sort out what's causing your bladder to behave so erratically.

Treating incontinence

Estrogen is very helpful as a treatment for incontinence because it restores the elasticity of your urethra just as it restores the vagina. Estrogen in pill, cream, or patch form will all have the same beneficial effects.

The *Kegel exercise* is also very helpful in strengthening the pubococcygeal muscle. The Kegel exercise is very convenient; you can do it in any position, anywhere, anytime: in an elevator, on the subway, in a movie theater, or while you're cooking, eating, or lying down! All you do is isolate the muscle that stops and starts your urinary stream. To isolate it, you can insert your finger into your vagina and try to squeeze your finger with your vaginal opening. Once you've isolated the muscle, just squeeze five times, and count five; squeeze five and count five. Or, squeeze ten and count ten. The key is to keep the muscles in shape. It's *that* simple, and it really helps. You can also do general exercises to firm up your abdomen and pelvis in conjunction with your Kegel exercises.

Being conscious of your diet and medications is also important. For example, certain drugs for high blood pressure or heart disease, sedatives, or tranquilizers can trigger bouts of incontinence. Ask your pharmacist about this. Some drugs or foods are diuretics, which will cause you to urinate more frequently. Caffeine and alcohol are classic diuretics you can easily cut out of your diet. Fruit juice and spicy foods can also irritate the bladder.

Overweight women are more likely to experience incontinence because the weight exerts pressure on the bladder, causing the muscles and urethra to be overworked. Weight loss may help to resolve the problem. (See chapter 2.)

More invasive treatments for incontinence include surgery that lifts and tightens the pelvic floor, or the use of a *pessary*, a stiff, doughnut-shaped rubber device (which needs to be fitted and sized) that fits into the top of the vagina, and holds it up slightly. This raises the neck of the bladder and helps to reposition it.

Some women choose to just live with the problem, and wear bladder control products (maxipads or diaperlike products) that protect them from the embarrassment of wetting themselves.

Uterine Prolapse: Is It Me, Or Is the Sky Falling?

This problem only affects women who still have a uterus. Basically, the problem is the uterus sagging or sinking, and literally falling down as one ages. When you experience a uterine prolapse, you may feel as though something is "falling out." You may also experience heaviness in your lower abdomen; constant lower back pain and pressure; menstrual-like cramps that seem to worsen after long intervals of standing; difficulty with penetration during intercourse; constipation combined with the urge to "bear down"; and urinary incontinence!

The different forms of prolapse

You can have a "straight line" prolapse, where the uterus falls down a little, or the entire length of the vagina can fall. In more severe cases, the cervix protrudes between the labia, making intercourse impossible. This is dangerous because the cervix can get infected through contact with urine or feces.

The uterus can also fall on an angle, pitching forward onto the bladder or back onto the bowel. This results in constant urination or chronic constipation. Because the uterus supports or rests on a variety of other organs, the main problem with a uterine prolapse is that it can cause *other* pelvic organs to fall down, making you experience:

- *Cystocele:* a falling bladder. You'll feel as though you can't empty your bladder completely, and will be plagued with frequent urinary tract infections. The urine may also stay in the bladder, causing stress, overflow, or urge incontinence.
- *Urethrocele:* in this case, the muscles supporting the urethra separate, and the urethra sags into the vagina, causing stress, urge, or overflow incontinence.
- *Rectocele:* here, the rectum falls into the vagina, causing severe constipation. Your stools may also pack into a "pouch," forming a bulging rectum.
- *Enterocele:* this is when the small intestine falls into the back of the vagina, causing a host of gastrointestinal problems.

What causes prolapse?

Pregnancy and childbirth are major contributors to prolapse. The uterus and tissues expand to such an extent that they lose their elasticity and ability to retain normal positions. During labor, the muscles in the vagina and perineum can be torn. Nonmuscle tissue, ligaments, and fascia may not have the resiliency to retain their normal positions and shape. Women who have had ten or more children (not seen as much today as in the past) often have internal tearing that destroys their pelvic configuration.

Obesity and poor nutrition are another cause. Poor nutrition prevents tissues from getting enough blood supply and nutrients. In obese women, fat inside the abdomen hangs like an extra organ pushing directly on the pelvis, uterus, and bowels, or pushing the intestines into the pelvis, ruining normal bowel function. The constant pressure from this extra fat tears the tissue and damages elasticity.

Finally, estrogen loss after menopause causes the mucosal tissue of the ligaments and fascia to thin and weaken (just like the vagina). In this case, hormone therapy can alleviate the problem, combined with good nutrition and exercise.

Occasionally, a large fibroid can push down on the uterus and vaginal wall, causing a prolapse. The fibroid may also put pressure on the bladder and stretch tissues. Finally, simple aging—heredity and gravity—may be the culprit.

Increasing physical activity is not only one of the best ways to manage your Type 2 diabetes, but it will also help reduce your risk of heart disease, breast cancer, and osteoporosis. When it comes to Type 2 diabetes, exercise will allow your body to use the insulin you do make much more efficiently. In fact, many experts find that when their Type 2 diabetes patients stick to their meal plans (see chapter 7) and incorporate regular exercise into their routines, they may not need any medications or insulin to manage their diabetes. The next chapter will tell you how to make your body into a "lean mean insulin machine."

CHAPTER 6

Women, Exercise, and Type 2 Diabetes

You are a "lean mean insulin machine" but you don't realize it yet. The purpose of this chapter is to explain how exercise affects your body when you have diabetes. It is not intended as a workout program, however. Anybody reading this chapter needs to design a *do-able* exercise program that is appealing and convenient; for most people, that will mean combining some kind of simple stretching routine with some aerobic activity. As one expert aptly put it on her video, the program you *can* do, is the one you *will* do.

Most people who have been sedentary most of their lives are intimidated by health and fitness clubs. Walking into a room full of complex machines populated by young, fit, supple bodies is not exactly an inviting atmosphere for somebody who's been inactive. And the "language" of exercise is intimidating, too. Not only do you need an anatomy lesson to understand which movements stretch which group of muscles, but you require a crash course in cardiology to know exactly how long you have to hyperventilate and have your pulse at X beats per minute, with the sweat pouring off you, before you burn any fat. The concept of "gaining muscle" over existing fat is also a hard one to grasp. (My stupid question is always, "How come, if I've been doing my program for six months, I weigh *more* than when I started?")

Aerobics classes are another problem; many women (like me) are uncomfortable with their lack of fitness in public. And many aerobics instructors assume you've had formal training with the American Ballet Theater; you need the grace of a dancer to perform half the moves! So let me stress something before you begin reading: you're wearing all the equipment you will ever need to exercise. If you can breathe, stretch, and walk, you can become a lean mean exercise machine without paying a membership fee.

WHAT DOES EXERCISE *REALLY* MEAN?

The Oxford dictionary defines exercise as "the exertion of muscles, limbs, etc., especially for health's sake; bodily, mental, or spiritual training." In the Western world, we have placed an emphasis on "bodily training" when we talk about exercise. We completely ignore mental and spiritual training. Only recently have Western studies begun to focus on the mental benefits of exercise. (It's been shown, for example, that exercise stimulates the production of endorphins, hormones that make us feel good.) But in the West we do not encourage meditation or other calming forms of mental and spiritual exercise, which have also been shown to improve well-being and health.

In the East, for thousands of years, exercise has focused on achieving mental and spiritual health *through* the body, using breathing and postures, for example. Fitness practitioner Karen Faye maintains that posture is extremely important for organ alignment. Standing correctly, with ears over shoulders, and shoulders over hips, with knees slightly bent, and head straight up naturally allows you to pull in your abdomen. According to Faye, many native populations who balance baskets on their heads or do a lot of physical work are noted for correct posture and low rates of osteoporosis. (See Table 6.1 for a list of activities suggested by Faye.)

Nor should we ignore the aboriginal rituals known to improve mental health and well-being, such as traditional dances, active

Table 6.1 Suggested Activities

More Intense	Less Intense
Skiing	
Running	Golf
Jogging	Bowling
Stair-Stepping or Stair-Climbing	Badminton
Trampolining	Cricket
Jumping rope	Sailing
Fitness walking	Strolling
Race walking	Stretching
Aerobic classes	
Roller skating	
Ice skating	
Biking	
Weight-bearing exercises	
Tennis	
Swimming	

Source: Karen Faye, L.P.N., A.F.F.A. fitness practioner.

prayers that incorporate physical activity, circles that involve community and communication, and even sweat lodges, believed to rid the body of toxins through sweating. These are all wellness activities that you should investigate.

The Meaning of Aerobic

If you look up the word *aerobic* in the dictionary, what you'll find is the chemistry definition: "living in free oxygen." This is certainly correct; we are all aerobes—beings that require oxygen to live. Some bacteria, for example, are anaerobic; they can exist in an environment without oxygen. All that jumping around and fast movement is done to create faster breathing, so we can take more oxygen into our bodies.

Why are we doing this? Because the blood contains *oxygen*! The faster your blood flows, the more oxygen can flow to your organs. When your health care practitioner tells you to "exercise," she's not referring solely to increasing oxygen, however, but to exercising the heart muscle. The faster the heart beats, the better a workout it gets (although you don't want to overwork your heart, either).

Why we want more oxygen

When more oxygen is in our bodies, we burn fat (see below), our breathing improves, our blood pressure improves, and our hearts work better. Oxygen also lowers triglycerides and cholesterol, increasing our high-density lipoproteins (HDL), or "good" cholesterol, while decreasing our low-density lipoproteins (LDL), or "bad" cholesterol. This means that your arteries will unclog and you may significantly decrease your risk of heart disease and stroke. More oxygen makes our brains function better, so we feel better, too. Studies show that depression is decreased when we increase oxygen flow into our bodies. Ancient techniques such as yoga, which specifically improve mental and spiritual well-being, achieve this by combining deep breathing and stretching, which improves oxygen and blood flow to specific parts of the body.

With Type 2 diabetes, more oxygen in the body increases your cells' sensitivity to insulin, causing your blood glucose levels to drop. More oxygen can also improve the action of insulin-producing cells in the pancreas. As you continue to do aerobic exercise, your blood sugar levels will become much easier to manage. You can also use exercise to decrease blood sugar levels in the short term, over a twenty-four-hour period. People who are taking oral hypoglycemic pills may find that their dosages need to be lowered, as they get into shape, or that they no longer need the medication.

Exercise has been shown to dramatically decrease the incidence of many other diseases, including cancer. Some research suggests that cancer cells tend to thrive in an oxygen-depleted environment. The more oxygen in the bloodstream, the less hospitable you make your body to cancer. In addition, since many cancers are related to fat-soluble toxins, the less fat on your body, the less fat-soluble toxins your body can accumulate.

Burning fat

The only kind of exercise that will burn fat is aerobic exercise because *oxygen burns fat.* If you were to go to your fridge and pull out some animal fat (chicken skin, red-meat fat, or butter), throw it in the sink, and light it with a match, it will burn. What makes the flame yellow is oxygen; what fuels the fire is the fat. That same process goes on in your body. The oxygen will burn your fat, no matter how you increase the oxygen flow in your body (through jumping around and increasing your heart rate or employing an established deep-breathing technique).

Of course, when you burn fat, you lose weight, which can cause your body to use insulin more efficiently, and lower your blood sugar levels. It may also allow your doctor to lower your dosage of oral hypoglycemics or stop your medication altogether.

The Western definition of aerobic

In the West, an exercise is considered aerobic if it makes your heart beat faster than it normally does. When your heart is beating fast, you'll be breathing hard and sweating and will officially be in your "target zone" or "ideal range" (the kind of phrases that turn many people off).

There are official calculations you can do to find this target range. For example, by subtracting your age from 220, then multiplying that number by 60 percent, you will find your recommended "threshhold level"—which means, "Your heart should be beating X beats per minute for twenty to thirty minutes." If you multiply the number by 75 percent, you will find your "ceiling level"—which means, "Your heart should not be beating faster than X beats per minute for twenty to thirty minutes." This is only an example. If you are on heart medications (drugs that slow down your heart, known as beta blockers), you'll want to make sure you discuss what "target" to aim for with your health care professional.

Finding your pulse

You have pulse points all over your body. The easiest ones to find are those in your neck, at the base of your thumb, just below your earlobe, or on your wrist. To check your heart rate, look at a watch or clock and begin to count the beats for fifteen seconds (if the second hand is on the twelve, count until it reaches fifteen). Then multiply by four to get your pulse.

Borg's Rate of Perceived Exertion (RPE)

This doesn't refer to the Borg on Star Trek, but to the "Borg Scale of Perceived Exertion." This is a way of measuring exercise intensity without finding your pulse, and because of its simplicity, it is now the recommended method for judging exertion. This "Borg scale," as it's dubbed, goes from 6 to 20 (shown in Table 6.2). Extremely light activity may rate a 7, for example, while a very, very hard activity may rate a 19. Exercise practitioners recommend that you do a "talk test" to rate your exertion level, as well. If you can't talk without gasping for air, you may be working too hard. You should be able to carry on a normal conversation throughout your activity. What's crucial to remember about RPE is that it is extremely individual; what one person judges a 7, another may judge a 10.

Other ways to increase oxygen flow

There is welcome news to people who have limited movement due to joint problems, arthritis, or other diabetes-related complications, ranging from stroke to kidney disease. You can increase the flow of oxygen into your bloodstream without exercising your

Table 6.2 Sample Borg Rate of Perceived Exertion Scales

Sample A		Sample B	
6		0	Nothing at all
7	Very, very light	0.5	Very, very weak
8		1	Very weak
9	Very light	2	Weak
10		3	Moderate
11	Fairly light	4	Somewhat strong
12		5	Strong
13	Somewhat hard	6	
14		7	Very strong
15	Hard	8	
16		9	Very, very strong
17	Very hard	10	Maximum
18			
19	Very, very hard		
20			

Source: Adapted from Lea and Febiger, *Guidelines for Exercise Testing and Prescription* (American College of Sports Medicine, 1991: 70).

heart muscle, by learning how to breathe deeply through your diaphragm. There are many yogalike programs and videos available which can teach you this technique, which does not require you to jump around. You can increase the oxygen flow into your bloodstream with these techniques. Though this will not strengthen your heart, it is better than doing nothing at all, and has many health benefits, according to a myriad of wellness practitioners.

"Aerobic" activity versus active living

The phrase "aerobic activity" means that the *activity* causes your heart to pump harder and faster, and makes you breathe faster, increasing oxygen flow. Activities such as cross-country skiing, walking, hiking, and biking are all aerobic.

But exercise professionals hate the terms *aerobic activity* and *aerobics program* because this is not about what people do in their daily lives. Health promoters are replacing these terms with the phrase "active living"—because that's what becoming unsedentary is all about. There are many ways you can adopt an active lifestyle. Here are some suggestions:

- If you drive everywhere, pick the parking space farthest away from your destination so that you can work some daily walking into your life.
- If you take public transit everywhere, get off one or two stops early so that you can walk the rest of the way to your destination.
- Choose stairs more often over escalators or elevators.
- Park at one side of the mall and then walk to the other.
- Take a stroll around your neighborhood after dinner.
- Volunteer to walk the dog.
- On weekends, go to the zoo or get out to flea markets, garage sales, and so on.

What About Muscles?

Forty percent of your body weight is made from muscle, where sugar is stored. The muscles use this sugar when they are being worked. When the sugar is used up, the muscles, in a healthy body, will drink in sugar from your blood. After exercising, the muscles will continue to drink in glucose from your blood to replenish the glucose that was lost through exercise.

But when you have insulin resistance, glucose from your blood has difficulty getting inside your muscles; the muscles act like a brick wall. As you begin to use and tone your muscles, they will become more receptive to the glucose in your blood, allowing the glucose in. Studies show that the muscles specifically worked out in a given exercise take up glucose far more easily than other muscles in the same body.

Doing weight-bearing activities is also encouraged because it builds bone mass and uses up calories. Building bone mass is particularly important; as Karen Faye says, "If you want a strong house, you need a strong frame!" Women who are vulnerable to osteoporosis (loss of bone mass) as a result of estrogen loss after menopause will benefit from these activities. The denser your bones, the harder they are to break. As we age, we are all at risk for osteoporosis unless we've been building up our bone mass for years, or are maintaining current bone mass. For information on osteoporosis, call the National Osteoporosis Foundation, listed at the back of this book, and consult chapter 5.

By increasing muscular strength, we increase flexibility and endurance. For example, you'll find that the first time you ride your bike from home to downtown, your legs may feel sore. Do that same ride ten times, and your legs will no longer be sore—you have built muscle endurance. Of course, you won't be as out of breath, either, which means you've built cardiovascular endurance.

Hand weights or resistance exercises (using rubber-band devices or pushing certain body parts together) help increase what's called "lean body mass"—body tissue that is not fat. This is why many people find their weight does not drop when they begin to exercise. Yet, as your muscles become bigger, your body fat decreases.

Sugar and muscle

When you think "muscle," think "sugar." Every time you work any muscle in your body, either independent of, or during, an aerobic activity, your muscles use up glucose from your bloodstream as fuel. People with high blood sugar prior to muscle toning will find that their blood sugar levels are lower after the muscle has been worked.

On the downside, if you have normal blood sugar levels prior to working a muscle, you may find that your blood sugar goes too low after you exercise *unless* you eat something; this should be carbohydrates. In fact, your muscles prefer to use carbohydrates rather than fat as fuel. When your muscles use up all the sugar in your blood, your liver will convert glycogen (excess glucose it stores up for these kinds of emergencies) back into glucose and release it into your bloodstream for your muscles to use.

To avoid this scenario, eat before and after exercising if your blood sugar level is normal. How much you eat prior to exercising largely depends on what you're doing and how long you're going to be doing it (see Table 6.3). The general rule is to follow your meal plan, eating smaller, more frequent meals throughout the day to keep your blood sugar levels consistent.

Athletes without diabetes generally consume large quantities of carbohydrates before an intense workout. In fact, it's a known strategy in the athletic world to eat 40 to 65 grams of carbohydrates per hour to maintain blood glucose levels to the point where performance is improved. It's also been shown that glucose, sucrose, maltodextrins, or high-fructose corn syrup during exercise can increase endurance. After a training session, athletes typically consume more carbohydrates to replenish their energy and carry them throughout the day.

Athletes who have Type 1 diabetes do exactly the same thing, except they must be more careful about timing their food intake with insulin to avoid either too low or too high blood sugar.

If your blood sugar is low, don't exercise at all, as it may be life threatening. Do not resume exercise until you get your blood sugar levels under control.

Exercises that can be hazardous

Some activities, such as wrestling or weightlifting, are usually of short duration but very intense. As a result, unless you fuel up ahead of time, they will force your body to use glycogen (see chapter 1), which is the stored glucose your liver keeps handy. When you have diabetes, it's a bad idea to force your liver to give up that glycogen. This can actually increase your blood pressure and put

Table 6.3 Grams of Carbohydrate Used per Hour in Different Exercises

Activity	Your Weight		
	100 Lb	150 lb	200 lb
Basketball	43	58	73
Bicycling 10 mph	33	45	57
Bicycling 15 mph	56	77	98
Carpentry	38	52	66
Disco dancing	26	36	46
Square dancing (fast)	32	44	56
Eating	6	8	10
Golfing (pull cart)	26	36	46
Jogging 5 mph	33	45	57
Ice/roller skating	25	34	43
Mowing (power)	16	22	28
Racquetball	66	90	114
Raking leaves	22	30	38
Running 7 mph	56	77	98
Running 9 mph	76	103	130
Scrubbing floors	18	25	32
Shoveling snow	33	45	57
Skiing	55	75	95
Softball	189	25	32
Swim 20 yds/min	26	36	46
Tennis (doubles)	21	28	35
Tennis (singles)	28	38	48
Walking 3 mph	15	21	27
Waterskiing	32	44	56

Source: Lois Jovanovic-Peterson, June Biermann, and Barbara Toohey, *The Diabetic Woman* (New York: Putnam, 1996), 44.

you at risk for other health problems, including hypoglycemia. To avoid this, you'll need to eat some carbohydrates prior to this type of exercise, which will provide enough fuel to the muscles.

A word about leg cramps

When your blood sugar is unstable, concentrations of sodium, potassium, and calcium can also "swing," which can cause leg cramps. Some things which aggravate leg cramps include:

- Diuretics, which can cause you to lose muscle potassium;
- Too much or too little intake of calcium;
- Sitting too long;
- Wearing high boots or knee highs; and
- Varicose veins or pregnancy.

Modify or avoid any of these factors that you can if you suffer from leg cramps. Experts suggest that increasing your potassium intake and stretching your leg muscles before going to bed can help to alleviate cramping.

LET'S GET PHYSICAL

More than 50 percent of all people with diabetes exercise less than once a week, and 56 percent of all diabetes-related deaths are due to heart attacks. This is terrible news, considering how beneficial and life-extending exercise can be. Reports from the United States show that one out of three American adults is over-weight, a sign of growing inactivity. But, as mentioned earlier, the fitness industry has done an excellent job of intimidating inactive people. Some people are so put off by the health club scene, they become even more sedentary. This is similar to diet failure, where you become so demoralized that you cheated that you binge even more.

If you've been sedentary most of your life, there's nothing wrong with starting off with simple, even leisurely activities such as gardening, feeding the birds in a park, or a few simple stretches. Any step you take toward being more active is a crucial and important one.

Experts also recommend that you find a friend, neighbor, or relative to "get physical" with you. When your exercise plans include someone else, you'll be less apt to cancel plans or make excuses for not getting out there. Whomever you choose, teach your training partner how to recognize the signs of hypo-glycemia, just in case (see chapter 1).

Things to Do Before "Moving Day"

1. *Choose an activity that's right for you.* Whether it's walking, chopping wood, jumping rope, or folk dancing—pick something you enjoy. You don't have to do the same thing each time, either. Vary your routine to avoid monotony. Just make sure that whatever activity you choose is continuous for the duration of your workout. Walking for two minutes, then stopping for three isn't continuous. It's also important to choose an activity that doesn't aggravate a preexisting condition. Lowering your head in a certain way (as in touching your toes), or straining your upper body can increase blood pressure and/or aggravate eye problems. If foot problems are a concern, an activity that doesn't involve walking, such as canoeing, is better.

2. *Choose the frequency and duration.* Decide how often you're going to do this activity. (Twice, three, or four times a week? Or once a day?) Try not to let two days pass without doing something. Select a target duration, as well. If you're elderly or ill, even a few minutes is a good start. If you're sedentary but otherwise healthy, aim for twenty to thirty minutes.

3. *Choose the intensity level that's right for you.* This is easy to do by just setting the dial if you're using an exercise machine of some kind. If you're walking, intensity is how fast you are planning to walk, or how many hills you will climb. In other words, how fast do you want your heart to beat?

4. *Work your activity into your meal plan.* Once you decide what kind of exercise you'll be doing, and for how long, see your dietitian about working your exercise into your current meal plan. You may need a small snack prior to and after exercise if you're planning to be active longer than thirty minutes. If you are overweight, you do not need to consume extra calories before exercising unless your blood sugar level is low.

5. *Tell your doctor what you're doing.* Your doctor may want to monitor your blood sugar more closely (or want you to do so),

or adjust your medication. Don't do anything without consulting your doctor first.

Think Like a Cat

Ever watch a cat in action? Cats will never do anything before stretching. If stretching *is* your exercise, that's just fine; but if it's not the focus of your activity, do some stretching before and after you get really active to reduce muscle tightness.

When Not to Exercise

Everyone can and should exercise, but your diabetes may get in the way at times, especially if you're taking insulin. So here are some alarm bells to listen for; if they go off, skip your exercise and do what you have to do to get back on track:

- Keep track of where you're injecting insulin. Insulin injected into an arm or leg that is being worked out gets used up faster. Any signs of low blood sugar means STOP!
- Check your blood sugar after thirty minutes to make sure it's still normal. If it's low, eat something before you resume exercising. (Blood sugar below 70 mg/dl [<4 mmol/L] is low; anything that's 54 mg/dl [3 mmol/L] or less means you should stop exercising or not start exercising at all.)
- If your blood sugar level is high, exercise will bring it down, but if it's greater than 250 mg/dl (14 mmol/L), check your urine for ketones and don't exercise. When your body is stressed, your blood sugar level can go even higher.

Exercise Parental Duties

Obesity in childhood and adolescence is at an all-time high in North America. For example, the American National Health and Nutrition Examination Survey III (NHANES III) revealed that 21 percent of people aged twelve to nineteen were obese, while as many as 40 percent of those in that age group were physically unfit. It wasn't until 1995 that the Dietary Guidelines for Americans even recommended physical activity. If you have Type 2 diabetes, unless you can encourage them to modify their lifestyles early, your children will be at high risk for Type 2 diabetes as well. Old habits die hard—something you're learning the difficult way. By making sure that your children appreciate the value and benefits of getting physical, you can help them avoid going through what you are. In fact, why don't you encourage your children to exercise right along with you?

After all that exercise, you must be hungry! What to eat is discussed next.

CHAPTER 7

How Sweet It Is: Counting Sugar, Planning Meals

The diabetes meal plan is not just for people with diabetes; it's healthy eating that everyone in North America should be following. So when you begin your meal plan, your entire family will benefit. Through food, you'll be able to gain control of your condition, while the rest of your family may be able to prevent or delay it.

Only carbohydrates influence blood sugar levels, while cholesterol-containing foods increase blood *fat* levels—cholesterol and triglycerides. What lowers the sugar in your bloodstream are exercise and medications you may be taking, such as oral hypoglycemic pills or insulin. Ideally, by balancing your food intake with activity, most of you will be able to control your diabetes. How do you know if you're balancing well? And how do you know what to eat so that you can create all this balance? That's what this chapter is about.

A FEW GOOD FOODS

Before the discovery of insulin in 1921, there was the Allen Diet, a very low calorie diet that required small quantities of carbohydrates, followed by exercise.

Dr. Frederick Madison Allen, a leading diabetologist who spent four years working with diabetic patients at the Rockefeller Institute in New York City, published a 600-plus-page paper in 1919 called "Total Dietary Regulation in the Treatment of Diabetes." Allen's work showed that diabetes was largely a problem of carbohydrate metabolism. He introduced a radical approach to diabetes, the vestiges of which are still apparent in current meal planning. It was known as the starvation treatment; fasting followed by a gradual building up of diet. Allen's treatment also included exercise—now a vital aspect of diabetes treatment. The idea of emaciated patients fasting and exercising was controversial, but at the time it was the best treatment available without insulin. Although in some cases, Allen's patients did die of starvation, Allen ultimately prolonged the lives of many through his system of dietary regulation. Allen's diets were more tolerable than any of the fad diabetes diets that were popular in Allen's day. Doctors were doing everything from feeding patients with diabetes as much sugar as possible to compensate for the sugar lost in the blood, to putting them on low-carbohydrate diets, which were so unappetizing that most patients wouldn't stick to them. Oatmeal diets, milk diets, rice diets, and potato diets were also popular. The most logical diet, however, was the low-carbohydrate diet, which included recipes such as "thrice-boiled vegetables." Although this diet was effective in eliminating sugar from the urine (the same effect as food rationing), it didn't seem to help patients who had insulin-dependent, or Type 1 diabetes.

Allen and his predecessors understood something central to diabetes meal planning; *carbohydrates are key.* Allen recognized the ability of carbohydrates to convert into glucose. The timing of this glucose conversion will affect how quickly and how high blood glucose levels rise after eating. What's changed drastically since the Allen Diet is that variety, quantity, and timing of meals are crucial, too.

What to Eat

To live, you need three basic types of foods: carbohydrates, protein, and fat. Carbohydrates are the main source of fuel for muscles. Protein is the "cell food" that helps cells grow and repair themselves. Fat is a crucial nutrient that can be burned as an alternative fuel in times of hunger or famine. Simple sugars that do not contain any fat will convert quickly into energy or be stored as fat.

Your body will change carbohydrates into glucose for energy. If you eat more carbohydrates than you can burn, your body will turn the extra into fat. The protein your body makes comes from the protein you eat. As for fats, they are not broken down into glucose, and are usually stored as fat. The problem with fatty foods is that they have double the calories per gram as carbohydrates and protein, so you wind up gaining weight. Too much saturated fat, as discussed in chapter 10, can increase your risk of developing cardiovascular problems. What we also know is that the rate at which glucose is absorbed by your body from starch and sugars is affected by other components of your meal, such as protein, fiber, and fat. If you're eating only carbohydrates and no protein or fat, for example, your blood sugar will go up faster.

The American Diabetes Association guidelines state that a healthy diet should consist mainly of complex carbohydrates (roughly 50 percent) with about 30 percent of your energy from fat—and less than 10 percent from saturated fats, and less than 10 percent from polyunsaturated fats. (See chapter 10 for an explanation of fats.)

According to guidelines set out by the British Diabetic Association (BDA), at least 50 percent of each meal should be made up of complex carbohydrates (see Table 7.1). Canadian guidelines stipulate that your daily intake of protein (from animal products) shouldn't exceed 20 percent (BDA guidelines stipulate 15 percent). And if you have a sweet tooth, the BDA recommends using artificial sweeteners instead of sugar (see below).

Table 7.1   How Your Food Breaks Down

Complex Carbohydrates (digests more slowly)	Defined by ADA
fruits	Fruit List
vegetables (corn, potatoes, etc.)	Vegetables List or Starches List
grains (breads, pastas, and cereals)	Starches List
legumes (dried beans, peas, and lentils)	Starches List
Simple Carbohydrates (digests quickly)	**Defined by ADA**
fruits/fruit juices	Fruit List
sugars (sucrose, fructose, etc.)	Fruit/Other Carbohydrates/ Starches Lists
honey	Fruit/Other Carbohydrates/ Starches Lists
corn syrup	Fruit/Other Carbohydrates/ Starches Lists
sorghum	Fruit/Other Carbohydrates/ Starches Lists
date sugar	Fruit/Other Carbohydrates/ Starches Lists
molasses	Fruit/Other Carbohydrates/ Starches Lists
lactose	Dairy List
Proteins (digests slowly)	**Defined by ADA**
lean meats	Meat and Meat Substitutes List
fatty meats	Meat and Meat Sub/Fats Lists
poultry	Meat and Meat Substitutes List
fish	Meat and Meat Substitutes List
eggs	Meat and Meat Substitutes List
low-fat cheese	Meat and Meat Substitutes List
high-fat cheese	Dairy List or Fats List
legumes	Starches List
grains	Starches List
Fats (digests slowly)	**Defined by ADA**
high-fat dairy products (butter or cream)	Dairy List or Fats List
oils (Canola/Corn/Olive/ Safflower/Sunflower)	Fats List

lard	Fats List
avocados	Fats List or Vegetable List
olives	Fats List or Vegetable List
nuts	Fats List or Vegetable List
fatty meats	Fats/Meat and Meat Sub Lists
Fiber (doesn't digest; goes through you)	**Defined by ADA**
whole-grain breads	Starches List
cereals (i.e., oatmeal)	Starches List
all fruits	Fruit List
legumes (beans and lentils)	Starches List
leafy greens	Vegetable List
cruciferous vegetables	Vegetable List

Variety, variety, variety

Variety is the key to a good meal plan. If your meal contains mostly carbohydrates (50 to 55 percent), some protein (15 to 20 percent), not much fat (less than 30 percent), and limited sugar, you're eating well. See Table 7.1 for some examples of simple and complex carbohydrates, proteins, and fat. (I think you know what sugar is, but there are examples provided there, too.) If you imagine the outside aisles of a supermarket, those contain the food items you need to eat. It's the middle aisles that have all the extras we don't need.

How Much to Eat

Meal plans recommended by registered dietitians are tailored to your individual goals and medication regimen. Men and women will usually require different quantities of food. The goal is to keep the supply of glucose consistent by spacing out your meals, snacks, and activity levels accordingly. If you lose weight, this will allow your body to use insulin more effectively, but not all people with Type 2 diabetes need to lose weight. If you're on insulin, meals will have to be timed to match your insulin's peak (see chapter 3). A dietitian can be helpful by prescribing an individu-alized meal plan that addresses your specific needs (weight con-trol, shift-work, travel, and so on).

Anatomy of a carbohydrate

Carbohydrates are like people; they can be simple or complex. Simple carbohydrates are found in any food that has natural sugar (honey, fruits, juices, vegetables, milk) and anything that contains table sugar or sucrose.

Complex carbohydrates are more sophisticated foods that are made up of larger molecules, such as grain foods, starches, and foods high in fiber. High-fiber foods, both soluble and insol-uble (an important distinction), such as cereals, oatmeal, or legumes, are discussed in chapter 10.

All About Sugar

Human beings have always been attracted to sweet foods. This can be tracked back to our need for vitamin C, the source of which is often fruit. Sugars are found naturally in many foods you eat. Fructose (in fruits and vegetables), lactose (in milk prod-ucts), and maltose (in flours and cereals) are all naturally occur-ring sugars. What you have to watch out for is *added sugar*; these are sugars that manufacturers add to foods during processing or packaging. Foods containing fruit juice concentrates, invert sugar, regular corn syrup, honey, molasses, hydrolyzed lactose syrup, or high-fructose corn syrup (made out of highly concen-trated fructose through the hydrolysis of starch), all are added sugars. Many people don't realize, however, that pure, *unsweet-ened* fruit juice is still a potent source of sugar, even when it con-tains no added sugar. Extra lactose, dextrose, and maltose are also contained in many of your foods. In other words, products may have naturally occurring sugars anyway, and then *more*

SUGAR ON THE TABLE

What's in a sugar?

Fructose: a monosaccharide or single sugar. It combines with glucose to form sucrose and is 1½ times sweeter than sucrose.

Glucose: a monosaccharide or single sugar. It combines with fructose to form sucrose. It can also combine with glucose to form maltose, and with galactose to form lactose. Slightly less sweet than sucrose.

High fructose corn syrup (HFCS): a liquid mixture of about equal parts glucose and fructose from cornstarch. Same sweetness as sucrose.

Sucrose: a disaccharide or double sugar made of equal parts glucose and fructose. Known as table or white sugar, sucrose is found naturally in sugar cane and sugar beets.

---

sugar is thrown in to enhance consistency, taste, and so on. With the exception of lactose, which breaks down into glucose and galactose, all of these added sugars break down into fructose and glucose during digestion. To the body, no one sugar is more nutritious than another; everything is broken down into either single sugars (called monosaccharides) or double sugars (called disacharides), which are carried to cells through the bloodstream. See above for the complete sugar breakdown. The best way to know how much sugar is in a product is to look at the nutritional label for carbohydrates.

As far as your body is concerned, all sugars are nutritionally equal. Honey and table sugar, for instance, are nutritionally comparable. Ultimately, all the sugars from the foods you eat wind up as glucose; your body doesn't know whether the sugar started out as maltose from whole-grain breads or lactose from milk products. Glucose then travels through your bloodstream to provide energy. If you have enough energy already, the glucose is stored as fat, for later. Sugars and starches (in equal "doses") affect blood sugar differently because of the time frame involved in glucose conversion. Sugars are converted faster than starches, so it's important to discuss sugar conversion with your dietitian. (See the Glycemic Index as another source of "measuring sugar.")

How fast that sugar is ultimately broken down and enters the bloodstream greatly depends on the amount of fiber in your food, how much protein you've eaten, and how much fat accompanies the sugar in your meal.

Why is sugar added?

Sugar is added to food because it can change the consistency of foods and, in some instances, act as a preservative, as in jams and jellies. Sugar can increase the boiling point or reduce the freezing point in foods; sugar can add bulk and density, and make baked goods do wonderful things, including helping yeast to ferment. Sugar can also add moisture to dry foods, making them "crisp," or balance acidic tastes found in foods such as tomato sauce or salad dressing. Invert sugar is used to prevent sucrose from crystallizing in candy, while corn syrup is used for the same purpose.

Since the 1950s, a popular natural sugar in North America has been fructose, which has replaced sucrose in many food products in the form of high-fructose syrup (HFS) made from corn. HFS was developed in response to high sucrose prices, and is very inexpensive to manufacture. In other parts of the world, high-fructose syrup is made from local starches, such as rice, tapioca, wheat, or cassava. According to the International Food Information Council in Washington, D.C., the average North American consumes about 37 grams of fructose daily.

GOING SHOPPING

Food shopping can be daunting because most foods are not purely carbohydrate, protein, fat, or sugar, but a mixture of two or three. That's where the American Diabetes Association exchange lists can help. Instead of forcing you to eyeball the ingredients of your foods, the exchange lists on page 197 are designed to do this for you. If you can count, you can plan a meal that has everything you need. A good meal plan will ensure that you are getting enough nutrients to meet your energy needs, and that your food is spread out over the course of the day. For example, if your meal plan allows for three meals with one to two snacks, meals should be spaced four to six hours apart so that your body isn't overwhelmed. If you are obese, snacks will likely be discouraged; snacks can cause you to oversecrete insulin, and increase your appetite. A meal plan should also help you to eat consistently rather than bingeing one day and starving the next.

A good meal plan will also ensure that you're getting the vitamins and minerals you need without taking supplements, such as iron, calcium, folic acid, and vitamims A, B_1, B_2, B_3, C, D, and E. By consuming a variety of foods at every meal, you'll be meeting your vitamin and mineral requirements.

GOLDEN RULES OF DIABETES MEAL PLANS

- Eat three meals a day at fairly regular times (spaced four to six hours apart).
- Ask your dietitian to help you plan your snacks.
- Try to eat a variety of foods each day from all food groups.
- Learn how to gauge serving sizes, volume of bowls and glasses, and so on.
- Ask your dietitian or diabetes educator how to adjust your diet if you're traveling (accounting for your medication, where you're going, what foods will be available, and so on.)
- Draw up a sick days plan with your dietitian. This will depend on what your regular meal plan includes.
- Ask about any meal supplements, such as breakfast bars, sports bars, or meal replacement drinks. How will these figure into your meal plan?
- Choose lower-fat foods more often (see chapter 10).

THE GLYCEMIC INDEX AT A GLANCE

This glycemic index developed at the University of Toronto measures the rate at which various foods convert to glucose, which is assigned a value of 100. Higher numbers indicate a more rapid absorption of glucose. This is not an index of food energy values or calories.

Sugars

Glucose	100
Honey	87
Table sugar	59
Fructose	20

Snacks

Mars bar	68
Potato chips	51
Sponge cake	46
Fish sticks	38
Tomato soup	38
Sausages	28
Peanuts	13

Cereals

Cornflakes	80
Shredded wheat	67
Muesli	66
All Bran	51
Oatmeal	49

Breads

Whole wheat	72
White	69
Buckwheat	51

Fruits

Raisins	64
Banana	62
Orange juice	46
Orange	40
Apple	39

Dairy Products

Ice cream	36
Yogurt	36
Milk	34
Skim milk	32

Root Vegetables

Parsnips	97
Carrots	92
Instant mashed potatoes	80
New boiled potato	70
Beets	64
Yam	51
Sweet potato	48

Pasta and Rice

White rice	72
Brown rice	66
Spaghetti (white)	50
Spaghetti (whole wheat)	42

Legumes

Frozen peas	51
Baked beans	40
Chickpeas	36
Lima beans	36
Butter beans	36
Black-eyed peas	33
Green beans	31
Kidney beans	29
Lentils	29
Dried soybeans	15

The Exchange Lists

The first thing you need to learn before you shop for food is the exchange system, developed by the American Diabetes Association, which tells you how various foods can be incorporated into your meal plan. (This is different than the Food Choice Value System symbols used by the Canadian Diabetes Association, in case you're shopping in Canada; see Table 7.2 for a comparison.) There are seven exchange list categories:

   I.   **Starches List.** Includes: cereals, grains, pasta, breads, crackers, snacks, and starchy vegetables, such as legumes (peas and beans), potatoes, corn, and squash.
  II.   **Meat and Meat Substitutes List.** Includes: poultry, fish, shellfish, game, beef, pork, lamb, cheese, tofu, tempeh, low-fat cheeses, egg whites, and soy milk.
 III.   **Fruit List.** Includes fresh fruit, frozen fruit, canned fruit, dried fruit, and juice. *(Remember: fruit is any produce that grows on trees/vines/plants, such as tomatoes!)*
  IV.   **Dairy List.** Includes: most milk products.
   V.   **Vegetable List.** Includes: most vegetables from A (for artichoke) to Z (for zucchini), but does NOT include starchy vegetables. (See Starches List.)
  VI.   **Fats List.** Includes: monounsaturated fats, polyunsaturated fats, and saturated fats, based on the main type of fat any food contains.
 VII.   **Other Carbohydrates.** Includes: cakes, pies, puddings, granola bars, gelatin, and so on. This list includes any food that contains more fats and sugars than vitamins and minerals.

Your dietitian or diabetes educator will work with you to create an individual meal plan built around the above exchange lists. One person, for example, may eat for breakfast two items from List I, three items from List II, and two items from list VI; another person may require a completely different

Table 7. 2   Comparing the U.S. and Canadian Food Group Systems

American Diabetes Association Exchange System	Canadian Diabetes Association Choice System
1 Starch	1 Starch
1 Fruit	1½ Fruits & Vegetables
1 Vegetable	½ Fruits & Vegetables
1 Milk	2 Milk
(No equal food group)	Sugars
1 Lean Meat	1 Protein
1 Fat	1 Fats & Oils
Free Foods	Extra Vegetables

Source: Diabetes Dialog 42, 1: 19.

plan. I cannot tell you, in this book, how many items from the above lists you can have; I can only explain *how* the foods are categorized.

The best advice regarding exchange lists is to purchase the American Diabetes Association's *Exchange Lists for Meal Planning* (the exchange list bible). It can be ordered directly from the American Diabetes Association for $4.50 by calling 1-800-232-6733.

Your dietitian or diabetes educator should also teach you how to incorporate *carbohydrate counting* ("carb counting") into meal planning, which can be done by learning to read labels properly (see Inside Aisles section), setting goals for a certain number of carbohydrates per day, and keeping accurate records of your blood sugar levels.

The Outside Aisles

What you need for basic nutrition is usually found on the outside aisles of any supermarket or grocery store. Outside aisles usually display the foods you can buy at outdoor markets: fruits, vegetables, meat, eggs, fish, breads, and dairy products. Natural fiber (both soluble and insoluble), discussed in chapter 10, is also found in the outside aisles. Remember, however, foods you buy in the outside aisles can also be high in fat unless you select wisely, as discussed in chapter 10.

The Inside Aisles

These are the aisles of temptation and foods found here may have complicated food labels. (Use Table 7.3 for the FDA guidelines for nutritional claims.) Since 1993, food labels have adhered to strict guidelines set out by the Food and Drug Administration (FDA) and the U.S. Department of Agriculture's (USDA) Food Safety and Inspection Service (FSIS). All labels list "Nutrition Facts" on the side or back of the package. The "Percent Daily Values" column tells you how high or low that food is in various nutrients, such as fat, saturated fat, and cholesterol. A number of 5 or less is "low"— good news if the product shows <5 for fat, saturated fat, and cholesterol—bad news if the product is <5 for fiber. Serving sizes are also confusing. Foods that are similar are given the same *type* of serving size defined by the FDA. That means that five cereals that all weigh X grams per cup will share the same serving sizes.

Table 7.3 Commonly Used U.S. and Canadian Nutrient Claim Comparisons

Claim	U.S.	Canada
"Low Calorie"	40 calories or less per serving	50 percent less energy than a regular product and 15 calories or less per serving
"Low Fat"	3 grams of fat or less per serving	3 grams of fat or less per serving
"Low Cholesterol"	20 mg of cholesterol or less per serving (in addition to saturated fat and total fat restrictions)	20 mg of cholesterol or less per serving (in addition to the saturated fat restrictions only)

Calories (how much energy) and calories from fat (how much fat) are also listed per serving of food. Total carbohydrate, dietary fiber, sugars, other carbohydrates (which means starches), total fat, saturated fat, cholesterol, sodium, potassium, and vitamins and minerals are given in Percent Daily Values, based on the 2,000-calorie diet recommended by the U.S. government. (In Canada, Recommended Nutrient Intake [RNI] is used for vitamins and minerals, while ingredients on labels are listed according to weight, with the "most" listed first.)

That's not where the confusion ends—or *even begins*! You have to wade through the various claims and understand what they mean. For example, anything that says "X free" (sugar free, saturated fat free, cholesterol free, sodium free, calorie free, and so on) means that the product indeed has "no X" or that "X" is so tiny, it is dietarily insignificant. This is not the same thing as a label that says "95 percent fat free." In this case, the product contains relatively small amounts of fat, but still has fat. This claim is based on 100 grams of the product. For example, if a snack food contains 2.5 grams of fat per 50 grams, it can be said to be "95 percent fat free."

A label that screams "low in saturated fat"or "low in calories" is *not* fat free or calorie free. In potato-chip terms, for example, it means you can eat twelve potato chips instead of six. But if you eat a whole bag of low fat chips, you're still eating a lot of fat. Be sure to check serving sizes.

"Cholesterol free" or "low cholesterol" means that the product doesn't have any, or much, animal fat (hence, cholesterol). This doesn't mean "low fat." Vegetable oil doesn't come from animals but is pure fat!

"Less and more"

Then there are the "comparison claims" such as "fewer," "reduced," "less," "more," or my favorite, "light" (or worse, "lite"!). These words appear on foods that have been nutritionally altered from a previous version or a competitor's version. For example, *Brand X Potato Chips—Regular* may have much more fat than *Brand X Potato Chips—Lite* "with less fat than regular Brand X." That doesn't mean that Brand X Lite is fat free, or even low in fat. It just means it's *lower* in fat than Brand X Regular.

On the flip side, *Brand Y* may have a trace amount of calcium, while *Brand Y—"now with more calcium"* may still have a small amount of calcium, but 10 percent more than regular Brand Y. (In other words, you may still need to eat 100 bowls of Brand Y before you get the daily requirement for calcium!)

To be light or "lite," a product has to contain either one-third fewer calories or half the fat of the regular product. Something that is "light in sodium" means it has at least 50 percent less sodium than the regular product, such as canned soup.

Planning to pick up some cough syrup for your cold when you hit the pharmacy section? How about vitamin pills? Check the sugar content first. Your pharmacist can recommend sugar-free products.

"Sugar Free"

When a label says "sugar free," the product contains less than 0.5 grams of sugar per serving; a "reduced sugar" food contains at least 25 percent less sugar per serving than the regular product. If the label states that the product is not a reduced- or low-calorie food, or it is not for weight control, there's enough sugar in there to make you think twice.

Sugar free in the language of labels simply means "sucrose free." That doesn't mean the product is *carbohydrate free.* Check the labels for all things ending in "ose" (dextrose, lactose, fructose) to find out the sugar content; you're not just looking for sucrose. Watch out for "no added sugar," "without added sugar," or "no sugar added." This simply means, "We didn't put the sugar in, God did." Again, reading the number of carbohydrates on the nutrition information label is the most accurate way to know the amount of sugar in the product.

SWEETENERS

We gravitate toward sweet flavors because we start out with the slightly sweet taste of breast milk. A product can be sweet without containing a drop of sugar, thanks to the invention of artificial sugars and sweeteners. Artificial sweeteners will not affect your blood sugar levels because they do not contain sugar; they may contain a tiny number of calories, however. It depends on whether the sweetener is classified as nutritive or nonnutritive.

Nutritive sweeteners have calories or contain natural sugar. White or brown table sugar, molasses, honey, and syrup are all considered nutritive sweeteners. *Sugar alcohols* (see below) are also nutritive sweeteners because they are made from fruits or produced commercially from dextrose. Sorbitol, mannitol, xylitol, and maltitol are all sugar alcohols. Sugar alcohols contain only 4 calories per gram, like ordinary sugar, and will affect your blood sugar levels like ordinary sugar. It all depends on how much is consumed, and the degree of absorption from your digestive tract.

Nonnutritive sweeteners are sugar substitutes or artificial sweeteners; they do not have any calories and will not affect your blood sugar levels. Examples of nonnutritive sweeteners are saccharin, cyclamate, aspartame, sucralose, and acesulfame potassium.

The Sweetener Wars

The oldest nonnutritive sweetener is saccharin, which is what you get when you purchase Sweet'n Low, Sweet Magic, and Zero-Cal. Saccharin is roughly 300 times sweeter than sucrose (table sugar) but has a metallic aftertaste. At one point in the 1970s, saccharin was also thought to cause cancer, but this was never proven.

In the 1980s, aspartame was invented, which is sold as Equal, Sweetmate, and Spoonfuls. It was considered a nutritive sweetener because it was derived from natural sources (two amino acids, aspartic acid and phenylalanine), which means that aspartame is digested and metabolized the same way as any other protein food. For every gram of aspartame, there are 4 calories. But since aspartame is roughly 200 times sweeter than sugar, you don't need very much of it to achieve the desired sweetness. In at least ninety countries, aspartame is found in more than 150 product categories, including breakfast cereals, beverages, desserts, candy and gum, syrups, salad dressings, and various snack foods. An interesting point about aspartame is that it's not recommended for baking or any other recipe where heat is required. The two amino acids in it separate with heat and the product loses its sweetness. It's not harmful if heated, but your recipe won't turn out.

At present, aspartame is considered safe for everybody, including people with diabetes, pregnant women, and children. The only people cautioned against consuming it are those with a rare hereditary disease known as phenylketonuria (PKU) because aspartame contains phenylalanine, which people with PKU cannot tolerate.

Another common tabletop sweetener is sucralose, sold as Splenda. Splenda is a white crystalline powder, actually made from sugar itself. It's 600 times sweeter than table sugar but is not absorbed in your digestive system, so it has no calories at all. Splenda can be used in hot or cold foods, and is found in hot and cold beverages, frozen foods, baked goods, and other packaged foods.

You can also purchase cyclamate, a nonnutritive sweetener sold as Sucaryl or Sugar Twin. Cyclamate is the sweetener used in many weight-control products and is thirty times sweeter than table sugar, with no aftertaste. Cyclamate is fine for hot or cold foods.

The newest sweeteners

The newest addition to the sweetener industry is acesulfame potassium (Ace-K). About 200 times sweeter than table sugar, Ace-K is sold as Sweet One and Swiss Sweet and is found in beverages, fruit spreads, baked goods, dessert bases, tabletop sweeteners, hard candies, chewing gum, and breath fresheners. While no specific studies on Ace-K and diabetes have been done, the only people cautioned against ingesting Ace-K are those on a potassium-restricted diet or people who are allergic to sulfa drugs.

Researchers at the University of Maryland have discovered another sweetener specifically designed for people with diabetes. This sweetener is based on D-tagatose, a hexose sugar found naturally in yogurt, cheese, and sterilized milk. The beauty of this ingredient is that D-tagatose has no effect on insulin levels or blood sugar levels in people both with and without diabetes. Experts believe that D-tagatose is similar to acarbose (see chapter 8) in that it delays the absorption of carbohydrates.

D-tagatose looks identical to fructose, and has about 92 percent of the sweetness of sucrose, but only 25 percent of it will be metabolized. Currently, D-tagatose is being developed as a bulk sweetener. It is a few years away from being marketed and sold as a brand-name sweetener, however.

Sugar alcohols

Not to be confused with alcoholic beverages, sugar alcohols are nutritive sweeteners, like regular sugar. These are found naturally in fruits or manufactured from carbohydrates. Sorbitol, mannitol, xylitol, maltitol, maltitol syrup, lactitol, isomalt, and hydrogenated starch hydrolysates are all sugar alcohols. In your body, these types of sugars are absorbed in the lower digestive tract, and will cause gastrointestinal symptoms if you use too much. Because sugar alcohols are absorbed slowly, they were once touted as ideal for people with diabetes. But, since they are carbohydrates, they still increase your blood sugar—just like regular sugar. Now that artificial sweeteners are on the market in abundance, the only real advantage of sugar alcohols is that they don't cause cavities. The bacteria in your mouth doesn't like sugar alcohols as much as real sugar.

According to the FDA, even foods that contain sugar alcohols can be labeled "sugar free." Sugar alcohol products can also be labeled "Does not promote tooth decay," which is often confused with "low calorie."

AT THE LIQUOR STORE

One alcoholic beverage is as fattening as 2 Fat exchanges on List VI (see above), delivering about 7 calories per gram or 150 calories per drink. Many people with diabetes think they have to avoid alcohol completely because it converts into glucose. This is not so. Alcohol *alone* doesn't increase blood sugar since alcohol cannot be turned into glucose. It's the *sugar* in that alcoholic beverage that can affect blood sugar levels. The problem with alcohol is that it's so darned fattening, something people with Type 2 diabetes may need to watch for. That said, alcohol has been proven to raise your "good" cholesterol (HDL). This fact was discovered in the late 1980s when researchers probed why France, with all its rich food, had such low rates of heart disease. It was the wine; red wine, in particular, was shown to decrease the risk of cardiovascular disease. But any alcohol will do this. So it's okay to use it, so long as *you plan for it* with your dietitian, discuss it with your doctor, and *count it* as an actual food choice.

It's crucial to note that alcohol can cause hypoglycemia (low blood sugar) if you're on oral hypoglycemic agents or insulin.

Discuss the effects of alcohol and hypoglycemia with your health care team.

Fine Wine

Dry wines that have no added sugar are fine to ingest if you are diabetic. Wine is the result of natural sugar in fruits or fruit juices fermenting. Fermentation means that natural sugar is converted into alcohol. A glass of dry red or white wine has calories (discussed below) but *should* have no sugar (ask your liquor dealer or check the label). And unless extra sugar is added to the wine, there's no way that alcohol will change back into sugar, even in your digestive tract. The same thing goes for cognac, brandy, and dry sherry that contain no sugar.

On the other hand, a sweet wine contains roughly 3 grams of sugar per 3.5-oz portion. Dessert wines or ice wines are really sweet; they contain about 15 percent sugar or 10 grams of sugar for a 2-oz serving. Sweet liqueurs are 35 percent sugar.

A glass of dry wine with your meal adds about 100 calories. Half soda water and half wine (a spritzer) contains half the calories. When you cook with wine, the alcohol evaporates, leaving only the flavor. If your wine has no sugar, it counts as 2 Fat exchanges. If it has sugar, you may need to count it as an Other Carbohydrates exchange, on List VII, but check with your dietitian.

At the Pub

If you're a beer drinker, you're basically having some corn, barley, and a couple of teaspoons of malt sugar (maltose) when you have a bottle of beer. The corn and barley ferment into mostly alcohol and some maltose. That's about 150 calories per bottle plus 3 teaspoons of malt sugar. Beer can be defined as 2 Fat exchanges. A light beer has fewer calories but still contains at least 100 calories per bottle. Dealcoholized beer still has sugar, and counts as 2 Vegetable exchanges on List V.

The Hard Stuff

The stiffer the drink, the fatter it gets. Hard liquors such as scotch, rye, gin, and rum are made out of cereal grains; vodka, the Russian staple, is made out of potatoes. In this case, the grains ferment into alcohol. Hard liquor averages about 40 percent alcohol, but has no sugar. Nevertheless, you're looking at about 100 calories per small shot glass, so long as you don't add fruit juice, tomato or clamato juice, or sugary soft drinks. As bizarre as it sounds, a Bloody Mary or Bloody Caesar is actually 1 Fruit and 1 Starch exchange: potatoes and tomatoes!

The Glycogen Factor

Recall from chapter 1 that glycogen is the stored sugar your liver keeps handy for emergencies. If your blood sugar needs a boost, the liver will tap into its glycogen stores and convert it into glucose. Alcohol in the liver *blocks* this conversion process. So, if you've been exercising, and then go out with friends for a few drinks, unless you've eaten something after you exercise, you may need that glycogen. If you drink to the point of feeling tipsy, that glycogen can be cut off by the alcohol, causing hypoglycemia. What complicates matters even more is that your hypoglycemia symptoms can mimic drunkenness. This glycogen problem can affect people with both Type 1 or Type 2 diabetes because it can result when either insulin or oral hypoglycemic agents are used. (See chapter 1 for details on hypoglycemia, and below for the alcohol/diabetes rules.)

Don't Drink and Starve

If you're going to drink, EAT! Always have food with alcohol. Food delays absorption of alcohol into the bloodstream, providing you with carbohydrates and therefore preventing hypoglycemia. Experts also recommend the following:

- Avoid alcohol when your blood sugar is high.
- Remember that two drinks a day is okay for someone with a healthy liver, but less is recommended for liver health.
- Choose dry wines or alcoholic beverages with no sugar (or rum and diet cola versus rum and cola).
- Remember that juice has sugar; even tomato and clamato juice.
- Never substitute alcohol for food if you're taking insulin or pills.
- Don't be afraid to ask your dietitian about how to count your favorite wine or cocktail as a food choice. Again, as long as it's planned for, it's fine.
- Talk to your doctor about how to safely balance alcohol and insulin, and alcohol and oral hypoglycemic agents.

Having Type 2 diabetes is a twenty-four-hour, seven-day-a-week job. Despite this, 70 percent of people with Type 2 diabetes never receive any diabetes education whatsoever. Clearly, diabetes is taking its toll on our health care system. Experts predict that as more people age and are diagnosed with Type 2 diabetes, less education will be available as doctors and diabetes educators become overburdened with patients.

The next chapter focuses on how to maximize your relationships with all your health care providers. Developing a good relationship with your doctor means *helping your doctor help you*! Actively managing your diabetes involves keeping health logs; choosing the right doctor to begin with; knowing the right questions to ask your doctors, educators, and pharmacists; and avoiding duplication of efforts.

CHAPTER 8

Diabetes Doctors and Diabetes Medications

Ask any feminist about "women and doctors," and you'll get a lecture about how the medical system, designed by white men, is still in the business of servicing the white male body in a world designed to support white male society. (Working nine to five, for example, is not an ideal setup for a body that has a menstrual cycle, gives birth, looks after children, breastfeeds, and so forth.) There is a lot of evidence to support this claim. Much of what we know about general health is general health in a *white man's* body—because it was *that* body which was participating in clinical trials researching diseases, treatments, drug interactions, and so on. Therefore, the "norms" for a healthy body are often based on a healthy white male body—one that does not menstruate, get pregnant, breast-feed, or go through menopause. Many women die of curable diseases simply because they do not exhibit the same symptoms as men, and their symptoms are therefore missed by their doctors. Considering the fact that women use the medical system more often than do men, it is disturbing that so much information is unknown when it comes to how a given disease or drug "works" in a female body.

Many people forget why women were, until recently, excluded from clinical research trials. In the past, women, the elderly, minorities, and other vulnerable populations had a long history of being abused in medical research—to such an extent that public outcry demanded stronger regulations that sought to protect them. In response to the horrors of thalidomide, a "morning sickness" drug that was not properly tested prior to marketing (which caused severe limb deformities in the developing fetus), as well as DES (diethylstilbestrol), a "miscarriage prevention" drug which was later revealed to cause a rare form of vaginal cancer in "DES daughters," legislation was passed to protect pregnant women and women of childbearing potential. But the ethics of excluding women from medical research were questioned when basic diseases, such as heart disease (a real risk for women with Type 2 diabetes), were shown to manifest in completely different ways in men than in women. For example, because men suffer from heart attacks at a much earlier age than do women, heart disease suddenly became a "man's disease" even though it kills just as many women, and more women die from heart disease than any other disease. What we know about heart disease (symptoms, prevention, treatment, and so on), therefore, is based on a man's body. As I discuss in the next chapter, the symptoms of heart disease in women, and the age they "present" or manifest, are much different than in men. But until recently, few primary care doctors were able to recognize heart disease symptoms in women. Unfortunately, the same can be said for other complications of Type 2 diabetes. Only recently have studies begun to look at gender differences and this disease.

Women also report considerable psychological and emotional abuse by paternalistic male (and female) doctors—doctors that behave like parents, treating adult patients like children. For example, women's health complaints are often not taken seriously. Many women are given "fluffy" answers about their symptoms, told it is "PMS" or "menopause," or are sent to psychiatrists for physical symptoms.

How does all this affect women with Type 2 diabetes? Many of the doctors women will need to see when dealing with their diabetes are male. On the flip side, because of the traditional "sexist" roles played out in the health care system, most of the diabetes nurse educators and nutritionists are female, which sometimes creates a power struggle between "doctor's orders" and ". . . but my dietitian said . . ." Many women with diabetes find conflicting viewpoints from the "male" role in diabetes (the specialist) and the "female" role in diabetes (the nurse)—even when the actors in these roles may be female doctors and male nurses. The message is simple: Ask questions about how X or Y affects *YOU*. Whether that "you" is pregnant, going through menopause, taking hormone replacement therapy, or working shifts, only *you* can individualize your health care.

Diabetes is a major problem for the North American health care system. In the United States, for example, 14 percent of all health care dollars is spent on managing Type 2 diabetes. Canada reports similar statistics. As a result, there is really no such thing as one "diabetes doctor" who manages the disease completely. Your primary care physician often acts as overall supervisor of your condition, but ideally, this doctor should be working with a team of health care professionals, which includes:

- *An endocrinologist* (a doctor who specializes in the endocrine system, and understands how hormones work and interact with each other). Many endocrinologists subspecialize in various conditions. Some do more diabetes care (and may even call themselves *diabetologists*) than reproductive endocrinology, for example. As a woman with diabetes, whoever is your "hormone" doctor should understand how estrogen, insulin, and blood sugar interact. Don't assume your family doctor or gynecologist knows this information. (See page 218.)
- *A certified diabetes educator (CDE)*. CDEs come from a variety of backgrounds. They can be dietitians, nurses, pharmacists,

social workers, or any other professionals in the health care system who have an interest in diabetes education. CDEs are absolutely vital to managing diabetes. They will help you gain control of your disease by teaching you how to adjust your diet, incorporate physical activity into your routine, and test your blood and record the results, as well as manage any medication or insulin that's been prescribed. CDEs can be found through the American Diabetes Association or you can be referred through your primary care doctor or endocrinologist.

- *A dietitian:* In addition to a CDE, you should see a dietitian regularly during your first year with diabetes. If you learn to meal-plan properly, you may be able to control your diabetes without taking any medications.

- *An exercise/fitness instructor:* This is any professional who can tailor a fitness program to your lifestyle and level of ability. Check with your CDE, the American Diabetes Association, the YMCA, or your local community center for lists of fitness instructors. You do not need a referral; you can simply make an appointment independent of your doctor.

- *Community Health Representative (CHR):* This is someone from your community who works with you and your family, as well as with other health care professionals, to educate you about diabetes. CHRs are usually found in rural areas where access to doctors is poor. CHRs attend a four-day training session and complete a skills test. They are required to review and update their skills annually. CHRs are common in Native communities, and are provided by the Indian Health Service.

- *Other specialists:* These are discussed further on page 221.

- *Pharmacist:* Since you may be expected to do home glucose tests, your pharmacist will recommend the right glucose meter for you, and will become a valuable source of information on drug interactions and their effects on your blood sugar. A diabetes care center in your neighborhood is an ideal place to purchase your diabetes products and consult with a pharmacist.

While Type 2 diabetes is clearly treatable, it is a complex disease that can only be managed through a multilayered approach. The goal of treatment is not just to relieve symptoms, but to prevent a range of other diseases down the road. Self-managing your disease while maintaining your quality of life can only happen if you're willing to learn and to change. That means asking questions and participating in your treatment.

There are various stops along this treatment highway. How many times you stop depends on how well you can control your blood sugar. Some of you may be able to control diabetes solely through exercise and diet (chapters 6 and 7). Some of you may need to combine diet and lifestyle modification with diabetes pills, while others may need to use insulin to control the disease.

This chapter will guide you through the maze of treatments and health care professionals you'll encounter. It will also provide you with the right questions so you can get the right answers. Only then can you be expected to participate fully in decisions that affect your diabetes and the rest of your life.

THE RIGHT PRIMARY CARE DOCTOR

A primary care doctor is the doctor you see all the time. For example, you would see this doctor for a cold, flu, or an annual physical; this is the doctor who refers you to specialists.

Primary care doctors today are *general practitioners* (four years of medical school and one year of internship), *family practitioners* (four years of medical school and a two-year residency in family medicine), or *internists* (four years of medical school and a four-year residency in internal medicine). During medical training, rotations are done in a variety of specialties, such as psychiatry, endocrinology, obstetrics and gynecology, emergency medicine, and so on. A residency is spent in a teaching hospital, under the supervision of teaching faculty (assistant, associate, or full professors of medicine) who teach one specialty. The number of years spent in a residency program after four years of medical school varies with the university and specialty. To qualify as a specialist, such as an endocrinologist, a doctor must do a residency in endocrinology. After this, a fellowship year is required, and the doctor becomes eligible to take exams for Fellowship of the American College of Physicians/Surgeons. (The letters "F.R.C.P." stand for Fellow Royal College of Physicians; "F.R.C.S." stands for Fellow Royal College of Surgeons, for physicians who received training in Canada or the United Kingdom.) Eighty percent of all people with Type 2 diabetes are cared for by their primary care doctors, but the quality of care may vary. What you'll find today is that most primary care doctors in the United States become very good at treating a few conditions. Some see a lot of patients with diabetes; others see many pregnant women; still others see a number of elderly patients requiring palliative care. It all depends on the magic phrase "patient population." *Where* is the doctor's practice located? With *what* plan is that doctor listed? *Who* are the people in that neighborhood?

A primary care physician may not be the best doctor to manage your diabetes, if that doctor doesn't see many diabetes patients. Some doctors are also behind the times when it comes to diabetes, and do not immediately recognize early warning signs or high-risk groups. Nor do all primary care doctors counsel their patients about newer approaches to therapy, such as self-monitoring of blood glucose levels (see chapter 1).

When you're diagnosed with diabetes, ask your doctor the following questions. The answers will help determine whether you should stay with your doctor or look for another one:

1. *What is your philosophy about blood sugar monitoring?* Any doctor who does not discuss the option of your purchasing a glucose meter and self-monitoring your blood sugar levels may not be up to date. As discussed in chapter 1, the

American Diabetes Association recommends that people with Type 2 diabetes get into the habit of self-testing their blood sugar. A discussion about this with your doctor is warranted, even though self-testing remains optional. A good family doctor should present the facts to date: "Here's what some people think; here's what I think; here are my recommendations." (Ultimately, the decision is yours.)

2. *How often will you be checking my glycosylated hemoglobin or glycohemoglobin levels?* If your doctor says "Huh?" get out of there and find another doctor! This is a blood test (HBA_{1c}) that should be done every three to six months.

3. *Will you be referring me to a specialist?* The answer should be "Yes!" If you've been diagnosed with diabetes, you need to see other health care professionals as soon as possible: an endocrinologist who specializes in diabetes, a certified diabetes educator, a dietitian, and an opthalmologist (or optometrist if the former isn't available). If your doctor says, "I can manage your condition without referring you to others," get out of that office and go elsewhere.

4. *Where can I go for more information?* Any doctor who does not tell you to call the American Diabetes Association as soon as you're diagnosed with diabetes is not worth seeing.

The Alarm Bells

If you hear the following words come out of your doctor's mouth, go elsewhere:

- You have borderline diabetes or "just a touch of sugar." (There's no such thing. There used to be a diagnosis of impaired glucose tolerance, discussed in chapter 1, but that may be an outdated diagnosis as of September 1998. See chapter 1 for the new guidelines.)
- You don't need to change your diet; I'll just give you a pill. (In general, no medication should be prescribed until you've

been sent to a dietitian, who will work with you to modify your diet and lifestyle. In cases where medication is warranted immediately, you must still see a dietitian.)

- You don't need to see a specialist. (You *do* need to see a specialist.)
- You have a recurrent vaginal infection. This is perfectly normal. (Chronic vaginal yeast infections are a classic sign of diabetes in postmenopausal women.)

Your Rights

When it comes to your diabetes care, you have rights. Make sure whoever is on your diabetes health care team knows that you're entitled to:

- *As much information about your diabetes as you want.* Any doctor who is reluctant to give you literature, videos, and a referral to a diabetes educator and dietitian is not giving you proper care.
- *Answers to your questions about diabetes.* If there isn't time during an exam or checkup, make another appointment that serves as a question-and-answer period.
- *Regular assessments.* When you have diabetes, you should be seen at least every three months for a checkup or at regular intervals. It's important to ask how much advance booking time you need to get an appointment.
- *Participate in treatment plans.* You'll need to educate yourself about your diabetes before you can participate, but you have many options in treatment.
- *Decent emergency care and to meet your doctor's substitute.* Who looks after you when your doctor is on holidays or sick?
- *Privacy and confidentiality.* Diabetes often taints relationships with employers, coworkers, and insurance companies. Find out what your doctor's legal obligations are with respect to health records—and what are *yours*?

- *Know about fees and costs.* What is covered by your health plan and what is not? How much of your medication and equipment is covered by your health plan? Your doctor should be able to give you an estimate for your diabetes care products in case you are not covered. He or she should also be able to give you less expensive products if you cannot afford what is being prescribed. Pharmacists and the American Diabetes Association are also helpful.
- *Be seen on time.* If you're on time for an appointment, your doctor should be as well. Do you generally have to wait more than thirty minutes in the reception area before your doctor will see you? Although this sometimes can't be helped, the doctor should be aware that waiting creates anxiety, especially if appointments are timed close to meals, and you are taking insulin.
- *To switch doctors.* If you're unhappy with your current doctor, or simply need a change, you have every right to switch. Make sure you arrange for your records to be transferred. Some costs may be involved, however.
- *A second opinion, or a consultation with a specialist.* No family doctor should deny you a referral to a specialist.

Your Doctor's Rights

Your doctor has the right to expect the following from you:

- *Honesty.* If you're not being truthful about how often you're checking your blood sugar levels or what you're eating, or you are "cooking" your log to avoid a lecture, your doctor can't be blamed if your health deteriorates.
- *Courtesy and respect.* Treat your doctor like a business associate. If you make an appointment, show up; if you need to cancel, give twenty-four hours' notice. If you have a problem, go through reasonable channels; dial the after-hours emergency number the doctor leaves with the answering service, or call your doctor's office during business hours.

- *Good reporting.* Don't tell your doctor "you're not feeling well" and expect a diagnosis. Tell your doctor what your *specific symptoms* are. Better yet, write them down before you visit your doctor.
- *Questions.* If you don't ask a particular question, you can't blame your doctor for not answering it.
- *Follow-through.* If you don't follow your doctor's advice, you can't blame the doctor if you experience side effects to medications, or worsening symptoms. If you don't think your doctor's advice is reasonable, say so and discuss it. Maybe your doctor doesn't have a full understanding of your condition; maybe you don't have a full understanding of your doctor's suggestions.
- *Self-management.* Don't call your doctor ten times a day with every little change in your blood sugar levels. You should be able to monitor your blood sugar levels and adjust your diet and medication regimen accordingly. Emergencies or illness are different, however, and your doctor should be notified since even a common virus will elevate your blood sugar level.

YOUR DIABETES SPECIALIST

A diabetes specialist is an endocrinologist who subspecializes in diabetes. Endocrinologists are hormone specialists. Some see more thyroid patients than diabetes patients. Some specialize in reproductive endocrinology (male and female hormones). Therefore, it's important that you wind up with someone who almost exclusively manages diabetes patients. The shortest route to a diabetes specialist is to ask your primary care doctor for a referral. If your primary care doctor refuses to refer you (this, by the way, is not unusual), call the American Diabetes Association and ask for a list of endocrinologists in your area.

If you live in an underserviced area, ask people you know if they have friends or relatives with diabetes. And then, call them!

Who are *they* seeing? You may need to go outside your area to a larger city. But it's worth the trip to receive proper care.

Your primary care doctor can continue to manage the rest of your referrals to ophthalmologists for diabetes eye disease, podiatrists for foot care, and so on. (See chapter 9 for more details.)

Getting Along with Your Specialist

You may find your endocrinologist a little intimidating because he or she may be quite academic; he or she may use technical terms to explain your disease and treatment. Endocrinologists often teach or run residency programs, are active in research, frequently lecture, and regularly publish articles and books in their field. These doctors are usually harder to get in touch with; they may be booked months in advance. That's why it's crucial to maximize the time you *do* have. The best way to do this is to tape-record your appointment. That way, you can replay the information in the comfort of your own home. It's also important to take a list of questions with you. If there isn't time for all your questions to be answered, schedule a separate question-and-answer session. Finally, ask your specialist to draw you a picture of your condition. Visualizing your disease, and seeing how various medications may interact in your body, will help you understand what's going on and what's being recommended.

A dozen good questions to ask

Of course, it's difficult to prepare questions in advance when you don't know what to ask. So here are a few good questions to get you started:

1. How severe is my diabetes? (If you are experiencing other health problems as a result of your diabetes, the disease is likely more advanced.)
2. Does my hospital or treatment center have a multidisciplinary diabetes education care team? (This means that a number of

health care professionals—certified diabetes educators, clinical nurse specialists, dietitians, endocrinologists, and other relevant specialists—discuss your case together and recommend treatment options.)

3. What treatment do you recommend, and why? (For example, if insulin therapy is being recommended over oral hypoglycemic agents, find out why. And find out how this particular treatment will reduce the odds of complications.)

4. How will my treatment help the risks/side effects associated with diabetes and who will help me adjust my medications or insulin?

5. How long do you recommend this particular treatment? (Lifelong? On a wait-and-see basis?)

6. What if I forget to take a pill or insulin shot? What are the consequences?

7. What other health problems should I look out for? (You'll want to watch for symptoms of high or low blood sugar, as well as symptoms of long-term complications, such as eye problems or numbness in your feet.)

8. How can I contact you between visits?

9. Can I take other medications? How will my pills or insulin affect other medications I'm taking?

10. What about alcohol? How will alcohol consumption affect any pills or insulin I'm on? How do I compensate for it?

11. Will I be able to participate in studies or clinical trials using new drugs or therapies?

12. Are there any holistic approaches I can turn to as a complement to diabetes pills or insulin therapy?

Other Specialists

Since diabetes can involve a variety of complications down the road, you may need to consult some or all of the following specialists:

The following drugs may complicate your diabetes, diabetes medications, or insulin. Please discuss side effects with your doctor and pharmacist if you're taking any of the following:

- Estrogen; this raises blood sugars.
- Diuretics; they raise blood sugar.
- Beta blockers; they keep the body from releasing its own sugar in response to hypoglycemia (low blood sugar).
- Steroids; they raise blood sugar levels.
- Nonsteroidal anti-inflammatory drugs (NSAIDs); they raise blood sugar levels.
- Seizure medications; Some raise blood sugar.

Internist: This is a doctor who specializes in nonsurgical treatment of a variety of medical problems, including diabetes.

Ophthalmologist: This is an eye specialist, someone who will be able to monitor your eyes and make sure that you're showing no symptoms of diabetes eye disease (see chapter 9). If you are, this is the specialist who will treat your condition.

Cardiologist: This is a heart specialist. People with Type 2 diabetes are four times more likely to suffer from heart attacks. You may be sent here if you are experiencing symptoms of heart disease or angina. (See chapter 9.)

Nephrologist: This is a kidney specialist. Since kidney disease is a common complication of diabetes, you may be sent here if you're showing symptoms of kidney disease (protein in your urine).

Gastroenterologist: This is a G.I. (gastrointestinal) specialist. Diabetes often results in a number of chronic gastrointestinal ailments. You may be sent here if you have symptoms of chronic heartburn, reflux, and other gastric aches and pains.

Neurologist: This is a nerve specialist who will see you if you're experiencing nerve damage as a result of your diabetes.

Gerontologist: This is a doctor who specializes in diseases of the elderly. If you are over age sixty-five and have a number of other health problems, this doctor will help you balance your various medications and conditions, in conjunction with your diabetes.

Obstetrician/Gynecologist: If you develop diabetes during pregnancy, you'll need to be under the care of an obstetrician for the remainder of your pregnancy (see chapter 4). All women should see a gynecologist regularly for Pap smears, breast care, consultation regarding sexual health, contraception, and hormone replacement therapy after menopause. (See chapters 3, 4, and 5 for more details.)

Orthopedist: This is a doctor who can help you monitor "foot health." If you're experiencing severe problems with your feet (see chapter 9), your podiatrist may send you here.

When You Want a Second Opinion

Getting a second opinion means that you see two separate doctors about the same set of symptoms. If you answer "yes" to one of the questions below, you're probably justified in seeking a second opinion.

1. Is the diagnosis uncertain? If your doctor can't give you a straight answer about what's going on, you're justified in seeing someone else.
2. Is the diagnosis life threatening? In this case, hearing the same news from someone else may help you cope better with your illness, or come to terms with the diagnosis.
3. Is the treatment controversial, experimental, or risky? You might not question the diagnosis, but have problems with the recommended treatment. For example, if you're not comfortable with treatment approach A, perhaps another doctor can recommend treatment approach B.
4. Is the treatment not working? If your oral hypoglycemic agents can't seem to control your blood sugar levels, maybe

it's time for insulin. In this case, getting a second opinion may help to clear up the problem.

5. Are risky tests or procedures being recommended? If you find a particular test or procedure frightening, a second opinion will either help confirm your suspicions, or solidify your original doctor's recommendations.

6. Do you want another approach? If you have poor control over your diabetes, your doctor may want you to begin taking insulin, while another doctor may prescribe dietary changes along with antidiabetic medication.

7. Is the doctor's competence in question? If you suspect that your doctor doesn't know what he or she is doing, go somewhere else to either reaffirm your faith in your doctor, or confirm your original suspicions.

SELF-SERVICE

Doctors cannot treat your diabetes; you have to do this yourself. That means you need to adjust your diet and lifestyle habits, quit smoking, and so on. You should also begin a health diary, in which you record any unusual symptoms and the times and dates those symptoms occur. Without your diary or health record, your doctors are working in the dark and may not be able to design the right therapy program for you.

Control Yourself

Healing yourself may start with tight control over your blood sugar levels. A healthy pancreas measures its owner's blood sugar levels once a second or 3,600 times an hour. It then produces exactly the right amount of insulin for that second. In light of this, testing your blood sugar (see chapter 1 for details on blood sugar testing) may prove useful, and for now is an option that the

American Diabetes Association thinks is worth considering for people with Type 2 diabetes.

What Your Health Diary Should Reveal

The most important information your health diary will contain is the pattern of your blood sugar's peaks and valleys. Dates and times of these peaks and valleys are important clues. Your meal plan, exercise routine, and medication regimen should be tailored to anticipate these peaks and valleys. You may need to incorporate a snack to prevent a low, or go for a twenty-minute walk after dinner to prevent a high. Since there are a variety of factors that can affect your blood sugar levels, your diary should also record:

- where you are in your menstrual cycle;
- any medication you're taking;
- unusually high or low readings that fall outside your pattern;
- stressful life events or situations;
- illness;
- out-of-the-ordinary happenings (no matter how insignificant);
- changes in your health insurance or status;
- severe insulin reactions (if you're taking insulin);
- general medical history (surgeries, tests you've had done, allergies, past drug reactions).

When to Call Your Doctor

As discussed in chapter 1, if you have Type 2 diabetes, it's important to call your doctor whenever you're sick with even just a cold or flu. Fighting off even the most common viruses will elevate your blood sugar levels and require some juggling of your regular routine.

Until you can get in to see your doctor, stay on your meal plan. If that's not possible, drink about a half cup of calorie-free broth or diet or regular soda every hour you are awake. Over-the-counter medications may alter your blood sugar levels unless they are sugar free. You should also test your blood sugar every four hours when you're ill to accommodate higher blood sugar levels. If you're taking any medication, take it as prescribed at the usual times. You may need to go on insulin temporarily if your blood sugar levels remain high. This should not be the case with a cold, but may be necessary if you're laid up with the flu.

When you're not ill, but you have an unusually high blood sugar reading (over 200 mg/dl (11.1 mmol/L), it's time to see your doctor, too.

WHAT THE DOCTOR ORDERS

Throughout the year, your managing doctor (primary care physician or endocrinologist) should be ordering a variety of blood tests to make sure that your blood sugar levels are as controlled as they can be, and that no complications from diabetes are setting in.

The Hemoglobin A_{1c} (HbA_{1c}) test

The most important test is one that checks your glycolsylated hemoglobin levels, known as the hemoglobin A_{1c} test or the HbA_{1c} test. Hemoglobin is a large molecule that carries oxygen to your bloodstream. When the glucose in your blood comes in contact with the hemoglobin molecule, it conveniently sticks to it. The more glucose stuck to your hemoglobin, the higher your blood sugar is. The HbA_{1c} test actually measures the amount of glucose stuck to hemoglobin. And since each hemoglobin molecule stays in your blood about three to four months before it is replaced, this test can show you the average blood sugar level over the last three to four months. This test is recommended at least every six months. If you have cardiovascular problems, you will need to have the HbA_{1c} test more often.

A similar test, known as a fructosamine test, can show the amount of glucose stuck to a molecule in your blood known as albumin. Albumin is replaced every four to six weeks, however, so this test can therefore give you an average of blood sugar levels only over the last four to six weeks.

What's a good HbA$_{1c}$ result?

Just like your glucose monitor at home, the goal of the HbA$_{1c}$ test is to make sure that your blood sugar "average" is as close to normal as possible. Again, the closer to normal it is, the less likely you are to experience long-term diabetes complications.

This test result is slightly different than your glucose meter result. For example, an HbA$_{1c}$ level of 7.0 percent is equal to 144 mg/dl (8 mmol/L) on your blood glucose meter. A result of 9.5 percent is equivalent to 234 mg/dl (13 mmol/L) on your blood glucose meter. In a person without diabetes, an HbA$_{1c}$ ranges from 4 to 6 percent. The results are often expressed as percentages of "normal" such as <110 percent, 111–140 percent, or >140 percent. (See Table 8.1.)

The new guidelines stipulate that values of 6 percent or less are good results and mean that your blood sugar is perfectly under control. Meanwhile, anything higher than 8.4 percent is alarming; this would be a poor result and means that your diabetes is not under control. Studies show that when your HbA$_{1c}$ result is 8.4 percent or higher, you have a greater chance of developing long-term complications. In fact, for every 10 percent drop in your HbA$_{1c}$ average (that is, 7.1 percent down from 8.1 percent), the risk of long-term complications falls by about 40 percent.

Problems with the HbA$_{1c}$ test

If your child came home with a report card showing a B average, it doesn't mean your child is getting a B in every course; it means

Table 8.1 What's a Good Glycosylated Hemoglobin Test (HbA$_{1c}$) Result?*

Nondiabetic Range	Optimal	Suboptimal	Poor Control
4–6.0%	<7.0%	7.0–8.4%	>8.4%
≤100%	≤115%	116–140%	>140%

*Based on fasting blood glucose levels.

Source: Canadian Medical Association Journal 159(8 Suppl 1998):S12.

that he or she could have received a D in one course and an A+ in another. Similarly, the HbA$_{1c}$ test is just an "average mark." You could have a decent result, even though your blood sugar levels may be dangerously low one day and dangerously high the next.

If you suffer from sickle-cell disease or other blood disorders, the HbA$_{1c}$ results will not be accurate. In this case, you may wind up with either false high or false low readings.

Any time, if your home blood sugar tests (if you've opted for self-testing) over the past two or three months do not seem to match the results of the HbA$_{1c}$ test, be sure to check the accuracy of your meter, and perhaps show your doctor or Certified Diabetes Educator how you are using the meter in case your technique needs some refining.

Other Important Tests

It's important to have the following routine tests done at least once a year, and more often if you are at high risk for complications.

Glucose meter checkup

If you've opted to test your own blood sugar, it's important to compare your home glucose meter's test results to a laboratory blood glucose test. In fact, it's a good idea to do this every six months. All you do is bring your meter to the lab when you're having a blood glucose test done. After the lab technician takes your blood, do your own test within about five minutes and record the result. Your meter is working perfectly as long as your result is within 15 percent of the lab test (if your meter is testing whole blood, as opposed to plasma).

Blood pressure

As discussed in chapter 1, high blood pressure can put you at greater risk for cardiovascular problems. Diabetes can also cause high blood pressure. That's why it's important to have your blood pressure checked every four to six months.

Kidney tests

One of the most common complications of diabetes is kidney disease, known in this case as *diabetic nephropathy* (diabetic kidney disease). This condition develops slowly over the course of many years, but there are usually few symptoms or warning signs. To make sure no damage to the kidneys has occurred, it's important to have your urine tested regularly to check the health of your kidneys.

Cholesterol

As discussed in chapter 1, high cholesterol is a problem for people with diabetes, while diabetes can also trigger high cholesterol. Your cholesterol is checked through a simple blood test that should be done once on diagnosis, and once a year thereafter.

Foot Exam

When you have diabetes, nerve damage and poor circulation can wreak havoc on your feet. Be sure to have a thorough foot exam each year to check for reduced sensation or circulation and evidence of calluses or sores. See chapter 9 for more details.

Eye Exam

Since diabetes can cause what's known as diabetes eye disease or diabetic retinopathy (damage to the back of your eye), annual eye exams are crucial. Your eye exam should also rule out cataracts and glaucoma.

When caught early, laser treatment can be used to treat diabetes eye disease and prevent blindness. If your exam results in the term *absent* on your chart, it means your retina is just fine. If you see the word *background,* it means that mild changes have occurred to your eye(s) and that you need more regular monitoring. If the terms *preproliferative* or *proliferative* are used, it means that there is some damage to one or both eyes and you will require treatment and regular exams. See chapter 9 for more details.

WHEN YOUR DOCTOR TELLS YOU TO TAKE A PILL

When diet and lifestyle changes make no impact on your blood sugar levels, you may be prescribed pills. This section provides you with an overview of the kinds of pills prescribed for Type 2 diabetes, who should take these pills, appropriate dosages, side effects, and questions to ask your doctor and/or pharmacist.

Before you fill your prescription for antidiabetic pills, you should know that between 40 and 50 percent of all people with Type 2 diabetes require insulin therapy after ten years. Continuing insulin resistance may cause you to stop responding to oral medications. Furthermore, these pills are meant to *complement* your meal plan, exercise routine, and glucose monitoring; they are not a substitute.

Bear in mind, too, that physicians who prescribe the medications discussed in this section without also working with you to modify your diet and lifestyle are not managing your diabetes properly. These medications should be prescribed only after you've been unsuccessful in managing your Type 2 diabetes through lifestyle modification and frequent blood sugar testing.

If you cannot get down to a healthy body weight, you are probably a good candidate for antidiabetic medication. And anyone with Type 2 diabetes who cannot control her blood sugar levels *despite* lifestyle changes is also a good candidate.

There are four kinds of medications that may be prescribed to you. It's crucial to note, however, that these medications can only be helpful to people who still produce insulin. They have no effect on people with Type 1 diabetes, or insulin-dependent diabetes.

Oral Hypoglycemic Agents (OHAs)

Sulphonylureas are pills that help your pancreas release more insulin. These pills are known as oral hypoglycemic agents (OHAs) and account for about 75 percent of all prescriptions for people with Type 2 diabetes. This medication can make your insulin-producing cells more sensitive to glucose, and stimulate them to secrete more insulin, which will lower your blood sugar.

Biguanides are pills that help your insulin work better. These pills primarily stop your liver from producing glucose, which will help to lower your blood sugar levels and increase glucose uptake by your muscle tissue. These pills also help your tissues respond better to your insulin. Ultimately, biguanides can lower premeal and postmeal blood sugar levels in about 75 to 80 percent of people with Type 2 diabetes. This medication also seems to lower "bad" cholesterol levels. These pills do not increase insulin levels and will not directly cause low blood sugar.

Initially, 75 percent of people with Type 2 diabetes will respond well to sulphonylureas, while biguanides will lower blood sugar in 80 percent of people with Type 2 diabetes. But about 15 percent of all people treated with OHAs fail to respond to them at all, while 3 to 5 percent will stop responding to them each year. So don't get too comfortable on these pills.

Sulphonylureas are generally the initial oral agent of choice in people who are not obese and/or have high blood sugar levels (or suffer from symptoms of high blood sugar). A biguanide is appropriate in people who *are* obese and have milder levels of high blood sugar. That's because biguanides do not result in the weight gain typically associated with sulphonylurea and insulin therapy.

Dosages for sulphonylureas

There is no fixed dosage for sulphonylureas; it all depends on the brand. For example, it's perfectly common to take anything from 80 to 320 mg a day. If you are taking a dosage higher than the recommended initial dose, indicated in Table 8.2, you should divide your dose into two equal parts. Your pills should be taken before or with meals, and your doctor should start you on the lowest effective dose. If your blood sugar levels are high when you start your pills, it's a good idea to have a short trial period of about six to eight weeks to make sure your drug is working.

Dosages for biguanides (Metformin)

Metformin works by decreasing glucose production in the liver and increasing glucose uptake into muscle cells. In this case, the usual dose is 500 mg three or four times a day or 850 mg two or three times a day. Your dose should not exceed 2.5 grams a day. If you're elderly, a lower dose will probably be prescribed.

When OHAs should not be used

If you've had Type 2 diabetes longer than ten years, this is not the time to start OHAs. And, of course, nobody with Type 1 or insulin-dependent diabetes (IDDM) should ever take OHAs; they will not work. OHAs should never be taken under the following conditions, as well:

- alcoholism;
- pregnancy;
- kidney or liver failure (Metformin only).

Table 8.2 Sulphonylureas, a Common Class of Oral Hypoglycemic Agent

	Daily/mg	Initial	Per day
*Acetohexamide	250–1,500	250	1–2
*Chlorpropamide	100–500	250	1
†Glimepiride	1–8	1	1
†Glipizide	5–40	10	1–2
†Glyburide	2.5–20	5	1–2
*Tolbutamide	500–3,000	1,000	1–3
*Tolazamide	100–1,000	100	1–2

*First generation—not prescribed very much.
†Second generation—more commonly prescribed.

Sources: Compendium of Pharmaceuticals and Specialities, 1996; Drum and Zierenberg, *The Type II Diabetes Sourcebook* (Los Angeles: Lowell House, 1998, 186–87).

Side effects

Sixty percent of people taking OHAs continue to have high blood sugar levels two hours after meals. These pills can also cause increased appetite and weight gain. The main side effect with first generation OHAs, however, is hypoglycemia (low blood sugar), which occurs in one in five people treated with OHAs. If you're over age sixty, hypoglycemia may occur more often, which is why it's dangerous for anyone over age seventy to take certain OHAs.

About one-third of all people taking OHAs will experience gastrointestinal side effects (no appetite, nausea, abdominal discomfort and, with Metformin, diarrhea). Adjusting dosages and taking your pills with your meals or afterward often clears up these symptoms.

OHAs and hypoglycemia

About 15 to 30 percent of all people taking sulphonylureas are vulnerable to hypoglycemia because this drug stimulates the pancreas to produce insulin. This is synonymous with taking an insulin injection. Furthermore, if you lose weight after you begin taking sulphonylureas, but don't lower your pill dosage, you could also experience hypoglycemic episodes. That's because losing weight will make your body more responsive to insulin.

Biguanides do not typically cause hypoglycemic episodes, since they work by preventing the liver from making glucose rather than stimulating the production of insulin. Similarly, acarbose (see further on) does not, by itself, cause hypoglycemia. It works by delaying the breakdown of starch and sucrose into glucose. That's not to say, however, that hypoglycemia can't happen to you if you're taking biguanides or acarbose; you can still develop it if you miss meals or snacks or overexercise without compensating for it, although this is rare.

Your diabetes pills may also interact with other medications. For example, some of the older oral hypoglycemic agents may work less or more effectively when combined with certain medications, including blood thinners (anticoagulants), oral contraceptives, diuretics, steroids, aspirin, and various anticonvulsive or antihypertensive medications.

Another factor is the half-life of your oral medication. By knowing when the drug peaks in your body, you'll be able to prevent hypoglycemia from occurring. For example, tolbutamide is a short-acting oral hypoglycemic agent. It begins to work about an hour after you take it and lasts for about twelve hours, peaking from five to six hours after you ingest it. Acetohexamide starts working about an hour after you take it, and stays in your body for about fourteen hours and peaks at about five hours. Glyburide goes to work in about one and a half hours, stays in your body for twenty-four hours, and peaks at about three hours. Finally, chlorpropamide has the longest half-life. It starts to work an hour after you take it, stays in your body for seventy-two hours, and peaks within thirty-five hours.

Roughly 40 percent of all people taking a combination of oral hypoglycemic agents experience hypoglycemic episodes, while 33 to 47 percent of people who combine insulin with sulphonylureas experience hypoglycemic episodes. These are higher odds than if you were taking one oral hypoglycemic agent only.

Acarbose (Alpha-Glucosidase Inhibitors)

Alpha-glucosidase inhibitors (acarbose) are pills that delay the breakdown of sugar in your meal. Introduced in 1996, acarbose is the first antidiabetic medication to come along since the mid-1950s, when sulphonylureas and biguanides were developed. Acarbose is very similar in structure to the sugars found in foods. The main sugar in blood, glucose, is a *simple sugar* that is made from starch and sucrose (table sugar). Starch and sucrose are turned into glucose by enzymes in the lining of the small intestine called alphaglucosidases. What acarbose does is stall this process by forcing the starch and sugar you eat to "take a number" before they're converted into glucose. Why do this? This slows down the absorption of glucose into the cells, preventing a rise in blood glucose after a meal. In order to work, acarbose must be taken with the first bite of each main meal. You'll also need to test your blood sugar two hours after eating to see how well you're responding to the medication.

Acarbose is prescribed to people who cannot seem to get their after-meal (that is, postmeal or postprandial) blood sugar down to acceptable levels. A major benefit of acarbose is that it may reduce the risk of hypoglycemic episodes during the night, particularly in insulin users. Investigators are studying whether acarbose may be used one day as a substitute for that "morning insulin." The usual rules apply here: Acarbose should complement your meal plan and exercise routine; it is not a substitute or a way out, and does not, by itself, cause hypoglycemia.

Who should take acarbose?

Anyone who
- cannot control her blood sugar through diet and lifestyle modification alone;

- is on OHAs but is still experiencing high blood sugar levels after meals;
- cannot take OHAs and for whom diet/lifestyle modification has failed;
- is not doing well on an OHA who wants to prevent the advent of insulin treatment.

Who should not take acarbose?

Anyone with the following conditions should not be taking this drug:
- inflammation or ulceration of the bowel (inflammatory bowel disease, ulcerative colitis, or Crohn's disease);
- any kind of bowel obstruction;
- any gastrointestinal disease;
- kidney or liver disorders;
- hernias;
- pregnancy or lactation; or
- Type 1 diabetes.

Dosage

The usual starting dosage for acarbose is 25 mg (half of a 50 mg tablet), with the first bite of each main meal. After four to eight weeks, your dosage may be increased to 50 mg, three times a day. Or you may start by taking one 50-mg tablet once daily with supper. If that's not working, you'll move up to two 50-mg tablets twice daily with your main meals or three 50-mg three times daily with main meals. The maximum dosage of acarbose shouldn't go beyond 100 mg three times a day.

For best results, it's crucial that you take acarbose with the first bite of each main meal. In fact, if you swallow your pill even five to ten minutes before a meal, acarbose will pass through your digestive system and have no effect. It's also important that you take acarbose with a carbohydrate; the medication doesn't work if there are no carbohydrates in your meal. You shouldn't take acarbose between meals, either; it won't work. Nor should acarbose be used as a weight-loss drug.

Side effects

The good news is that acarbose doesn't cause hypoglycemia. Since you may be taking this drug along with an OHA, however, you may still experience hypoglycemia, as acarbose doesn't prevent it, either. (See chapter 1 for warning signs and treatment for hypoglycemia.)

The only side effects acarbose, by itself, causes are gastrointestinal: gas, abdominal cramps, softer stools, or diarrhea. Acarobose combined with Metformin can produce unacceptable gastrointestinal symptoms. You'll notice these side effects after you've consumed foods that contain lots of sugar. Avoid taking antacids; they won't be effective in this case. Adjusting the dosage and making sure you're taking acarbose correctly will usually take care of the side effects.

Thiazoladinediones (Troglitazone or Rezulin)

Thiazoladinediones (troglitazone or Rezulin) are pills that make your cells more sensitive to insulin, thereby improving insulin resistance. When this happens, more glucose gets into your tissues, and less glucose hangs around in your blood. The result is that you'll have lower fasting blood glucose levels, without the need to increase insulin levels. Troglitazone works by stimulating muscle tissue to "drink in" glucose. It also decreases glucose production from the liver, and makes fat tissue more receptive to glucose. This drug is reserved for people with Type 2 diabetes who must take insulin to reduce their blood sugar levels (see next section). Troglitazone is being touted as a wonder drug because you only need one tablet a day for the pill to work. Researchers are currently investigating troglitazone to delay or prevent the onset of Type 2 diabetes altogether. Clinical trials suggest that troglitazone is effective in just a single daily dose of 200-, 400-, 600- or 800-mg tablets. You can also split a dosage into two, such as 200 or 400 mg twice daily.

One study showed that one 400-mg tablet every morning for a six-week period improved blood sugar to normal readings in 75 percent of study participants. After twelve weeks of treatment, 80 percent of study participants with high blood sugar showed normal glucose levels.

It may all be too good to be true. Unfortunately, warnings about troglitazone have been issued because it can cause liver failure. In early studies (these were controlled trials), 1.9 percent of people in the trial developed mild liver problems. But as soon as the drug was more widely prescribed, the U.S. Food and Drug Administration received reports of several cases of severe liver disease that led to death or the need for a liver transplant. For example, in one case, after a fifty-five-year-old woman using insulin took a daily dose of 400 mg of troglitazone for about three months, she developed liver failure. Please ask your doctor about the risks of this drug if it's prescribed. If you've ever had hepatitis (A, B, or C), you should not take this drug. There are a number of other factors in your history that may prevent you from using it, which you must discuss with your doctor.

Other side effects

When taken at doses of 600 and 800 mg a day, troglitazone can raise LDL ("bad") cholesterol. Anyone with cardiovascular problems should not be on this drug. White blood cell counts also went down in people taking the highest dosage of 800 mg daily. Therefore, high doses of this drug are not recommended for people who are immune suppressed for any reason; the drug may also trigger an infection in healthy people. Headaches were also reported in some users, but for the most part, troglitazone is a well-tolerated drug with a low incidence of adverse side effects.

Natural alternatives

If you don't like the idea of taking pills to control your diabetes, you can try to incorporate more natural methods to see if you can prevent taking medication. You'll have to discuss this approach with your doctor, of course, but there are some options.

Guar gum is a high source of fiber (a polysaccharide—see glossary), made from the seeds of the Indian cluster bean. When you mix guar with water, it turns into a gummy gel, which slows down your digestive system, similar in effect to acarbose (see above). Guar has often been used to treat high blood sugar as well as high cholesterol. Guar can cause gas, stomachaches, nausea, and diarrhea. (These are also side effects of acarbose, discussed above.) The problem with guar is that there are no scientific studies to date concluding that it improves blood sugar control. Nevertheless, most experts agree that it can certainly provide at least some marginal benefits.

Delay glucose absorption by eating more fiber, avoiding table sugar (sucrose), and eating smaller meals more often to space out your calories. Meal planning is discussed in detail in chapter 7.

Questions to Ask About Diabetes Drugs

Before you fill your prescription, it's important to ask your doctor or pharmacist the following:

1. What does this drug contain? If you are allergic to particular ingredients, such as dyes, it's important to find out the drug's components before you take it.
2. Are there any medications I shouldn't combine with this drug? Be sure to ask about interactions with cholesterol or

hypertension medications, as well as any antidepressants or antipsychotics.

3. If this drug doesn't work well, am I a candidate for combination therapy? This means that your drug could be combined with another drug. Common combinations include a sulphonylurea and biguanide, and acarbose and an OHA. The first drug you started is raised to its maximum dosage, before the second drug is started at its lowest dosage; or both drugs are started at their lowest dosages and then raised gradually.

4. If this drug doesn't work well, would insulin ever be prescribed along with this pill? Some studies have shown that there is some benefit to this combination, but it remains controversial.

5. How will you measure the effectiveness of your drug? You should be testing your blood sugar with a glucose monitor, particularly two hours after eating, to make sure that the lowest effective dose is prescribed. Your doctor should also be doing a glycosylated hemoglobin or HbA_{1c} test two to three times per year (see above).

6. How should I store my drugs? All pills should be kept in a dry place at a temperature between 59°F (15°C) and 77°F (25°C). Keep these drugs away from children, don't give them out as "samples" to your sister-in-law, and don't use tablets beyond their expiration dates.

7. What symptoms should I watch out for while on these drugs? You'll definitely want to watch for signs of high or low blood sugar.

WHEN YOUR DOCTOR PRESCRIBES INSULIN

Let me dispel a common fear about insulin: Since insulin is not a blood product, you don't have to worry about being infected with a blood-borne virus such as HIV or hepatitis.

Many doctors delay insulin therapy for as long as possible by giving you maximum doses of the pills discussed above. This isn't considered good diabetes management. If you need insulin, you should take insulin. The goal is to get your disease under control. Therefore, anyone with the following conditions is a candidate for insulin:

- high blood sugar levels, despite maximum doses of oral hypoglycemic agents;
- fasting glucose levels consistently over 162 mg/dl (9 mmol/L);
- illness or stress (insulin may be needed until you recover);
- major surgery;
- complications of diabetes (see chapter 9); or
- pregnancy (insulin may be temporary).

If going on insulin will affect your job security, you should discuss this with your doctor so that appropriate notes or letters can be drafted to whom it may concern. You should also keep in mind that if insulin therapy does not bring your diabetes under control within six months of treatment, it may be necessary to return to your drug therapy after all.

Right now, 40 to 50 percent of all people with Type 2 diabetes require insulin injections to manage their condition. Until troglitazone is more widely prescribed and in use, this is the reality. Insulin resistance eventually may lead to requiring insulin from an outside source. You'll need to discuss the various insulins available with your doctor, as well as be trained in giving yourself insulin injections.

The Right Insulin

The newest insulin is known as insulin lispro, an insulin analog ("copycat"). This is a synthetic insulin that does not have an animal or human source. It's made by reversing the order of two amino acids (LYS and PRO) in the human insulin molecule.

With traditional human insulins (animal insulin is not readily available, but is discussed further on), you need to be extremely good at calculating when you're going to eat, how much you're going to eat, and how much insulin to inject. Basically, you need to be in excellent control of your diabetes. The problem with traditional, longer-acting insulin is that you can wind up with too much of it in your system, which can cause insulin shock, or hypoglycemia (low blood sugar—see chapter 1). Insulin lispro is a very short-acting insulin, which means that you inject it about fifteen minutes before you eat (while you're cooking dinner or when ordering food in a restaurant). Therefore, some experts consider it an easier insulin with which to work.

That said, insulin is highly individualized. It's simply not possible for me to tell you in this book which insulin you need to be on any more than I can tell you what, exactly, you need to *eat* each day. This is why a diabetes health care team is so crucial. Your meal plans, medications, and insulin (when needed) is tailored to suit YOU. And that has everything to do with who you are, not which brand of insulin is popular.

The goal of a good insulin program is to try to mimic what your pancreas would do if it were working properly. Blood sugar rises in a sort of "wave" pattern. The big waves come in after a big meal; the small waves come in after a small meal or snack. The insulin program needs to be matched to your own particular wave pattern. So what you eat—and when—has a lot to do with the right insulin program. The right insulin for someone who eats three square meals a day may not be appropriate for someone who tends to "graze" all day. And the right insulin for an active forty-seven-year-old man in a stressful job may not be the right insulin for a sixty-seven-year-old woman who does not work, and whose heart condition prevents her from exercising regularly.

You and your health care team will also need to decide how much control you need over your blood sugar. Insulin "recipes" depend on whether you need tight control, 60–120 mg/dl (3.3–6.6 mmol/L); medium control, 72–180 mg/dl (4–10 mmol/L); or even loose control, 140–234 mg/dl (11–13 mmol/L). Loose control is certainly not encouraged, but on rare occasions, when a person is perhaps quite elderly and suffering from a number of other health problems, it is still "done." To determine the appropriate insulin recipe for you, your health care team should look at who you are as a person—what you eat, where you work, your willingness to change your eating habits, and other lifestyle factors.

There are many kinds of insulins available. Every manufacturer has a different brand of insulin, and a separate letter code for the insulin action. To make things as easy to understand as possible, I've provided a translation of all these codes on page 243. Once you and your diabetes health care team choose the right insulin for you, you will need to take a minicourse on how to use and inject insulin. This is usually done by a certified diabetes educator (CDE).

Human insulin

All human insulin is biosynthetic, which means that the biochemically created "product" normally made by the human pancreas has been re-created in a test tube through DNA technology.

Today, most manufacturers produce only these insulins, which are considered the purest form of insulin available. Human insulins come in three different actions: short acting (clear fluid), intermediate acting (cloudy fluid), and long acting (cloudy fluid). Short acting means that it stays in your body for the shortest duration of time; long acting means that it stays in your body for the longest duration of time. (See Table 8.3 for details.)

Beef/Pork insulin

The only people who should be on animal insulin are people who began using it years ago. These are likely people with Type 1 diabetes who developed a rhythm with their animal insulin and are reluctant to switch to human insulin or an insulin analog. If

BREAKING THE CODES

R: This stands for "regular" biosynthetic human insulin. Regular means that it is short-acting insulin.

"ge' Toronto: "ge" is the name Connaught-Novo gives to all of its biosynthetic insulin. It stands for "genetically engineered." Toronto is the brand name of this company's short-acting insulin, like "Kraft" or "President's Choice."

Insulin Lispro: This is a very new and "super short-acting" insulin under the brand name Humalog, which starts to work in fifteen to thirty minutes. It is a biosynthetic insulin made from two amino acids, LYS and PRO. It's ideal for people with Type 1 diabetes.

N or NPH: NPH is simply the initials of the man who invented this type of insulin, which is an intermediate-acting insulin that is said to have an "abrupt" peak ("ge"-NPH stands for genetically engineered NPH).

L or Lente: This is also an intermediate-acting insulin which is very similar to NPH except it has a more "lumbering" peak ("ge"-Lente stands for genetically engineered Lente).

Beef/Pork: This is animal insulin made from cows or pigs. It's still available in Canada from Eli Lilly but isn't readily available at most pharmacies unless special ordered.

Humulin 10/90: This is a premixed insulin, meaning that it is 10 percent regular and 90 percent NPH. Also available in 20/80, 30/70, 40/60, and 50/50. (Note: Many people with Type 2 diabetes do well on 30/70.)

Novolin 10/90 'ge': Exactly the same as above, except "ge," which stands for genetically engineered.

Novolin ultra 'ge': Connaught-Novo's long-acting insulin which starts acting in four hours, peaks within eight to twenty-four hours, and exits within twenty-eight hours. Again, "ge" stands for genetically engineered.

Ultra Lente 'ge': The same as above except it peaks in ten to thirty hours and exits in thirty-six hours.

Semi Lente-NPH: This is a very long-acting insulin that is rarely used. Most diabetes educators haven't seen someone on this stuff for years!

Table 8.3 Getting to Know Your Insulin

Short-Acting Insulin (This is the "hare." It gets there fast but tires easily.)

Starts working in: 30 minutes (Insulin Lispro: <15–30 minutes)

Peaks in: 2 to 4 hours (Insulin Lispro: 30 minutes–2.5 hours)

Duration of action: 6 to 8 hours (Insulin Lispro: 3–4 hours)

When to eat: within 30 minutes of injecting

Peak effect (maximum action): 1½ to 5 hours

Exits body in: 8 hours

Appearance: Clear. Don't use if cloudy, slightly colored, or if solid chunks are visible.

Intermediate-Acting Insulin (This is the "tortoise." It gets there at a slower pace, but it lasts longer.)

Starts working in: 1 to 2 hours

Peaks in: 4 to 12 hours (usually around 8 or less)

Duration of action: 24 hours (or less)

When to eat: within 2 hours

Exits body in: 24 hours

Appearance: Cloudy. Do not use if the white material remains at the bottom of the bottle after mixing, leaving a clear liquid above; or if clumps are floating in the insulin after mixing, or if it has a "frosted" appearance.

Long-acting insulin (This is the "two-legged turtle." It's *really* slow. And it hangs around for a long time.)

Starts working in: 8 hours

Peaks in: 18 hours

Duration of action: 36 hours

When to eat: within 8 hours

Exits body in: 36 hours or more

Appearance: Cloudy. Do not use if the white material remains at the bottom of the bottle after mixing, leaving a clear liquid above; or if clumps are floating in the insulin after mixing, or if it has a "frosted" appearance.

For information about brand names, premixed insulins, and specific products, consult your doctor, pharmacist, diabetes educator, or insulin manufacturer.

you're newly diagnosed with Type 2 diabetes, or you have just started to take insulin, this is not the right insulin for you. Animal insulin is less pure and causes a higher incidence of hypo-glycemia. If you're currently on animal insulin and would like to switch, you must discuss this with your managing physician first. On the flip side, you shouldn't feel pressured into switching insulins if you're happy on animal insulin.

Premixed insulin

Premixed insulin means that both short-acting insulin and inter-mediate-acting insulin are mixed together. These are extremely popular insulins for people with Type 2 diabetes for reasons explained in Table 8.3. These work well for people who have a very set routine and don't want to take more than one or two insulin injections daily.

Both human and animal insulin are available in premixed for-mats. They are labeled as 10/90 (10 percent short acting; 90 percent intermediate acting), 20/80, 30/70, 40/60, and 50/50. Premixed insulin is always cloudy. It's also possible to mix together short act-ing with long acting, or long acting with intermediate acting.

Your insulin gear

If you've graduated to insulin therapy, here's what you'll need to buy:

- a really good glucose monitor that is made for people who test frequently (see chapter 1);
- lancets and a lancing device for testing your blood sugar (see chapter 1);
- insulin pens and cartridges (this is far easier) or traditional needles and syringes (a diabetes educator will need to walk you through the types of products available);
- the right insulin brand for you.

Learning to Use Insulin

Insulin must be injected. It cannot be taken orally because your own stomach acids digest the insulin before it has a chance to work. Your doctor, pharmacist, CDE, or someone at a diabetes care center will teach you how to inject yourself painlessly. Don't inject insulin by yourself without a training session. The most convenient way to use insulin is with an insulin pen. In this case, your insulin (if human or biosynthetic) will come in a cartridge. If you decide against a pen, your insulin will come in a bottle and you will need a needle and syringe. Always know the answers to these questions before you inject your insulin:

1. How long does it take before it starts to work? (Known as the *onset of action*.)
2. When is this insulin working the hardest? (Known as the *peak*.)
3. How long will my insulin continue to work? (Known as the *duration of action*.)

How many injections will I need?

This really depends on what kind of insulin you're taking and why you're taking it. A sample routine may be to take an injection in the morning, a second injection before supper, and a third before bed. What you want to prevent is low blood sugar while you're sleeping. You may need to adjust your insulin if there is a change in your food or exercise routine (which could happen if you're sick). Your insulin schedule is usually carefully matched to your meal times and exercise periods.

Where to inject it

The good news is that you do not have to inject insulin into a vein. As long as it makes it under your skin or in a muscle, you're fine. Thighs and tummies are popular injection sites. These are also large enough areas that you can vary your injection site. (You should space your injections about 2 to 3 cm apart.) Usually you establish a little rotating pattern. Other injection sites are the upper outer area of the arms, the upper outer surfaces of the buttocks, and lower back areas. Insulin injected in the abdomen is absorbed more quickly than insulin injected in the thigh. In addition, strenuous exercise will speed up the rate of absorption of insulin if the insulin is injected into the limb you've just "worked out." Other factors that can affect insulin's action are the depth of injection, your dose, the temperature (it should be room temperature or body temperature) and what animal your insulin came from (human, cow, or pig).

Experts also suggest you massage the injection site to increase the rate of insulin absorption. If you notice a hardening of skin due to overuse, this will affect the rate of absorption. Your doctor or CDE will show you how to actually inject your insulin (angles, pinching folds of skin, and so on). There are lots of tricks of the trade to optimize comfort. With the fine needle points available today, it doesn't have to be an uncomfortable ordeal.

Side Effects

The main side effect of insulin therapy is low blood sugar, which means that you must eat or drink glucose to combat symptoms. This side effect is also known as insulin shock. Low blood sugar, or hypoglycemia is discussed in chapter 1.

You may also notice something called *lipodystrophy* (a change in the fatty tissue under the skin) or *hypertrophy* (an enlarged area on your skin). Rotating your injection sites will prevent these problems. A sunken area on your skin surface may also occur, but it is usually only present with animal insulin. Rashes can sometimes occur at injection sites, too, but less than 5 percent of all insulin users notice these problems.

Questions to Ask About Insulin

The answers to these questions will depend on your insulin brand. Pharmacists and doctors should know the answers to all these questions, but if they don't, I recommend calling the customer care 1-800 number provided by your insulin manufacturer.

- How do I store this insulin?
- What are the characteristics of this insulin (that is, onset of action, peak, and duration of action)?
- When should I eat after injecting this insulin?
- When should I exercise after injecting this insulin?
- How long are opened insulin bottles/cartridges safe at room temperature?
- What about the effect of sunlight or extreme temperatures on this insulin?
- Should this insulin be shaken or rolled?
- What should I do if the insulin sticks to the inside of the vial/ cartridge?
- Should this insulin be clear or cloudy? What should I do if the appearance looks "off" or has changed?
- What happens if I accidentally inject out-of-date insulin?
- What other medications can interfere with this particular brand?
- Who should I see about switching insulin brands?
- If I've switched from animal to human insulin, what dose should I be on?

Traveling with insulin

When traveling, you'll need to make sure you pack enough insulin for your trip, as well as identification (a doctor's note) that clearly states you have diabetes, so you don't get harassed over carrying needles, syringes, and vials. In fact, many experts suggest that for a trip, you switch to an insulin pen, which is far easier to carry and less obvious. In some cases, even lancets and a glucose meter may be suspect without identification. Experts recommend the following supplies for travel:

- a backup supply of insulin *on you,* as well as extra cartridges, needles, syringes, and testing supplies; vials break, baggage gets lost, and planes, trains, and buses get delayed;
- a doctor's written prescription for your insulin and a doctor's note explaining why you're carrying your equipment;
- a Medic Alert tag or card stating that you have diabetes;
- a day's supply of food (especially if you're flying);
- an extra sugar source, such as dextrose tablets;
- a list of hospitals in your travel destination areas.

It's also important never to part with your insulin; always carry it with you in carry-on baggage. Dividing your supplies between two bags is best in case vials break. If you're flying, drink lots of liquids prior to boarding, as well as one glass of nonalcoholic liquid for every hour of flight. And don't order a special meal; these have a nasty habit of never making it to your plane. Bring food with you and pick at the airline food you're served. You should also stroll up and down the cabin as much as possible to avoid high blood sugar. (This bit of exercise will use up some sugar.) If you're traveling to a different time zone, consult your doctor or diabetes educator about adjusting insulin injections to the new time zone.

Why are you going through the maze of information in this chapter? To prevent further complications of diabetes, and to prepare yourself for dealing with even *more* doctors and medications should complications happen down the road—the topic of the next chapter.

CHAPTER 9

Women Down the Diabetes Road

Why is it so important to manage your diabetes as well as possible? Many of the preexisting conditions that led to your diabetes (see chapter 1) can cause other complications down the road. In addition, higher than normal blood sugar levels can lead to even more complications.

At least 40 percent of all people with Type 2 diabetes will develop another disease as a result of their diabetes. Many of you may already be affected by some of the conditions discussed in this chapter. If you've been newly diagnosed with Type 2 diabetes, however, you may not realize exactly how many other diseases it can trigger; after all, you may feel fine now. The purpose of this chapter is to simplify the complex language of "complications" so that you can see what may be waiting down the road, clearly read the road signs, and perhaps take a different route. You'll find out why diabetes leads to other diseases, the diagnosis and treatment of those diseases, and what can be done to prevent complications.

MACRO VERSUS MICRO

The most important point to grasp about diabetes complications is that two different kinds of problems can lead to similar diseases. The first kind of problem is known as a *macrovascular complication.*

The prefix *macro* means large, as in macroeconomics (studying an entire economic system as opposed to one company's economic structure). The word *vascular* means blood vessels—your veins and arteries, which carry the blood back and forth throughout your body. Put it together and you have "large blood vessel complications." A plain-language interpretation of macrovascular complications is: "BIG problems with your blood vessels."

If you think of your body as a planet, a macrovascular disease would be a disease that affects the whole planet; it is bodywide, or systemic. Cardiovascular disease is a macrovascular complication, which can cause heart attack, stroke, high blood pressure, and bodywide circulation problems, clinically known as peripheral vascular disease (PVD). So your body, head to toe, is affected (see Head to Toe section, p. 254).

A second type of problem is known as a *microvascular complication*. Micro means tiny, as in microscopic. Microvascular complications refer to problems with the smaller blood vessels (capillaries) that connect to various body parts. A plain-language interpretation of microvascular complications is "Houston, we've got a problem." In other words, the problem *is* serious, but it's not going to affect the whole planet, just the spacecraft in orbit. Eye disease (clinically known as retinopathy) is a microvascular complication. Blindness is a serious problem, but you won't die from it. Nerve damage (neuropathy) is a microvascular complication that can affect your whole body—feet, eyes, sexual functioning, skin—but, again, you won't die from it.

The Combo Platter

Complications get really complicated to understand when macro *and* micro converge. This is what happens with kidney disease (clinically known as renal disease nephropathy). The high blood pressure that is caused by macrovascular complications, combined with the small blood vessel damage caused by microvascular complications, together can cause kidney failure—something you *can* die from unless you have dialysis (filtering out the body's waste products through a machine) or a kidney transplant.

Who Gets Macrovascular Complications?

Macrovascular complications are caused, not only by too much blood sugar, but also by preexisting health problems. People with Type 2 diabetes are far more vulnerable to macrovascular complications because they usually have contributing risk factors, such as high cholesterol and high blood pressure (both of which are discussed in chapter 1). Obesity, smoking, and inactivity can then aggravate those problems, resulting in major cardiovascular disease.

Warning signs of macrovascular complications

If you are obese, inactive, and have Type 2 diabetes as well as high blood pressure and/or high cholesterol, you are at high risk for macrovascular problems. The bomb is ticking. In this case, you should be working *right now* on making changes in your diet and lifestyle, and discussing whether you're a candidate for blood pressure–lowering or cholesterol-lowering medication with your doctor. If you're a woman entering menopause, you should definitely consider hormone replacement therapy, which offers protection from heart disease, balancing the benefits of that against other risks. (See chapters 3 and 5 for more information.) You may also want to look into more effective strategies to manage your obesity, discussed in chapter 2.

You also need to stay alert to signs of circulation problems, heart attack, and stroke, discussed in detail below.

Who Gets Microvascular Complications?

People with Type 1 diabetes are very vulnerable to microvascular complications, but a number of people with Type 2 diabetes suffer from them, too. Microvascular complications are known as sugar-related complications. Small blood vessel damage is caused by high blood sugar levels over long periods of time. The Diabetes Control and Complications Trial, referred to throughout this book and discussed in detail at the end of this chapter, showed that by keeping blood sugar levels as normal as possible, *as often as possible,* through frequent self-testing, microvascular complications can be prevented.

Warning signs of microvascular problems

Numbness in arms, face, or legs, vision problems, bladder infections, and other bladder problems are warning signs of microvascular problems. Specific alarm signals for each microvascular problem are discussed separately in the next section.

FROM HEAD TO TOE

It's important to understand which parts of the body are vulnerable to macrovascular problems, microvascular problems, or both. Therefore, each subheading in this section will indicate "macro," "micro," or "both." People with Type 2 diabetes are far more likely to experience problems with areas sensitive to "macro" and "both"; people with Type 1 diabetes are far more likely to suffer problems with areas vulnerable to "micro."

Your Brain (Macro)

Cardiovascular disease puts you at risk for a stroke, which occurs when a blood clot (a clog in your blood vessels) travels to your brain and stops the flow of blood and oxygen carried to the nerve cells in that area. When that happens, cells may die or vital functions controlled by the brain can be temporarily or permanently damaged. Bleeding or a rupture from the affected blood vessel is very serious and can lead to death. People with Type 2 diabetes are two to three times more likely to suffer a stroke than people without diabetes.

Since the 1960s, the death rate from strokes has dropped by 50 percent. This drop is largely due to public awareness campaigns regarding diet and lifestyle modification (quitting smoking, eating low-fat foods, and exercising), as well as the introduction of blood pressure–lowering drugs and cholesterol-lowering drugs.

Strokes can be mild, moderate, severe, or fatal. Mild strokes may affect speech or movement for a short period of time only; many people recover from mild strokes without any permanent damage. Moderate or severe strokes may result in loss of speech, memory impairment, and paralysis; many people learn to speak again and can function with partial paralysis. How well you recover depends on how much damage was done. It's never too late to reduce the risk of stroke by quitting smoking and making even small changes in diet and lifestyle. Discuss with your doctor whether you're a candidate for medications to control your blood pressure and cholesterol levels. Aiming for normal blood sugar levels as often as possible is also important. A considerable amount of research points to stress as a risk factor for stroke. The Heart section on page 261 suggests ways to cut down on stress.

Signs of a stroke

Recognizing the key warning signs can make a difference in preventing a major stroke or in the severity of a stroke.

Call 911 or get to Emergency if you suddenly notice one or more of the following symptoms:

- weakness, numbness, and/or tingling in your face, arms, or legs (this may last only a few moments);
- loss of speech or difficulty understanding somebody else's speech (this may last only a short time);
- a severe headache that feels different than any headache you've had before;
- feeling unsteady, falling a lot.

Alzheimer's disease

According to new research done at the Mayo Clinic and Mayo Foundation in Rochester, Minnesota, family members should become acquainted with early signs of Alzheimer's disease. This study showed that people with Type 2 diabetes were 66 percent more likely to develop Alzheimer's disease than those in the general population. The risk was more than double in men, and more than one-third in women. It was unclear why there were gender differences, but the overall increase in Alzheimer's disease among people with Type 2 diabetes may be the result of common genetic predispositions. In other words, there may be some genes that go together in diabetes and Alzheimer's disease.

Your Nerves (Micro)

When your blood sugar levels are too high for too long, you can develop a condition known as diabetic neuropathy or nerve disease. Somehow, the cells that make up your nerves are altered in response to high blood sugar. This condition can lead to foot amputations in people with diabetes. See the Feet section on page 269 for more details.

There are different groups of nerves that are affected by high blood sugar; keeping your blood sugar levels as normal as possible is the best way to prevent many of the following problems. Drugs that help to prevent chemical changes in your nerve cells can also be used to treat nerve damage.

Some nerve diseases

Polyneuropathy is a disease that affects the nerves in your feet and legs. The symptoms are burning, tingling, and numbness in the legs and feet.

Autonomic neuropathy is a disease that affects the nerves you don't notice; the nerves that control your digestive tract (see Stomach section on page 264), blood pressure, sweat glands, overall balance, and sexual functioning (see Sexual Organs section on page 268). Treatment varies depending on what's affected, but there are drugs that can help individual parts of the body, such as the digestive tract.

Proximal motor neuropathy is a disease that affects the nerves that control your muscles. This can lead to weakness and burning sensations in the joints (hands, thighs, and ankles are most commonly affected). These problems can be individually treated with physiotherapy and/or specific medication. When the nerves that control the muscles in the eyes (see Eye section below) are involved, you may experience problems such as double vision. Finally, nerve damage can affect the spine, causing pain and loss of sensation to the back, buttocks, and legs.

Your Eyes (Both)

Diabetes is the leading cause of new blindness in adults. Seventy-eight percent of people with Type 2 diabetes experience diabetes eye disease, clinically known as diabetic retinopathy. Microvascular complications damage the small blood vessels in the eyes. High blood pressure, associated with macrovascular complications, also damages these blood vessels.

While 98 percent of people with Type 1 diabetes will suffer from eye disease within fifteen years of being diagnosed, in Type 2 diabetes, eye disease is often diagnosed *before* the diabetes. In other words, many people don't realize they have diabetes until their eye doctors ask, "Have you been screened for diabetes?" In fact, 20 percent of people with Type 2 diabetes already have diabetes eye disease before their diabetes is diagnosed.

What happens to the eyes?

Eighty percent of all eye disease is known as nonproliferative eye disease, meaning "no new blood vessel growth" eye disease. This is also called background diabetic eye disease. In this case, the blood vessels in the retina (the part of your eyeball that faces your

brain, as opposed to your face) start to deteriorate, bleed, or hem-
orrhage (known as microaneurysms) and leak water and protein
into the center of the retina, called the macula; this condition is
known as macular edema, and causes vision loss, which sometimes is only temporary. Without treatment, however, more permanent vision loss will occur.

Proliferative eye disease means "new blood vessel growth" eye
disease. In this case, your retina says, "Since all my blood vessels
are being damaged, I'm just going to grow *new* blood vessels!"
This process is known as neovascularization. The problem is that
these new blood vessels are deformed, or abnormal, which makes
the problem worse, not better. These deformed blood vessels look
a bit like Swiss cheese; they're full of holes and have a bad habit of
suddenly bleeding, causing severe damage without warning. They
can also lead to scar tissue in the retina, retinal detachments, and
glaucoma, greatly increasing the risk of blindness.

Symptoms

In the early stages of diabetes eye disease, there are no symptoms. That's why you need to have a thorough eye exam every six
months. As eye damage progresses, you may notice blurred
vision. The blurred vision is due to changes in the shape of the
eye's lens. During an eye exam, your ophthalmologist may notice
yellow spots on your retina, signs that scar tissue has formed on
the retina from bleeding. If the disease progresses to the point
where new blood vessels have formed, vision problems may be
quite severe, as a result of spontaneous bleeding or detachment
of the retina. Other diabetes-related eye problems that may affect
vision include cataracts and glaucoma.

How to protect yourself from diabetes eye disease

Early detection is your best protection! Using Type 1 rules is the
best way to detect diabetes eye disease early and prevent vision

loss. In other words, it's crucial to have frequent eye exams. Teens or young adults diagnosed with Type 1 diabetes should have semi-annual or annual eye exams. This way, eye disease can be detected before it affects vision permanently. The average person has an eye exam every five years. If you have undiagnosed Type 2 diabetes, you could also have early signs of diabetes eye disease. So as soon as you're diagnosed with Type 2 diabetes, get to an eye specialist for a complete exam and make it a yearly "gig" from now on.

During an eye exam, an ophthalmologist will dilate your pupils with eyedrops, and then use a special instrument to check for:

- tiny red dots (signs of bleeding);
- a thick or "milky" retina, with or without yellow clumps or spots (signs of macular edema);
- a "bathtub ring" on the retina—a ring shape that surrounds a leakage site on the retina (also a sign of macular edema);
- "cottonwool spots" on the retina—small fluffy white patches (signs of new blood vessel growth, or more advanced eye disease).

Today, it's estimated that if everyone with impaired glucose tolerance (see chapter 1) went for an eye exam once a year, blindness from diabetes eye disease would drop from 8 percent in this group to 1 percent.

Can you treat diabetes eye disease?

Diabetes eye disease is only somewhat treatable. A procedure known as laser photocoagulation can burn and seal off the damaged blood vessels, which stops them from bleeding or leaking. In the earlier stages of eye disease, this procedure can restore your vision within about six months. In most cases, however, laser surgery only slows down vision loss, rather than restoring vision. In other words, without treatment, your vision will get worse; with treatment, it will stay the same.

If new blood vessels have already formed, a series of laser treatments are performed to purposely scar the retina. Since a scarred retina needs less oxygen, blood vessels stop reforming, reducing the risk of further damage.

In more serious cases, surgery known as a vitrectomy is performed. In this procedure, blood and scar tissue on the retina are surgically removed.

If you're suffering from vision loss, a number of visual aids can help you perform daily tasks more easily. See the Resources section at the back of this book for more details.

A word about smoking

Because smoking damages blood vessels, and diabetes eye disease is a blood vessel disease, smoking will certainly aggravate the problem. Quitting smoking may help to reduce eye complications.

Eye infections

High blood sugar can predispose you to frequent bacterial infections, including conjunctivitis (pinkeye). Eye infections can also affect your vision. To prevent eye infections, make sure to wash your hands before you touch your eyes, especially before you handle contact lenses.

Your Teeth (Micro)

High blood sugar levels get into your saliva, and then into your teeth. Cavities are caused by bacteria in plaque, which breaks down the starches and sugars to form acids that eventually deteriorate your tooth enamel.

Moreover, damage to the blood vessels in your gums can lead to periodontal problems, while blood sugar levels naturally rise when you're fighting a gum infection (known as a periodontal infection), such as an abscess. Preventing dental problems means the usual: regularly "rubber tipping" (massaging your gums with that rubber tip at the end of your toothbrush, or buying a separate rubber-tip instrument at the drugstore); flossing regularly; brushing regularly; and rinsing regularly with a mouthwash that kills plaque and bacteria. You may also wish to use a fluoride rinse every night. Have your teeth cleaned at least every six months, have an annual dental exam, and avoid sugary foods (which you should be doing anyway) that can increase cavities.

Your Heart (Macro)

Type 2 diabetes is often called "a heart attack about to happen." When large blood vessels are damaged, it means cardiovascular disease (heart disease). When blood vessels become blocked due to hardening of the arteries (clinically known as arteriosclerosis), not enough blood gets to the heart muscle, causing it to die. That's what a heart attack is.

Peripheral vascular disease (meaning "fringe" blood flow problems) is part of the heart disease story. PVD occurs when blood flow to the limbs (arms, legs, and feet) is blocked, which creates cramping, pain, or numbness. *In fact, pain and numbing in your arms or legs may be signs of heart disease or even an imminent heart attack.* A 1992 study reported that 20 percent of all women over age sixty suffered from PVD.

One way for women to prevent heart disease and peripheral vascular disease is to consider hormone replacement therapy (HRT) after menopause. Estrogen protects women against heart disease, but after menopause, the rates of heart disease in women soar as a result of estrogen loss. HRT is thoroughly discussed in chapters 3 and 5. Modifying your lifestyle (stop smoking, eat less fat, get more exercise) is another way of preventing heart and peripheral vascular disease. Blood pressure-lowering medication and cholesterol-lowering drugs are also an option if you have high blood pressure and/or high cholesterol. And, finally, heart surgery is a possibility, which includes angioplasty, laser treatment, and bypass surgery. Smoking, high blood pressure, high blood sugar, and high cholesterol (called the "catastrophic quartet" by one diabetes specialist) will greatly increase your risk of heart disease. These problems are discussed in detail in chapter 1.

Women and heart disease

Heart disease is currently the number one cause of death in post-menopausal women; more women die of heart disease than of lung cancer or breast cancer. Half of all North Americans who die from heart attacks each year are women.

One of the reasons for such high death rates from heart attacks among women is medical ignorance; most studies examining heart disease excluded women (see Introduction), which led to a myth that more men than women die of heart disease. The truth is, more men die of heart attacks before age fifty, while more women die of heart attacks after age fifty, as a direct result of estrogen loss. Moreover, women who have had oopherectomies (removal of the ovaries) prior to natural menopause increase their risk of a heart attack by *eight times*. Since more women work outside the home than ever before, a number of experts cite stress as a huge contributing factor to increased rates of heart disease in women.

Another problem is that women have different symptoms than men when it comes to heart disease. The "typical" warning signs we know about in men—angina, or chest pains—often never appear in women. In fact, chest pains in women are almost never related to heart disease. For women, the symptoms of heart disease, or even an actual heart attack, can be much more vague—seemingly unrelated to heart problems. Signs of heart disease in women include some surprising symptoms:

- Shortness of breath and/or fatigue
- Jaw pain (often masked by arthritis and joint pain)
- Pain in the back of the neck (often masked by arthritis or joint pain)
- Pain down the right or left arm

- Back pain (often masked by arthritis and joint pain)
- Sweating (have your thyroid checked—this is a classic sign of an overactive thyroid gland; also test your blood sugar—you may be low)
- Fainting
- Palpitations (again, have your thyroid checked; this is also a classic symptom of an overactive thyroid)
- Bloating (after menopause, would you believe this is a sign of coronary artery blockage?)
- Heartburn, belching, or other gastrointestinal pain (this is often a sign of an actual heart attack in women)
- Chest "heaviness" between the breasts—this is how women experience chest pain; some describe it as a sinking feeling or burning sensation, an aching, throbbing, or a squeezing sensation, hot poker tab between the breasts, or feeling like your heart jumps into your throat
- Sudden swings in blood sugar
- Vomiting
- Confusion

Clearly, there are lots of other causes for the symptoms on this list, including low blood sugar. But it's important that your doctor includes heart disease as a possible cause, rather than dismissing it because your symptoms are not "male" (which your doctor may refer to as "typical"). Bear in mind that if you're suffering from nerve damage, you may not feel a lot of these symptoms. Therefore, you should take extra care to be suspicious of anything feeling out of the ordinary.

Diagnostic tests that can confirm heart disease in women include a manual exam (doctor examining you with a stethoscope), an electrocardiogram, an exercise stress test, an echocardiogram, and a myriad of imaging tests that may use radioactive substances to take pictures of the heart.

If you're diagnosed with heart disease, the "cure" is prevention through diet, exercise, and protection through hormone replacement therapy (see chapters 3 and 5).

If you're premenopausal . . .

If you have diabetes that is not well controlled, the high blood sugar will cancel out the protective effects of estrogen against heart disease even if your ovaries are still making estrogen. Therefore, stay alert to the symptoms above. Keeping your blood sugar levels in the normal range will help to restore estrogen's protective properties.

Your Stomach (Micro)

When high blood sugar levels affect your nerve cells, this can include the nerves that control your entire gastrointestinal tract. In fact, 30 to 50 percent of people with diabetes suffer from dysmotility, when the muscles in the digestive tract become uncoordinated, causing bloating, abdominal pain, and reflux (heartburn). In this case, your doctor may prescribe a motility drug known as a pro-kinetic agent, a medication which can restore motility. See *The Gastrointestinal Sourcebook* (1998) for more information.

Your Kidneys (Both)

Both micro- and macrovascular complications can lead to kidney problems. High blood pressure and high blood sugar can be a dangerous combination for your kidneys. About 15 percent of people with Type 2 diabetes will develop kidney disease, known as either renal disease or nephropathy. In fact, diabetes causes 40 percent of all end-stage renal disease (ESRD), the term used to describe kidney failure. Roughly 40 percent of all dialysis patients have diabetes.

What do your kidneys do all day?

Kidneys are the public servants of the body; they're busy little bees! If they go on strike, you lose your water service, garbage pickup, and a few other services you don't even appreciate.

Kidneys regulate your body's water levels; when you have too much water, your kidneys remove it by dumping it into a large storage tank: your bladder. The excess water stays there until you're ready to "pee it out." If you don't have enough water in your body (or if you're dehydrated), your kidneys will retain the water for you to keep you balanced.

Kidneys also act as your body's sewage filtration plant. They filter out all the garbage and waste that your body doesn't need and dump it into the bladder; this waste is then excreted into your urine. The two waste products your kidneys regularly dump are *urea* (the waste product of protein) and *creatinine* (waste products produced by the muscles). In people with high blood sugar levels, excess sugar will get sent to the kidneys, and the kidneys will dump it into the bladder, too, causing sugar to appear in the urine. The kidneys also balance calcium and phosphate in the body, needed to build bones.

The kidneys operate two little side businesses on top of this— they make hormones. One hormone, called renin, helps to regulate blood pressure. Another hormone, called erythropoetin, helps bone marrow make red blood cells.

Macrovascular complications

When you suffer from cardiovascular disease, you probably have high blood pressure. High blood pressure damages blood vessels in the kidneys, which interferes with their job performance. As a result, they won't be as efficient at removing waste or excess water from your body. And if you are experiencing poor circulation, which can also cause water retention, the problem is further aggravated.

Poor circulation may cause your kidneys to secrete too much renin, which is normally designed to regulate blood pressure, but in this case, increases it. All the extra fluid and the high blood pressure places a heavy burden on your heart—and your kidneys. If this situation isn't brought under control, you'd likely suffer from a heart attack before kidney failure, but kidney failure is inevitable.

Microvascular complications

High blood sugar levels affect the small blood vessels, including the small blood vessels in the kidney's filters (called the nephrons). This condition is known as *diabetic nephropathy*. In the early stages of nephropathy, good, usable protein is secreted in the urine. That's a sign that the kidneys were unable to distribute usable protein to the body's tissues. (Normally, they would excrete only the waste product of protein—urea—into the urine.)

Another microvascular problem affects the kidneys: nerve damage. The nerves you use to control your bladder can be affected, causing a sort of sewage backup in your body. The first place that sewage hits is your kidneys. Old urine floating around your kidneys is not healthy. The kidneys can become damaged as a result, aggravating all the conditions discussed so far in this section.

Infection

There's a third problem at work here. If you recall, frequent urination is a sign of high blood sugar. That's because your kidneys help to rid the body of too much sugar by dumping it into the bladder. You're not the only one who likes sugar; bacteria, such as *e. coli* (the "hamburger bacteria"), like it, too. In fact, they thrive on it. So all that sugary urine sitting around in your bladder and passing through your ureters and urethra can cause this bacteria to overgrow, resulting in a urinary tract infection (UTI) such as cystitis (inflammation of the bladder lining). The longer your urethra is, the more protection you have from UTIs. Men have long urethras; women have very short urethras, however, and in the best of times are prone to these infections—especially after a lot of sexual activity, thus the term *honeymoon cystitis*. Sexual intercourse can introduce even more bacteria (from the vagina or rectum) into a woman's urethra due to the close space the vagina and urethra share. Women who wipe from back to front after a bowel movement can also introduce fecal matter into the urethra, causing a UTI.

Any bacterial infection in your bladder can travel back up to your kidneys, causing infection and inflammation and aggravating all the other problems.

Smoking

In the same way that smoking contributes to eye problems (see eye section on page 257), it can also aggravate kidney problems. Smoking causes small blood vessel damage throughout your body.

Signs of diabetic kidney disease

Obviously, there are a lot of different problems going on when it comes to diabetes and kidney disease. If you have any of the following early warning signs of kidney disease, see your doctor as soon as possible:

- high blood pressure (see chapter 1);
- protein in the urine (a sign of microvascular problems);
- burning or difficulty urinating (a sign of a urinary tract infection);
- foul-smelling or cloudy urine (a sign of a urinary tract infection);
- pain in the lower abdomen (a sign of a urinary tract infection);
- blood or pus in the urine (a sign of a kidney infection);
- fever, chills, or vomiting (a sign of *any* infection);
- foamy urine (a sign of kidney infection);
- frequent urination (a sign of high blood sugar and/or urinary tract infection).

Treating kidney disease

If you have high blood pressure, getting it under control through diet, exercise, or blood pressure-lowering medication will help to save your kidneys. If you have high blood sugar, treating any UTI as quickly as possible with antibiotics is the best way to avert kidney infection, while drugs known as ACE inhibitors can help to control small blood vessel damage caused by microvascular complications.

If you wind up with kidney failure or end-stage renal disease, dialysis, or in the worst-case scenario, a kidney transplant, are the only treatments. (Perhaps some day, cloning technology can be used to clone replacement organs, such as kidneys.)

Your Sexual Organs (Both)

The discussion here focuses on sexual dysfunction in women that is *directly* related to diabetes.

Diabetes can cause sexual dysfunction in the form of vaginal dryness due to high blood sugar levels. High blood sugar levels can also cause chronic yeast infections (the fungus *candida albicans* will overgrow when there is sugar), as well as urinary tract infections (see Kidney section, page 264), which can make sexual intercourse uncomfortable. (Diabetes will indirectly affect your sex life if your partner is suffering from diabetes-related impotence; for more information, consult *The Fertility Sourcebook*, 2d edition (1998).

Since Type 2 diabetes often coincides with menopause, many women notice a compromised libido. It may be more difficult to become aroused or achieve orgasm. There is no clear evidence whether diabetes contributes to a reduced libido, or if this is due to hormonal changes. Talking about the problem with a good sexual counselor and using vaginal lubricants or estrogen creams can work wonders. As discussed in chapter 1, women with diabetes are very susceptible to vaginitis (vaginal inflammation caused by an infection—usually fungal). High blood sugar levels can definitely aggravate vaginitis, which will compromise your sex life. Signs of vaginitis include a foul-smelling vaginal discharge, which may be brown or deep yellow in color, with the consistency of cottage cheese. You will also notice itching and burning.

If you're suffering from any kind of vaginal infection, it's important to be evaluated by a gynecologist, and be cultured for the specific organism causing the infection. That way, you can be treated with the right medication. Douching is not recommended, and can actually drive the infection higher up the reproductive tract.

Nerve damage can also affect your sex life. Special nerve fibers and blood vessels connect to the clitoris, vaginal wall, and vulva, necessary for achieving orgasm and lubrication. If you have sustained nerve damage, you may notice a loss of sensation in your genital area, which can be a frustrating experience. Estrogen therapy and lubricants may help, as well as trying different positions to increase arousal. Asking your partner to touch you "with the intent to arouse or gratify" may also work wonders.

Your Feet (Both)

Foot complications related to diabetes were dramatized in the mid-1980s film *Nothing In Common,* in which Jackie Gleason plays the ne'er-do-well diabetic father, and Tom Hanks plays the son who cannot accept him. In a heartbreaking scene, Tom Hanks is shocked to discover how ill his father really is when he finally sees his feet; they are swollen, purple, and badly infected. Ultimately, the story ends with the father and son coming to terms as Gleason must undergo surgical amputation.

I share this example with you because many of us are used to ignoring and abusing our feet. We wear uncomfortable shoes, we pick at our calluses and blisters, we don't wear socks, and so on. You can't do this anymore. Your feet are the targets of both macrovascular (large blood vessel) and microvascular (small blood vessel) complications. In the first place, peripheral vascular disease affects blood circulation to your feet. In the second place, the nerve cells in your feet, which control sensation, can be altered through microvascular complications. Nerve damage can also affect your feet's muscles and tendons, causing weakness and changes to the foot's shape.

The combination of poor circulation and no feeling in your feet means that you can sustain an injury to your feet and not know about it. For example, you might step on a piece of glass or badly stub your toe, and not realize it. If an open wound becomes infected, and you have poor circulation, the wound doesn't heal properly and infection could spread to the bone or gangrene could develop. In this situation, amputation may be the only treatment. Also, without sensation or proper circulation, your feet are far more vulnerable to frostbite or exposure than they would be otherwise.

Diabetes accounts for approximately half of all nonemergency amputations, but experts agree that doing a foot self-exam every day (see below) can prevent most foot complications from becoming severe. Those at most risk for foot problems are people who smoke (smoking aggravates *all* diabetic complications), are overweight (more weight on the feet), are over age forty, or have had diabetes for more than ten years. It's important to note that at least 90 percent of people with diabetes who require amputations are smokers. Quitting smoking can greatly reduce your risk of amputation.

Signs of foot problems

The most common symptoms of foot complications are burning, tingling, or pain in your feet or legs. These are all signs of nerve damage. Numbness is another symptom, which could mean nerve damage or circulation problems. If you do experience pain from nerve damage, it usually gets worse with time (as new nerves and blood vessels grow), and many people find that it's worse at night. Bed linens can actually increase discomfort. Some people only notice foot symptoms after exercising or a short walk. But many people don't notice symptoms until they've lost feeling in their feet.

Other symptoms are frequent infections (caused by blood vessel damage), hair loss on the toes or lower legs, or shiny skin on the lower legs and feet.

When you knock your socks off

When you take off your socks at the end of the day, get in the habit of doing a foot self-exam. This is the only way you can have damage control on your feet. You're looking for signs of infection or potential infection triggers. If you can avoid infection at all costs, you will be able to keep your feet. Look for the following signs:

- reddened, discolored, or swollen areas (blue, bright red, or white areas mean that circulation is impaired);
- pus;
- temperature changes or "hot spots" in the feet;
- corns, calluses, and warts (potential infections could be hiding under calluses; do not remove these yourself—see a podiatrist);
- toenails that are too long (your toenail could cut you if it's too long);
- redness where your shoes or socks are rubbing due to a poor fit (when your sock is scrunched inside your shoe, the folds could actually rub against the skin and cause a blister);
- toenail fungus (under the nail);
- fungus between the toes (this is athlete's foot, common if you've been walking around barefoot in a public place);
- breaks in the skin (especially between your toes), or cracks, such as in calluses on the heels; this opens the door for bacteria.

If you find an infection, wash your feet carefully with soap and water; *don't use alcohol.* Then see your doctor or a podiatrist (a foot specialist) as soon as possible. If your foot is irritated but not yet infected (redness, for example, from poor-fitting shoes but no blister yet), simply avoid the irritant—the shoes—and it should clear up. If not, see your doctor. If you're overweight and have trouble inspecting your feet, get somebody else to check them for the signs listed above. In addition to doing a self-exam, see your doctor to have the circulation and reflexes in your feet checked four times a year.

Foot rules to live by

- Walk a little bit every day; this is a good way to improve blood flow and get a little exercise!
- Don't walk around barefoot; wear proper-fitting, clean cotton socks with your shoes daily, and get in the habit of wearing slippers around the house and shoes at the beach. If you're swimming, wear some sort of shoe (plastic "jellies" or canvas running shoes).
- Before you put on your shoes, shake them out in case your (grand)child's Lego piece, a piece of dry catfood, or a pebble is in there.
- Wash your feet and lower legs every day in lukewarm water with mild soap. Dry them really well, especially between the toes.
- Trim your toenails straight across to avoid ingrown nails. Don't pick off your nails.
- No more "bathroom surgery" on your feet, which may include puncturing blisters with needles or tweezers, shaving your calluses, and the hundreds of other crazy things people do to their feet (but never disclose to their spouses).
- Baby your feet. When the skin seems too moist, use baby powder or foot powder recommended by your doctor or pharmacist (especially between the toes). When your feet are too dry, moisturize them with a lotion recommended by your doctor or pharmacist. The reason is simple: breaks in the skin happen if feet are too moist (such as between the toes) or too dry (such as

---

HOW TO SHOE SHOP FOR HEALTH

To save your feet, you may not be able to save on your next pair of shoes. These are shoe-shopping rules:

- Shoe-shop at the time of day when your feet are most swollen (such as the afternoon). That way, you'll purchase a shoe that fits you in "bad times" as well as good.
- Don't even think about high heels or any type of shoe that is not comfortable or that doesn't fit properly. Say good-bye to thongs. That strip between your toe can cause too much irritation.
- Buy leather; avoid shoes with the words "man-made upper" or "man-made materials" on the label; this means the shoes are made of synthetic materials and your foot will not breathe. Cotton or canvas shoes are fine, as long as the insole is cotton, too. Man-made materials on the very bottom of the shoe are fine as long as the upper—the part of the shoe that touches your foot—is leather, cotton/canvas, or something breathable.
- Remember that leather does, indeed, stretch. When that happens, the shoe could become loose and cause blisters. On the other hand, if the shoe is too tight and the salesperson tells you the shoe will stretch, forget it. The shoe will destroy you in the first few hours of wear.
- If you lose all sensation and cannot "feel" whether the shoe is fitting, make sure you have a shoe salesperson fit you.
- Avoid shoes that have been on display. A variety of people try on these shoes; you never know what bacteria and fungi these previously tried-on shoes harbor.

---

cracking). Use a foot buffing pad on your calluses after bathing.
- When you're sitting down, feet should be flat on the floor. Sitting cross-legged can cut off your circulation—and frequently does in people without diabetes.
- Wear comfortable, proper-fitting footwear. See above for tips about shoe shopping.

Treatment for open wounds on the feet or legs

To heal cuts, sores, or any open wound, your body normally manufactures macrophages, special white blood cells that fight infection, as well as special repair cells, called fibroblasts. These "ambulance cells" need oxygen to live. If you have poor circulation, the situation is akin to an ambulance not making it to an accident scene in time because it gets caught in a big traffic jam.

When wounds don't heal, gangrene infections can set in. Until recently, amputating the infected limb was the only way to deal with gangrene. But there is a new therapy available at several hospitals throughout North America called Hyperbaric Oxygen Therapy (HBO). The procedure involves placing you in an oxygen chamber or tank and feeding you triple the amount of oxygen you'd find in the normal atmosphere. To heal gangrene on the feet, you'd need about thirty treatments (several per day for a week or so). The result is that your tissues become saturated with oxygen, enabling the body to heal itself. In one research trial, 89 percent of diabetics with foot gangrene were healed, compared to 1 percent of the control group. This treatment is expensive, but it's much cheaper than surgery, which is why HBO is catching on.

Not everybody is an HBO candidate; and not everybody has access to this therapy. But if you're being considered for surgical amputation, you should definitely ask about HBO first.

Your Skin (Micro)

High blood sugar levels, combined with poor circulation, puts the skin—on your whole body—at risk for infections ranging from yeast to open wound-related infections. You may form scar tissue, develop strange, yellow pimples (a sign of high fat levels in the blood), boils, or a range of localized infections. Yeast can develop not just in the vagina, but in the mouth, under the arms, or anyplace where there are warm, fatty folds. And all skin, whether on the feet or elsewhere, can become dry and cracked, requiring a daily regimen of cleaning, moisturizing, and protecting.

PREVENTING COMPLICATIONS

Earlier chapters referred to a study known as the Diabetes Control and Complications Trial (DCCT). This study involved 1,441 people with Type 1 diabetes, who were randomly managed according to one of two treatment philosophies: "intensive" treatment and "conventional" treatment. Intensive treatment means frequently testing your blood sugar, and adding a short-acting insulin that requires three to four injections daily, or one dose of longer-acting insulin. The goal of this type of management is to achieve blood sugar levels that are as normal as possible as often as possible. Conventional treatment means controlling your diabetes to the point where you avoid feeling any symptoms of high blood sugar, such as frequent urination, thirst, or fatigue, without doing very much, if any, self-testing.

The Results

The results of the DCCT were pretty astounding, so much so that the trial, planned for a ten-year period, was cut short—a rare occurrence in research trials. The DCCT results were unveiled in 1993, at the American Diabetes Association's annual conference.

The people who were managed with intensive therapy were able to reduce microvascular complications (all the conditions labeled "micro" or "both" above) between 39 and 76 percent. Specifically, eye disease was reduced by 76 percent, kidney disease by 56 percent, nerve damage by 61 percent, and high cholesterol by 35 percent. Those are very significant results. Statistically, anything over 1 percent is considered clinically significant. The overwhelming consensus among diabetes practitioners is that intensive therapy for people with Type 1 diabetes prolongs health and greatly reduces complications. Conventional therapy for Type 1 diabetes is now considered archaic, and even detrimental.

The National Institute of Diabetes and Digestive and Kidney Diseases (NIDDK) in the United States reported similar findings. NIDDK research found that with intensive therapy, eye disease was reduced by 76 percent, kidney disease by 50 percent, nerve disease by 60 percent, and cardiovascular disease (a macrovascular complication) by 35 percent.

What the DCCT Means for Type 2 Diabetes

The DCCT did not look at blood sugar control and macrovascular complications—the cardiovascular complications for which people with Type 2 diabetes are most at risk—even though it showed a significant reduction in cholesterol levels. In fact, the priorities of many specialists treating Type 2 diabetes are weight control, *not* sugar control. (A cholesterol-lowering drug can have far greater effects on cholesterol levels than the DCCT showed.)

For several years, the DCCT was an area of controversy for Type 2 specialists. Should people with Type 2 diabetes be counseled to *intensively* control their blood sugar? Many specialists said, "No—losing weight and getting the diet under control is hard enough. Asking people to self-test their blood sugar three to four times per day is too much for most people with Type 2 diabetes." In other words, what's the point of avoiding microvascular complications when you're about to drop dead from a massive heart attack or stroke? Nevertheless, many specialists felt that since the DCCT showed such overwhelming reductions in complications for Type 1 diabetes, until more data was available, people with Type 2 diabetes should be intensively controlling their blood sugar.

The British Study

As of this writing, the results of a long-awaited British study have been published (September 15, 1998). Known as the United Kingdom Prospective Diabetes Study (UKPDS), this study sought to determine whether blood sugar control reduces macro-vascular complications in Type 2 diabetes, together with lowering blood pressure.

The results show that frequent blood sugar testing can reduce the risk of blindness and kidney failure in people with Type 2 diabetes by 25 percent. In those Type 2s with high blood pressure, lowering blood pressure reduced the risk of stroke by 44 percent and heart failure by 56 percent. And, for every 1 percentage point reduction in the value of the HbA_{1c} test (see chapter 8), there was a 35 percent reduction in eye, kidney, and nerve damage, and an overall 25 percent reduction in diabetes-related deaths. The bottom line is that the UKPDS shows that frequently self-testing blood sugar can prevent long-term diabetes complications for people with Type 2 diabetes, although there was not a direct link between lowering blood sugar and reducing macro-vascular complications.

In addition, preventing complications for Type 2 diabetes revolves around blood sugar control, exercise, and low-fat eating (chapters 6 and 7)—the same things that can prevent Type 2 diabetes in the first place.

CHAPTER 10

Prevention: Low-Fat and Healthful Eating

If you are at risk for Type 2 diabetes and want to prevent it, the best thing to do is pretend you have the disease right now and design a meal plan in accordance with the Canadian Diabetes Association's guidelines. These guidelines will help you eat a balanced diet and reduce your fat intake, which will dramatically lower the risk of Type 2 diabetes (see chapter 1) or the risk of macrovascular complications (see chapter 9) if you have already been diagnosed. Studies show that reducing dietary fat may also prevent various cancers, such as colorectal cancer and estrogen-dependent cancers such as breast cancer.

When you begin to conscientiously eat a balanced diet and reduce your fat intake, you'll notice that you're much more aware of what goes into your mouth, be it animal, vegetable, or mineral. Almost without exception, people who adopt a lower-fat diet will begin to incorporate less animal products and more vegetable products into their diets. This, by itself, makes a significant contribution to the environment. And once you begin to eat more fruits and vegetables, you may want to know whether they are organically grown or laden with pesticides. Therefore, this chapter includes information on organic produce. (Don't forget, many of those animals we eat are grazing on pesticides, which remain in their fat, which then winds up in ours!)

THE COSTS OF HIGH-FAT EATING

Our entire agricultural economy is designed to support livestock and animal products, which we consume in huge quantities. This is making us too fat, requires a large amount of resources to support its production, and is ruining our environment. Land-animal food production uses:

- 85 percent of all cropland and 55 percent of all agricultural land in the United States;

- forest-land and rangeland, through erosion and depletion;

- 80 percent of all piped water in the United States;

- pesticides, which pollute two-thirds of U.S. waters and more than half of U.S. lakes and streams;

- wildlife, through conversion and preemption of forest and rangeland habitats and through poisoning and trapping of predators;

- 14 percent of the U.S. energy budget, greater than twice the energy supplied by all our nuclear power stations;

- large amounts of scarce raw materials, such as aluminum, copper, iron, steel, tin, zinc, potassium, rubber, wood, and petroleum products, used for processing, storing, and packaging;

- 90 percent of our grains and legumes, and half of our fish catch to feed livestock;

- our incomes: meats cost five to six times as much as foods with equivalent amounts of vegetable protein; the average household spends roughly $7,500 annually on meat;

- 50 percent of the world's tropical forests to expand land for cattle production; the average hamburger is made from meat imported from Central or South America, representing the loss of 55 square feet of rainforest;

- our ozone layer: the rainforest is the "lungs of the planet"; it absorbs excess carbon dioxide and clears methane, a greenhouse gas. Cattle, however, produce methane, while the clearing of rainforest interferes with our ecosystem;

- arable land: cloud seeding, which upsets natural atmospheric weather patterns and weather cycles, results in rapid loss of arable land and the spread of desert regions across Africa, Central Asia, and parts of Latin America.

Despite all the information you may read here, you may be unable to change your eating habits. That's because you may not fully understand *why* you're eating. I recommend you review chapter 2 for some insight into women and food.

THE SKINNY ON FAT

Fat is technically known as *fatty acids*, which are crucial nutrients for our cells. We cannot live without fatty acids, or fat. Fat is therefore a good thing—in moderation. But like all good things, most of us want too much of it. Excess dietary fat is by far the most damaging element in the Western diet. A gram of fat contains twice the calories as the same amount of protein or carbohydrate. Decreasing the fat in your diet and replacing it with more grain products, vegetables, and fruit is the best way to lower your risk of Type 2 diabetes, cardiovascular problems, and a host of other diseases. Fat in the diet comes from meats, dairy products, and vegetable oils. Other sources include coconuts (60 percent fat), peanuts (78 percent fat), and avocados (82 percent fat). There are different kinds of fatty acids in these sources: saturated, unsaturated, and trans-fatty acids (transfat), which is a saturated fat in disguise. Some fats are harmful while others are beneficial to your health.

Understanding fat is a complicated business. This section explains everything you need to know about fat, and a few things you probably don't *want* to know.

Saturated Fat

Saturated fat is solid at room temperature and stimulates cholesterol production in your body. In fact, the way the fat looks prior to ingesting it is the way it will look when it lines your arteries. Foods high in saturated fat include processed meat, fatty meat, lard, butter, margarine, solid vegetable shortening, chocolate, and tropical oils (coconut oil is more than 90 percent saturated). Saturated fat should be consumed only in very low amounts.

Unsaturated Fat

Unsaturated fat is partially solid or liquid at room temperature. This group of fats includes monounsaturated fats, polyunsaturated fats, and omega-3 oils (fish oil), which even protect you against heart disease (see below). Sources of unsaturated fats include vegetable oils (canola, safflower, sunflower, corn) and seeds and nuts. To make it easy to remember, unsaturated fats come from plants, with the exception of tropical oils, such as coconut. The more liquid the fat, the more polyunsaturated it is, which *lowers* your cholesterol levels. If you have familial hyperlipidemia (high cholesterol), however, which often occurs in conjunction with diabetes, unsaturated fat may not make a difference in your cholesterol levels.

What Is a Triglyceride?

Each fat molecule is a link chain made up of glycerol, carbon atoms, and hydrogen atoms. The more hydrogen atoms that are on that chain, the more saturated or solid the fat. If you looked at each fat molecule carefully, you'd find three different kinds of fatty acids on it: saturated (solid), monounsaturated (less solid, with the exception of olive and peanut oils), and polyunsaturated (liquid) fatty acids, or three fatty acids plus glycerol, chemically known as triglycerides (see chapter 1).

The liver breaks down fat molecules by secreting bile (stored in the gallbladder)—its sole function. The liver also makes cholesterol (see chapter 1). Too much saturated fat may cause your liver to overproduce cholesterol, while the triglycerides in your bloodstream will rise, perpetuating the problem. Too much cholesterol can clog your blood vessels, get into the bile, and crystallize, causing gallstones and gallbladder disease.

Fish Fat (Omega-3 Oils)

The fat naturally present in fish that swim in cold waters, known as omega-3 fatty acids (crucial for brain tissue), or fish oils, are all polyunsaturated. They lower your cholesterol levels, and protect against heart disease. These fish have a layer of fat to keep them warm in cold water. Mackerel, albacore tuna, salmon, sardines, and lake trout are all rich in omega-3 fatty acids. In fact, whale meat and seal meat, once the staples of the Inuit diet, are enormous sources of omega-3 fatty acids. Overhunting and federal moratoriums on whale and seal hunting have dried up this once-vital source of food for the Inuit, which clearly offered real protection against heart disease.

Man-Made Fats

An assortment of man-made fats have been introduced into our diet, courtesy of food producers who are trying to give us the taste of fat without the calories or harmful effects of saturated fats. Unfortunately, man-made fats offer their own set of damages.

Trans-fatty acids (hydrogenated oils)

These are harmful fats that not only raise the level of "bad" cholesterol (LDL) in your bloodstream, but lower the amount of "good" cholesterol (HDL) that's already there. Trans-fatty acids are what you get when you make a liquid oil, such as corn oil, into a more solid or spreadable substance, such as margarine. Trans-fatty acids are the "road to hell, paved with good intentions." Someone, way back when, thought that if you could take the "good fat"—unsaturated fat—and solidify it so it could double as butter or lard, you would not miss the spreadable fat. That sounds like a great idea. Unfortunately, to make an unsaturated liquid fat more solid, you have to add hydrogen to its molecules.

This is known as *hydrogenation,* the process that converts liquid fat to semisolid fat. That ever-popular chocolate bar ingredient, hydrogenated palm oil, is a classic example of a trans-fatty acid. Hydrogenation also prolongs a fat's shelf life, preventing it from becoming rancid. Deep-frying oils used in restaurants are generally hydrogenated.

Trans-fatty acid is sold as polyunsaturated or monounsaturated fat with ads such as "Made from polyunsaturated vegetable oil." Except your body treats it as a saturated fat. This is why trans-fatty acids are saturated fat in disguise. The advertiser may say that the product contains "no saturated fat" or is "healthier" than the comparable animal or tropical oil product. So be careful and READ YOUR LABELS. The magic word you're looking for is hydrogenated. If the product lists a variety of unsaturated fats (monounsaturated X oil, polyunsaturated Y oil, and so on), keep reading. If the word hydrogenated appears, count that product as a saturated fat; your body will!

Margarine versus butter

There's an old tongue twister: "Betty Botter bought some butter that made the batter bitter; so Betty Botter bought more butter that made the batter better." Are we making our batters bitter or better with margarine? It depends.

Since the news of trans-fatty acids broke in the late 1980s, margarine manufacturers began to offer some less "bitter" margarines; some contain no hydrogenated oils, while others have much smaller amounts. Margarines with less than 60 to 80 percent oil (9 to 11 grams of fat) will contain 1 to 3 grams of trans-fatty acids per serving, compared to butter, which is 53 percent saturated fat. You might say it's a choice between a bad fat and a *worse* fat.

It's also possible for a liquid vegetable oil to retain a high concentration of unsaturated fat when it's been partially hydrogenated. In this case, your body will metabolize this as some saturated fat and some unsaturated fat.

Fake fat

We have artificial sweeteners; why not artificial fat? This question has led to the creation of an emerging yet highly suspicious ingredient: *fat substitutes,* designed to replace real fat and hence reduce calories without compromising taste. This is accomplished by creating a fake fat that the body cannot absorb.

One of the first fat substitutes was Simplesse, an all-natural fat substitute made from milk and egg-white protein, which was developed by the NutraSweet Company. Simplesse apparently adds 1 to 2 calories per gram instead of the usual 9 calories per gram from fat. Other fat substitutes simply take protein and carbohydrates and modify them in some way to simulate the textures of fat (creamy, smooth, and so on). All these fat substitutes help to create low-fat products, discussed in chapter 7.

The calorie-free fat substitute now being promoted is called olestra, developed by Procter and Gamble. It's currently being test-marketed in the United States in a variety of snacks such as potato chips and crackers. Olestra is a potentially dangerous ingredient that most experts feel can do more harm than good. Canada has not yet approved it.

Olestra is made from a combination of vegetable oils and sugar. It tastes just like real fat, but the biochemical structure is a molecule too big for your liver to break down. So, olestra just gets passed into the large intestine and is excreted. Olestra is more than an "empty" molecule, however. It causes diarrhea and cramps and may deplete your body of vital nutrients, including vitamins A, D, E, and K, necessary for blood clotting. If the FDA approves olestra for use as a cooking-oil substitute, you'll see it in every imaginable high-fat product. The danger is that instead of encouraging people to choose nutritious foods such as fruits, grains, and vegetables over high-fat foods, products like these encourage a high-*fake*-fat diet that's still too low in fiber and other essential nutrients. These people could potentially wind up with a vitamin deficiency, as well. Products such as olestra should make you nervous.

THE INCREDIBLE BULK

For every action, there is an equal and opposite reaction. When you decrease your fat intake, you should increase your bulk intake, or fiber. As discussed in chapter 7, complex carbohydrates are foods that are high in fiber. Fiber is the part of a plant your body can't digest, which comes in either water-soluble fiber (which dissolves in water) and water-insoluble fiber (which does not dissolve in water, but instead absorbs water); this is what's meant by *soluble* and *insoluble* fiber.

Soluble Versus Insoluble Fiber

Soluble and insoluble fiber do differ, but they are equally good. Soluble fiber somehow lowers the "bad" cholesterol, or LDL, in your body. Experts aren't entirely sure how soluble fiber works its magic, but one popular theory is that it gets mixed into the bile the liver secretes, and forms a type of gel that traps the building blocks of cholesterol, thus lowering your LDL levels. It's akin to a spider web trapping smaller insects. Sources of soluble fiber include oats or oat bran, legumes (dried beans and peas), some seeds, carrots, oranges, bananas, and other fruits. Soybeans are also high in soluble fiber. Studies show that people with very high cholesterol levels have the most to gain by eating soybeans. Soy is also a *phytoestrogen* (plant estrogen) that is believed to lower the risks of estrogen-related cancers (for example, breast cancer), as well as reduce the incidence of estrogen-loss symptoms associated with menopause.

Insoluble fiber doesn't affect your cholesterol levels at all, but it regulates your bowel movements. How does it do this? As the insoluble fiber moves through your digestive tract, it absorbs water like a sponge and helps to form your waste into a solid form faster, making the stools larger, softer, and easier to pass. Without insoluble fiber, your solid waste just gets pushed down to the colon or lower intestine as always, where it is stored and dries out until you're ready to have a bowel movement. High-starch foods are associated with drier stools. This is exacerbated when you "ignore the urge," as the colon will dehydrate the waste even more until it becomes harder and more difficult to pass, a condition known as constipation. Insoluble fiber helps to regulate your bowel movements by speeding things along. It is also linked to lower rates of colorectal cancer. Good sources of insoluble fiber are wheat bran and whole grains, skins of various fruits and vegetables, seeds, leafy greens, and cruciferous vegetables (cauliflower, broccoli, and Brussels sprouts).

Fiber and Diabetes

Soluble fiber helps delay glucose from being absorbed into your bloodstream, which not only improves blood sugar control but helps to control postmeal peaks in blood sugar, which stimulate the pancreas to produce more insulin. Fiber in the form of all colors of vegetables will also ensure that you're getting the right mix of nutrients. Experts suggest that you eat different colors of vegetables daily—for example, carrots, beets, and spinach. An easy way to remember what nutrients are in which vegetable is to remember that all green vegetables are for cellular repair; the darker the green, the more nutrients the vegetable contains. All red, orange, and purplish vegetables contain antioxidants (vitamins A, C, and E), which boost the immune system and fight off toxins. Studies suggest that vitamin C, for example, is crucial for people with Type 2 diabetes because it helps to prevent complications as well as rid the body of sorbitol, which can increase blood sugar. (Another study suggests that vitamin E helped to prevent heart disease in people with Type 2 diabetes by lowering levels of "bad" cholesterol, but this isn't yet conclusive.) Other minerals, such as zinc and copper, are essential for wound healing. By eating all colors of vegetables in ample amounts you will get your vitamins, minerals, and dietary fiber. This makes sense when you understand diabetes as a disease of starvation. In starvation, there are naturally lower levels of nutrients in your body that can only be replenished through excellent sources of food.

Breaking Bread

For thousands of years, cooked whole grains were the dietary staple for all cultures: rice and millet in the Orient; wheat, oats, and rye in Europe; buckwheat in Russia; sorghum in Africa; barley in the Middle East; and corn in pre-European North America.

Whole-grain breads are good sources of insoluble fiber (flax bread is particularly good because flaxseeds are a source of soluble fiber, too). The problem is understanding what is truly "whole grain." For example, there is an assumption that because bread is dark or brown, it's more nutritious; this isn't so. In fact, many brown breads are simply enriched white breads dyed with molasses. ("Enriched" means that nutrients lost during processing have been replaced.) High-fiber pita breads and bagels are available, but you have to search for them. A good rule is to simply look for the phrase "whole wheat," which means that the wheat is, indeed, whole.

FOOD PILLS

In countries where high-fiber and plant-rich diets are the norm, there are far lower rates of cancer, heart disease, and diabetes. This fact has led to research into specific foods or food ingredients that you can now buy in pill or capsule form: garlic capsules, broccoli pills, and hundreds of other food supplements have sprung onto the health food market. Should you be taking supplements or simply eating a healthy diet? The answer is boring, and not one you want to hear: eat a variety of good foods that are high in fiber and low in fat! The problem with taking a "plant pill" instead of eating the plant is that by taking the pill, you're missing out on other benefits, such as fiber, taste, or the biochemical reaction that results from dozens of unknown ingredients in the plant.

Phytochemicals

Phytochemicals, or "plant chemicals" (*phyto* is Greek for "plant") are the natural ingredients found in plant foods such as tomatoes, oats, soy, oranges, and broccoli. As researchers strive for some magic wellness ingredient, they're finding all kinds of disease-fighting chemicals in common fruits and vegetables. While phytochemicals, such as *isoflavones* (found in soybeans), *allylic sulphides* (found in garlic, onions, and chives), *isothiocyanates* (found in cruciferous vegetables such as Brussels sprouts, cabbage, and cauliflower), *saponins* (in spinach, potatoes, tomatoes, and oats), *lignin,* and *alphalinolenic* acid (flaxseeds) sound exotic, you can easily get them by simply eating a variety of fruits, grains, and vegetables.

Another hot phytochemical right now is *betaglucan* (found in legumes, oats, and other grains). Betaglucan is believed to help prevent diabetes by delaying gastric emptying and by slowing down glucose absorption in the small intestine.

In fact, biologically engineered foods, which alter the natural genetic codes in vegetables (see below) may interfere with these natural phytochemicals.

Functional foods

Functional foods are foods that have significant levels of biologically active disease-preventing or health-promoting properties.

Tomatoes, oatmeal, soy, and garlic are all examples of functional foods because they contain phytochemicals. Functional foods are therefore different than nutraceuticals (from the words *nutrition* and *pharmaceutical*), which are manufactured health foods, such as dietary fiber drinks or Zbars™, discussed in chapter 1.

In the next few years, you may even see tomato sauces or canned goods with a functional food label, touting, for example, that the food "may prevent prostate cancer" because it contains lycopene (a phytochemical in tomatoes, red peppers, and red grapefruit).

CHANGING YOUR DIET (AND HELPING THE ENVIRONMENT, TOO!)

It's difficult enough to stick to a meal plan (see chapter 7) without having to worry about pesticides, toxins, and "saving the world" all at the same time. Yet since many people reading this book are concerned about healthful eating, it's important to have some of this "nice to know" versus "need to know" information at hand, in case, someday, you *want* to know. I present this data based on numerous published works on healthful eating so you can make informed choices about your diet. But if you were to put down this book right now, rest assured that everything women need to know about managing Type 2 diabetes has now been provided. For those of you stopping here, thank you for taking this journey with me. For those of you continuing on . . .

The American Association of Advancement of Science states that a diet centered on whole-grain cereals and vegetables rather than meat, poultry, and dairy would benefit our entire way of life, making more land, water, fuel, and minerals available, which would in turn have positive effects on inflation, employment, and international trade. For example, in 1991, researchers at the California Institute of Technology reported that a meat-based

FAT TIPS

- Whenever you refrigerate foods (such as soups, stews, or curry dishes), skim the fat from the top before reheating and reserving. A gravy skimmer will also help skim fats; the spout pours from the bottom, and oils and fats coagulate on top.
- Use substitutes for butter: yogurt (great on potatoes) or low-fat cottage cheese, or, at dinner, just dip your bread in olive oil with some garlic, Italian style. For sandwiches, any condiment except butter, margarine, or mayonnaise is fine—mustards, yogurt, and so on.
- Powdered nonfat milk is in vogue again; it's high in calcium, low in fat. Substitute it in any recipe calling for milk or cream.
- Dig out fruit recipes for dessert. Sorbet with low-fat yogurt topping can be elegant. Remember that fruit must be planned for in a diabetes meal plan.
- Season low-fat foods well. That way, you won't miss the flavor fat adds.
- Lower-fat protein comes from vegetable sources (whole grains and bean products); higher-fat protein comes from animal sources.

MEAT TIPS

- Broil, grill, or boil meat instead of frying, baking, or roasting it. (If you drain fat and cook in water, baking/roasting is fine.)
- Trim off all visible fat from meat before and after cooking.
- Frying lean meat in flour, breadcrumbs, or other coatings adds fat.
- Try substituting low-fat turkey meat for red meat.

MILK TIPS

In North America, we consume a lot of milk. Know what you're getting:
- Whole milk contains 48 percent calories from fat.
- 2% milk gets 37 percent of its calories from fat.
- 1% milk gets 26 percent of its calories from fat.
- Skim milk is completely fat free.
- Cheese gets 50 percent of its calories from fat, unless it's skim-milk cheese.
- Butter gets 95 percent of its calories from fat.
- Yogurt gets 15 percent of its calories from fat

HOW TO GET MORE FRUITS AND VEGETABLES*

- Go for one or two fruits at breakfast, one fruit and two vegetables at lunch and dinner, and a fruit or vegetable snack between meals.
- Consume many differently colored fruits and vegetables. For color variety, select at least three differently colored fruits and vegetables daily.
- Put fruit and sliced veggies in an easy-to-use, easy-to-reach place (sliced vegetables in the fridge; fruit out on the table).
- Keep frozen and canned fruit and vegetables on hand to add to soups, salads, or rice dishes.

*Fruits and vegetables must be planned for in a diabetes meal plan.

Source: Adapted from "Beyond Vitamins: Phytochemicals to Help Fight Disease," *Health News*, June 1996, Volume 14, No. 3, by June V. Engel, Ph.D.

---

diet was actually ruining the environment. According to research, cooking meat contributes to air pollution by releasing hydrocarbons, furans, steroids, and pesticide residues. Interestingly, a major source of smog in Los Angeles is smoke from *barbecued beef*! On Earth Day 1992, an international coalition of environmental groups pledged to help lower beef consumption by 50 percent by the year 2002. The plan is to move toward a diet centered on whole grains and vegetables.

Animal Farm

See page 280. If those numbers don't make an impact on your food-buying habits, here are some other things to consider about animal farms.

Sulphonamides and penicillin, first used to a limited extent in the 1930s and 1940s, were routinely added to feed by the late 1950s, when farmers began raising animals in concentrated areas to meet increased demands. (Tight quarters triggered the spread of disease, necessitating antibiotics.) Today, antibacterial, antiparasitic drugs, and hormones are in widespread use on meat-producing farms. Anabolic hormones or steroids are used to increase growth and muscle in cattle (so we can have our thick, juicy steaks). A few years ago, the European Community banned the raising or importing of any animal that was given hormones. The United States and Canada continue to use growth hormones, however.

When you see statements such as "low incidence" or "acceptable levels" of drug residue in animals, it means that the meat or milk has drugs in it. It's like saying "acceptable levels of toxins," when, in fact, NO LEVEL of toxin should be acceptable! The U.S. Food and Drug Administration has defined "no residue" as a drug level that presents no more than a one-in-a-million risk of cancer over a lifetime; that's not the same thing as "no level of drug."

Bovine somatotropin (BST)

It gets worse. Bovine somatotropin, or BST, is a hormone that causes cows to overproduce milk. When that happens, the cows can become engorged and develop a bacterial infection called mastitis, necessitating the use of even more antibiotics. Although the FDA has concluded that milk and meat from BST-treated cows are safe for human consumption, Canada has not yet approved it. We don't know whether BST can cross over into humans and affect our own lactation hormones, nor do we know what effect "mastitis milk" may have on us, or the antibiotics used to treat mastitis. Clear labeling guidelines for BST milk products must also be introduced before it is sprung onto unsuspecting milk consumers.

Mad cows

An almost biblical lesson in eating foods that are not indigenous can be seen with the revolting tale of mad cow disease, or *bovine spongiform encephalopathy* (BSE). BSE is an infectious disease that causes degenerative changes in the brains of cattle, and degenerative brain disease in humans who ingest "mad cow" brains. This is not old news, but ongoing news. BSE is passed on to the cow through other animal brains, commonly sheep with a sheep disease known as *scrapies* (although humans cannot get this disease by eating sheep with scrapies).

In nature, the only way a cow can contract this disease is to eat the brain of an infected animal, which wouldn't happen because cows are vegetarian. In the interest of cost-effective farming, agriculture began using animal parts (slaughterhouse waste, dead pets, and roadkill) in cattle feed. This brain disease was passed on to "Cow Zero" when Cow Zero unwittingly ate a piece of another animal brain, probably a sheep who was a carrier of the infection. Cow Zero gets slaughtered and becomes a hamburger. Its leftover brain parts get mixed into another sack of cattle feed and Cow Number 2 eats infected Cow Zero's brain parts and *also* becomes infected. The cycle continues as the cows eat one another's brains—something that Mother Nature never meant to happen. Ultimately, when a human being eats a hamburger made with ground beef, which may have some remnants of mad cow brains and spinal cords, she will contract mad cow disease as well.

What's truly frightening is that BSE has a five-year incubation period. So even if you became a vegetarian today, the hamburger you ate three years ago could still have infected you. And in that time period, BSE can spread to other animals in many other countries that use slaughtered-cattle products in their feed. Mad cows have been identified in Canada, Denmark, France, Germany, Ireland, the Netherlands, Oman, Portugal, and Switzerland.

One way to prevent BSE from spreading, or to prevent similar types of agricultural atrocities, is to stop eating cows. If you don't want to give up red meat, support organic growing, which is committed to ethical farming practices and raising cattle the old-fashioned way: feeding them good, organic feed—what Nature intended. (This is discussed in detail below.)

Vegging Out

By simply becoming more vegetarian, you can actually change the world, lessening the demand for meat. Cleaning up the environment starts at your own kitchen table, in your own house, not in the House of Representatives.

It's estimated that at least 7 to 10 percent of North Americans practice some form of vegetarianism. Semivegetarians, like myself, eat poultry, fish, eggs, and dairy foods. Pescovegetarians eat fish, eggs, and dairy foods; lacto-ovovegetarians eat eggs and dairy foods. Stricter forms of vegetarianism include ovovegetarians, who do not eat dairy but will consume eggs; lactovegetarians who will not eat eggs but will have dairy; and vegans, who will not eat any sort of animal-derived foods.

When you compare the health of vegetarians to that of the general population, vegetarians have lower rates of heart disease, colon cancer, colitis (inflammation of the colon), hypertension, Type 2 diabetes, and obesity. Keep in mind that becoming more vegetarian isn't a license to overdo it on high-fat, meatless food. You should still choose lower-fat dairy products if you eat dairy. See page 291 for details.

Indigenous Eating

Earlier, I discussed how the loss of ecology and environment has led to an epidemic of diabetes in Native Americans. There are many other reasons to support an indigenous diet. Eastern health practitioners (from Asia and India—*not* New England) maintain that the right diet is based on where you live. Americans need no further proof than to look at the traditional aboriginal diet. In hotter climates, such as India and other tropical regions, lighter diets based on grains and vegetables and even certain spices are conducive to good health.

Eating seasonally

Eating foods that are seasonal to our own habitat ensures that we are getting the most from our produce. Food begins to lose its natural phytochemicals (healthful properties) when it travels long distances in refrigeration units. Since most of us don't have the luxury of living on a farm, we haven't much choice in controlling the produce that is in our local grocery stores. But is it natural for those in Chicago to eat tropical fruits in January, or for Tokyo to turn into a steak-and-potatoes society? What are the consequences of this?

For one thing, there may be some health-related reasons that we plant in the spring, harvest and preserve in the fall, and make soups in the winter. Eastern nutritionist Mushio Kushi advises against foods that are not in harmony with the seasons. In cold weather, for example, food that is cooked longer—soups and stews—is considered better than salads and tropical fruits; in summer, lighter fare is healthier than heavy meats and starches.

Epidemiologists observe that as we send our meat and dairy diet to vegetarian-based societies, we find that the incidence of Western diseases, such as Type 2 diabetes, rises. Yet as we meat-eaters adopt a more vegetarian diet, which need not mean tropical but rather *indigenous* fruits and vegetables and a wide variety of nuts we can grow right here in North America, we see a decrease in disease.

Discovering American roots

According to many horticulturists and organic growers, the future of farming is learning how to grow *native plants* from seed, which is called *sustainable farming*. This isn't anything new, but rather is centuries old. Sustainable farming creates a sustainable vegetation system or "web" that will keep rebuilding on itself for decades to come. Planting in this way helps to renew and protect soil, allowing a diverse range of organisms—some even pests—to coexist within the food chain. When the food chain is left intact, parasites are taken care of by their natural predators, or natural repellents. Organic farmers therefore practice what's known as *companion planting*, which is simply ethical biological pest management. In other words, if Vegetable A is always pestered by Beetle X, you simply plant Vegetable B next to it, which together with Vegetable A produces an odor that turns off Beetle X so that it doesn't go near either plant. Or you can plant Weed A next to Vegetable A, which is a more tempting treat for Beetle X. Vegetable A grows beautifully, Weed A gets devoured, and then you simply hand-pick Weed A and throw it out at the end of the season. Companion planting is used to confuse insects, repel them, or trap them. Companion planting is also used to make crops healthier. Vegetable A, for example, will grow better when it's beside Herb A for reasons not completely understood.

Why not just use pesticides?

Pesticides cause mutations in wildlife and humans, and have definitively and scientifically been shown to cause cancer. By mutating and destroying wildlife, pesticides are causing the food chain to die off, which has led to disastrous consequences for planetary health. The entire pesticide story is, however, another big book. For the purposes of this chapter, all you need to understand is that by eating more indigenous and seasoned foods, you are supporting an enormous network of organic growers and farmers, who, in the next century, will be leading the way for sustaining and maintaining life on earth. We simply cannot continue to eat as we once did. It makes us fat; it makes us sick; and it can trigger Type 2 diabetes if you are genetically predisposed. Not only that, it wastes billions of acres of arable farmland that could be used to grow nutritious foods; and it wastes billions of dollars of natural resources we can't afford to lose.

But I don't want to be a farmer!

You don't have to be a farmer to eat organic produce. Hundreds of organic farmers, united under the Organic Trade Association, will be happy to sell you their organic produce, from vegetables and beef to clothing (made with cotton that was grown without pesticides). By buying organic spinach instead of spinach that was sprayed with endosulphan (a pesticide), you are supporting organic farming, eating well, and saving the world, all at the same time. To find out where your organic farmers are, contact your local chapter of the Organic Trade Association, listed in the Resource section at the back of the book.

As for your supermarket's produce, many supermarkets are getting into the organic act. In fact, a chain of U.S. supermarkets, called Bread and Circus, sells only organic produce. To get your local supermarkets to disclose where your produce was grown and how it was raised, demand labeling that provides this information. You can exert your consumer power (and you do have power!) by contacting the corporate office of your supermarket and asking to speak to the head of consumer relations, public relations, or marketing. You can also exert pressure by calling manufacturers' 800/888 numbers that appear on your food labels; starting a newsgroup; or banning products to help change standards. You have a right to a label that reads, "This produce sprayed with pesticide A." In fact, by calling the Grocery Manufacturers of America at (202) 337-9400, you can find out:

- what animal sources have eaten, and whether they were injected with anything;
- what waters your fish has swum in; and
- with what your grown produce was sprayed.

In your own backyard

You may have a beautiful flower garden, which may be the envy of all your neighbors, but if you're using pesticides, you're part of the problem, not the solution. Contact the Organic Trade Association for literature on organic insecticides and fungicides for lawns and gardens, as well as for companion planting tips for the backyard (such as planting garlic beside roses).

You now know how to manage Type 2 diabetes, prevent further complications, and lower your risk of Type 2 diabetes. I've also assembled several useful tables and charts that can help you trim fat, lower cholesterol, and choose the least toxic vegetables. Don't forget to browse through the Glossary and Resources section. And don't forget exercise. I wish you all good luck, good health, and a long and happy life.

Note: This list is not exhaustive. These are not literal dictionary definitions, but rather definitions created solely for the context of this book.

Adrenaline: a hormone your body secretes that creates "fight-or-flight" symptoms of increased heart rate, sweating, nervousness, and dizziness.

Aerobic activity: any activity that makes the heart pump harder and faster, causing you to breathe faster, which increases the level of oxygen in the bloodstream.

Alpha-glucosidase inhibitor (acarbose or Precose): a drug that delays the breakdown of sugar in your meal.

Andrologist: a doctor who specializes in male reproductive problems.

Anorexia nervosa: "a loss of appetite due to mental disorder." People with anorexia refuse to eat any food at all, starving themselves.

Antioxidants: vitamins A, C, E, and beta carotene, found in colored (nongreen) fruits and vegetables. Antioxidants prevent the oxidation of cell membranes, which can lead to cancer.

Autoimmune disease: a disease in which the body produces antibodies to its own tissues, seen in Type 1 diabetes.

Betaglucan: a phytochemical found in legumes, oats, and other grains that is believed to help prevent diabetes by delaying gastric emptying and slowing down glucose absorption in the small intestine.

Biguanides (Metformin): oral hypoglycemic agents that help the body's insulin work better.

Binge-eating disorder: refers to compulsive overeating, or bingeing without purging.

Bulimia nervosa: bingeing followed by purging in the form of self-induced vomiting, laxative/diuretic abuse, or abusing other medications to induce weight loss.

Carbohydrates: the building blocks of most foods, which provide energy to the body to fuel the central nervous system; they help the body use vitamins, minerals, amino acids, and other nutrients.

Certified Diabetes Educator (CDE): a dietitian, nurse, pharmacist, social worker, or any other health care professional who has an interest in diabetes education, and who has taken a diabetes educator certification course; teaches diabetes patients about diet and management.

Cholesterol: a whitish, waxy fat made in vast quantities by the liver. (*See also* HDL; LDL)

Community Health Representative (CHR): Someone from the community who works with you and your family, as well as with other health care professionals, to educate you about various health issues, including diabetes.

Complex carbohydrates: sophisticated carbohydrate foods that contain larger molecules, such as grain foods and foods high in fiber.

Creatinine: waste product produced by the muscles and released by the kidneys.

Cystitis: urinary tract infection (UTI) resulting in an inflammation of the bladder lining.

Dextrose tablets: tablets that contain pure dextrose to boost the blood sugar level quickly, in case of hypoglycemia.

Diabetes: also known as hyperglycemia,which means high blood sugar, a condition where blood sugar levels are too high, usually defined by a fasting blood sugar level of over 7.8 mmol/L.

Diabetes specialist: an endocrinologist (hormone doctor) who subspecializes in diabetes.

Diabetic ketoacidosis (DKA): an emergency situation that can lead to death; signs of DKA include frequent urination, excessive thirst, excessive hunger, and a fruity smell to the breath.

Diabetic neuropathy: diabetic nerve disease; occurs when the cells that comprise nerves are altered in response to high blood sugar.

Diabetic retinopathy: diabetes eye disease, characterized by damage to the back of the eye, or retina.

Diastolic pressure: one of the readings in a blood pressure measurement; the pressure occurring when the heart rests between contractions.

Dysmotility: occurs when the muscles in the digestive tract become uncoordinated, causing bloating, abdominal pain, and reflux (heartburn).

Edema: water retention.

End-stage renal disease: a term used to describe kidney failure.

Erythroepoetin: a hormone produced by the kidneys which helps bone marrow to make red blood cells.

Fasting blood glucose readings: what your blood sugar levels are before you've eaten.

Fatty acids: crucial nutrients for cells, which also regulate hormone production.

Fiber: part of a plant that cannot be digested, which can lower cholesterol levels or improve regularity; also causes a slower rise in glucose levels, which lowers the body's insulin requirements.

Fructose: a monosaccharide or single sugar that combines with glucose to form sucrose and is one and a half times sweeter than sucrose.

Functional foods: foods that have significant levels of biologically active disease-preventing or health-promoting properties.

Gastroenterologist: a doctor who is a G.I. (gastrointestinal) specialist.

Gerontologist: a doctor who specializes in diseases of the elderly.

Gestational diabetes mellitus (GDM): a type of diabetes that usually occurs between the twenty-fourth and twenty-eighth weeks of pregnancy; it simply means "diabetes during pregnancy" and generally takes the form of Type 2 diabetes.

Gestational hypertension: high blood pressure during pregnancy.

Glucagon: a hormone which, when injected under the skin, causes an increase in blood glucose concentration.

Glucose: a monosaccharide or single sugar that combines with fructose to form sucrose; can also combine with glucose to form maltose, and with galactose to form lactose; slightly less sweet than sucrose.

Glycosuria: sugary urine, a symptom of very high blood sugar.

Glycosylated hemoglobin levels: detailed blood sugar test that checks for glycosylated hemoglobin (glucose attached to the protein in red blood cells), known as glycohemoglobin or HbA$_{1c}$ levels; this test can determine how well blood sugar has been controlled over a period of two to three months by showing what percentage of it is too high.

Guar gum: a good source of fiber made from the seeds of the Indian cluster bean. When you mix guar with water, it turns into a gummy gel, which slows down the digestive system, similar to acarbose.

HDL: high-density lipoproteins, known as "good" cholesterol.

High-fructose corn syrup (HFCS): a liquid mixture of about equal parts glucose and fructose from cornstarch, which has the same sweetness as sucrose.

Human insulin: a type of insulin that is identical to the insulin normally produced by the human body.

Hydrogenation: a process that converts liquid fat to semisolid fat by adding hydrogen.

Hyperglycemia: high blood sugar, also known as diabetes; a condition where blood sugar levels are too high; defined by a fasting blood sugar level of over 7.8 mmol/L.

Hyperinsulinemia: when the pancreas produces too much insulin; a condition caused by insulin resistance.

Hypertension (high blood pressure): too much tension or force exerted on the artery walls; a condition that damages the small blood vessels as well as the larger arteries.

Hypertensive drug: a drug designed to lower blood pressure.

Hypoglycemia: means low blood sugar; defined by a blood sugar level less than 4 mmol/L, any time.

Impaired glucose tolerance (IGT): what many doctors refer to as the "gray zone" between normal blood sugar levels and full-blown diabetes.

Impotence: the inability to obtain or sustain an erection long enough to have intercourse, for a period of at least six months.

Insulin: a hormone made by the islets of Langerhans, small islands of cells afloat in the pancreas, which regulates blood sugar levels.

Insulin lispro: an insulin analog ("synthetic copycat") that is very short-acting.

Insulin resistance: occurs when the pancreas is making insulin but the cells are not responding to it.

Insulin shock: occurs when low blood sugar is caused by insulin therapy.

Intensive insulin therapy: a treatment program involving close monitoring of blood sugar levels combined with taking short-acting insulin prior to meals.

Islets of Langerhans: one of two cell systems located inside the pancreas, which secretes insulin.

Isokinetic exercise: an activity such as wrestling or weightlifting that is short but intense.

Ketones (ketone bodies): a poisonous by-product the body produces when there is not enough glucose in the cells, and the body burns fat as an alternate fuel; this situation can occur when blood sugar levels are 14 mmol/L at any one time.

Lancet: tiny needle used to prick the finger for a blood sample.

Laser photocoagulation: a procedure that can burn and seal off damaged blood vessels, stopping them from bleeding or leaking; this can restore vision in the earlier stages of diabetes eye disease.

LDL: low-density lipoproteins, known as "bad" cholesterol.

Lean body mass: body tissue that is not fat.

Leptin: a hormone currently being used to treat obesity (a leptin deficiency is thought to cause weight gain); also being tested as a preventive drug for Type 2 diabetes.

Macrosomia: a condition that occurs in gestational diabetes, when high blood sugar levels cross the placenta and feed the fetus too much glucose, causing it to grow too fat and large for its gestational age; technically defined by a birth weight greater than 4,000 grams; babies with macrosomia are usually not able to fit through the birth canal because their shoulders get stuck (known as shoulder dystocia).

Macrovascular complication: a large blood vessel complication, one that is bodywide, or systemic, such as cardiovascular problems.

Maturity-onset diabetes of the young (MODY): rare form of non-insulin-dependent Type 2 diabetes developed in a person under age thirty.

Mellitus: Latin for "honey"; added to the term *diabetes* because in the past, diabetes was diagnosed through sweet-tasting urine.

Microvascular complication: a problem with the smaller blood vessels (capillaries) that connect to various body parts, such as eyes.

Mmol: millimole, a unit of measurement that counts molecular volume per liter.

Modifiable risk factor: risk factor that can be changed by alterations in lifestyle or diet.

Monosodium glutamate (MSG): the sodium salt of glutamic acid; an amino acid that occurs naturally in protein-containing foods such as meat, fish, milk, and many vegetables.

Nephrologist: a kidney specialist.

Neurologist: a nerve and brain specialist.

Nonnutritive sweeteners: sugar substitutes or artificial sweeteners, such as saccharin and sucralose, that do not have any calories and will not affect blood sugar levels.

Nutritive sweeteners: sweeteners such as table sugar, molasses, and honey, which have calories or contain natural sugar.

Obesity: when you weigh more than 20 percent of your ideal weight for your age and height.

Omega-3 fatty acids: naturally present in fish that swim in cold waters; crucial for brain tissue are all polyunsaturated, and not only lower cholesterol levels, but protect against heart disease.

Ophthalmologist: an eye specialist.

Oral glucose tolerance test: standard method of diagnosing impaired glucose tolerance (IGT) or diabetes; blood sugar is tested every thirty minutes for two hours following a period of fasting.

Oral hypoglycemic agents (OHAs): drugs that help the pancreas release more insulin or help the insulin work more effectively.

Orlistat: an antiobesity drug that blocks the absorption of almost one-third of the fat one consumes.

Pancreas: a bird-beak–shaped gland situated behind the stomach.

Pancreatitis: inflammation of the pancreas; occurs when the pancreas's digestive enzymes attack itself.

Peripheral vascular disease (PVD): occurs when blood flow to the limbs (arms, legs, and feet) is blocked, causing cramping, pains, or numbness.

Phytochemicals: plant chemicals (*phyto* is Greek for "plant"); disease-fighting or protective chemicals found in plant foods such as tomatoes, oats, soy, oranges, and broccoli.

Polydipsia: excessive thirst.

Polyphagia: excessive hunger.

Polyuria: excessive urination.

Postprandial: postmeal or after a meal, as in postprandial blood sugar levels.

Premixed insulin: when both short-acting insulin and intermediate-acting insulin are mixed together.

Primary care doctor: the doctor you see for a cold, flu, or an annual physical; the doctor who refers you to specialists; general and family practitioners (GPs and FPs) or internists are common primary care doctors.

Renin: a hormone produced by the kidneys which helps to regulate blood pressure.

Risk marker: a risk factor that cannot be changed, such as age or genes.

Saturated fat: a fat that is solid at room temperature, from animal sources, that stimulates the body to produce LDL, or "bad" cholesterol.

Secondary diabetes: occurs when diabetes surfaces as a side effect of a particular drug or surgical procedure; also called iatrogenic or clinically caused diabetes.

Soluble fiber: fiber that is water soluble, or dissolves in water; forms a gel in the body that traps fats and lowers cholesterol.

Stroke: occurs when a blood clot travels to the brain and stops the flow of blood and oxygen carried to the nerve cells in that area, at which point cells may die or vital body functions controlled by the brain may be temporarily or permanently damaged.

Sucrose: A disaccharide or double sugar made of equal parts glucose and fructose; known as table or white sugar; found naturally in sugar cane and sugar beets.

Sugar alcohols: nutritive sweeteners that are half as sweet as sugar; found naturally in fruits or manufactured from carbohydrates (for example, Sorbitol).

Sulphonylureas: oral hypoglycemic agents that help the pancreas release more insulin.

Systolic pressure: one of the readings in a blood pressure measurement; the pressure occurring during the heart's contraction.

Thiazoladinediones (troglitazone or Rezulin): agents that make the cells more sensitive to insulin.

Traditional healer: a vital health care professional within the aboriginal population.

Trans-fatty acids (hydrogenated oils): harmful, man-made fats that not only raise the level of "bad" cholesterol (LDL) in the bloodstream, but lower the amount of "good"cholesterol (HDL) that's already there; produced through the process of hydrogenation.

Triglycerides: a combination of saturated, monounsaturated, and polyunsaturated fatty acids and glycerol.

Type 1 diabetes: insulin-dependent diabetes mellitus (IDDM), a disease usually diagnosed before age thirty, in which the pancreas stops producing insulin; Type 1 diabetes, also known as juvenile diabetes, requires daily insulin injections for life.

Type 2 diabetes: non-insulin-dependent diabetes mellitus (NIDDM), also called late-onset or mature-onset diabetes because it's usually diagnosed after age forty-five; the body is either not producing enough insulin or the insulin it does produce cannot be used efficiently.

Unsaturated fat: known as "good fat" because it doesn't cause the body to produce "bad" cholesterol and it increases the levels of "good" cholesterol; partially solid or liquid at room temperature.

Urea: the waste product of protein released by the kidneys.

Chronology: Diabetes to Date

1552 B.C.: Earliest-known record of diabetes noted on third dynasty Egyptian papyrus by physician Hesy-Ra; mentions polyuria (frequent urination) as a symptom.

First century A.D.: Diabetes described by Arateus as "the melting down of flesh and limbs into urine."

A.D. 164: Greek physician Galen of Pergamum mistakenly diagnoses diabetes as an ailment of the kidneys.

Up to eleventh century: Diabetes commonly diagnosed by "water tasters" who drank the urine of people suspected of having diabetes; the urine of people with diabetes was thought to be sweet tasting. *Mellitus,* the Latin word for honey (referring to its sweetness), is added to the term *diabetes* as a result.

1500s: Swiss-born alchemist and physician Paracelsus identifies diabetes as a serious general disorder.

Early 1800s: First chemical tests developed to indicate and measure the presence of sugar in urine.

1800s: French researcher Claude Bernard studies the workings of the pancreas and the glycogen metabolism of the liver.

1800s: Czech researcher I.V. Pavlov discovers the links between the nervous system and gastric secretion, making an important contribution to science's knowledge of the physiology of the digestive system.

Late 1800s: Italian diabetes specialist Catoni isolates his patients under lock and key in order to get them to follow their diets.

Late 1850s: French physician Priorry advises diabetes patients to eat extra large quantities of sugar as a treatment.

1869: Paul Langerhans, a German medical student, announces in a dissertation that the pancreas contains two systems of cells. One set secretes normal pancreatic juice; the function of the other was unknown. Several years later, these cells are identified as the islets of Langerhans.

1870s: French physician Bouchardat notices the disappearance of glycosuria in his diabetes patients during the rationing of food in Paris while under siege by Germany during the Franco-Prussian War; formulates idea of individualized diets for his diabetes patients.

1889: Oskar Minkowski and Joseph von Mering at the University of Strasbourg, Austria, first remove the pancreas from a dog to determine the effect of an absent pancreas on digestion. They proved that without its pancreas a dog becomes severely diabetic. They also showed through experiments with duct ligation (surgically tying off different parts of tissue) that the pancreas indeed had two secretions: the *external* (which fed directly into the bloodstream and regulated carbohydrate metabolism) and a mysterious *internal* secretion, which appeared to be the "missing secretion" in diabetics. This connection between diabetes and the pancreas resulted in a series of early experiments using pancreatic extracts to treat animals and humans. These experiments didn't work, however, and even served to challenge the entire hypothesis of internal secretion.

November 14, 1891: Frederick Banting born near Alliston, Ontario. His parents, devout Methodists, try to pressure their son into joining the ministry; however, Banting enrolls in medical school at the University of Toronto in 1912 instead.

February 28, 1899: Charles Best born in West Pembroke, Maine.

1900–1915: Fad diabetes diets include the oat cure (in which the majority of the diet was made up of oatmeal), the milk diet, the rice cure, potato therapy, and even the use of opium.

1906: German scientist Georg Zuelzer makes some interesting progress on June 21, 1906. He injects pancreatic extract under the skin of a comatose fifty-year-old diabetic. The man is momentarily revived, reinforcing the connection between pancreatic extract (pancreatic secretion) and diabetes. Zuelzer obtains funding from the Schering Drug Company to produce a viable extract for therapy. By 1907, he produces what appears to be a workable pancreatic extract, but the Schering company decides that the results of his work didn't justify their costs, and withdraws funding. (This was a shame, considering that Zuelzer's formula was the first pancreatic extract to suppress glycosuria [sugary urine]). Unfortunately, Zuelzer's extract also caused many toxic side effects—what we know today as insulin shock. What should have been a major breakthrough in research is viewed by pancreatic researchers as a setback. Caution still rules, and the risks of these toxic side effects interferes with many pancreatic extract experiments.

1910–1920: Frederick Madison Allen and Elliot P. Joslin emerge as the two leading diabetes specialists in the United States. Joslin believes diabetes to be "the best of the chronic diseases" because it is "clean, seldom unsightly, not contagious, often painless, and susceptible to treatment."

1913: After three years of diabetes study, Frederick Allen publishes *Studies Concerning Glycosuria and Diabetes,* a book that is significant for the revolution in diabetes therapy that developed from it. J. J. R. Macleod, a professor of medicine at the University of Toronto, publishes a book called *Diabetes: Its Pathological Physiology.* Library records show that Frederick Banting borrowed Macleod's book for his research in 1920.

1919: Frederick Allen publishes *Total Dietary Regulation in the Treatment of Diabetes,* citing exhaustive case records of 76 of the 100 diabetes patients he observed, and becomes the director of diabetes research at the Rockefeller Institute.

1919–1920: Frederick Allen establishes the first treatment clinic in the United States, the Physiatric Institute in New Jersey, to treat patients with diabetes, high blood pressure, and Bright's disease; wealthy and desperate patients flock to it.

July 1, 1920: Dr. Banting opens his first office in London, Ontario; he treats his first patient on July 29; total earnings for his first month of work are four dollars.

October 30, 1920: Dr. Banting conceives of the idea of insulin after reading Moses Barron's "The Relation of the Islets of Langerhans to Diabetes with Special Reference to Cases of Pancreatic Lithiasis" in the November issue of *Surgery, Gynecology and Obstetrics.* In fact, Banting's notebook from that night is fully preserved at the Academy of Medicine in Toronto. In it he writes: "Diabetus. Ligate pancreatic ducts of dogs. Keep dogs alive till acini degenerate leaving Islets. Try to isolate the internal secretion of these to relieve glycosurea."

November 1920: Banting approaches Dr. J. J. R. Macleod with his idea. In that meeting, Macleod apparently brings Banting up to date on a variety of research attempts in the area of pancreatic extract. Macleod concedes that no one thought about the fact that the digestive agents of the pancreas may be responsible for destroying the secretion made by the islets of Langerhans. Banting proposes to Macleod that by using duct-ligated pancreases to make an extract, which would destroy the digestive secretions, they could find a treatment for diabetes. (Macleod was apparently irritated by Banting's clear lack of knowledge in the area of diabetes. Nevertheless, he thought it a good idea! Macleod, it would appear, was sorry the idea never occurred to him.) For the next year, with the assistance of Charles H. Best, J. B. Collip, and J. J. R. Macleod, Dr. Banting continues his research using a variety of different extracts on depancreatized dogs.

December 30, 1921: Dr. Banting presents a paper entitled "The Beneficial Influences of Certain Pancreatic Extracts on Pancreatic Diabetes," summarizing his work to this point, at a session of the American Physiological Society at Yale University. Among the attendees are Frederick Allen and Elliot Joslin. Little praise or congratulation is received.

January 23, 1922: One of Banting's insulin extracts is first tested on a human being, a fourteen-year-old boy named Leonard Thompson, in Toronto; treatment considered a success by the end of the following February.

May 21, 1922: James Havens becomes the first American successfully treated with insulin.

May 30, 1922: Pharmaceutical manufacturer Eli Lilly and Company and the University of Toronto collaborate on the mass production of insulin in North America.

October 25, 1923: Dr. Banting and Dr. Macleod awarded the Nobel Prize for Medicine; Banting shares his award with Best; Macleod then shares his award with Collip. (History would not remember Macleod's nor Collip's role in the discovery of insulin. While Banting, Best, Collip, and Macleod privately acknowledged they were a team, they could never admit it to each other. For Banting's obituary tribute, Collip wrote that his own contribution to insulin was trivial compared to Banting's. Banting apparently admitted in his later years that he and Best wouldn't have "achieved a damned thing" without Collip.*)

1934: Dr. Banting is knighted; he becomes Sir Frederick Banting.

February 21, 1941: Sir Frederick Banting is killed in an airplane crash over Newfoundland while en route to England.

1971: Fiftieth anniversary of the discovery of insulin celebrated worldwide.

1996: Seventy-fifth anniversary of the discovery of insulin celebrated.†

---

* In 1978, Banting's first biographer, Lloyd Stevenson, published an article that contained Macleod's personal account of the insulin discovery. Although Macleod had died in 1935, the University of Toronto did not want to reopen old wounds and for many years prevented the publication of that account. Macleod's account was bitter. He left the University of Toronto in 1928, and returned to Scotland as Regius Professor at the University of Aberdeen; it is believed that he moved away from Toronto because he couldn't stand living in the shadow of Banting's idea.

Charles Best replaced Macleod as professor of physiology at the University of Toronto when he was just twenty-nine years old. He went on to enjoy a long, distinguished career, and received many awards and honors; he died in 1978. Best continued Macleod's work on the properties of insulin, and received delayed credit for insulin's discovery after Banting's death in 1941. The Best Institute was erected next door to the Banting Institute in 1953.

J. B. Collip attempted to invent another version of insulin he called *gluclokinin,* but then abandoned it. He is also known for pioneering work on parathyroid hormone. Collip received his M.D., and eventually became Chair of Biochemistry at McGill

University. He became a world-renowned endocrinologist in Canada, and in 1947 was made Dean of Medicine at the very university that triggered Banting's idea: the University of Western Ontario. Collip enjoyed a great career and died in 1965 at the age of seventy-two.

†New evidence challenges whether Canadians have the right to claim complete ownership of the insulin discovery at all. Romanian scientist Nicolas Paulesco, who was concentrating on measuring the impact of *his* pancreatic extract (called "pancreine") on blood sugar, likely would have been the discoverer of insulin had the Canadians not beaten him to human testing. In 1971, on the fiftieth anniversary of the discovery of insulin, a campaign was launched by Bucharest medical students to honor Paulesco's work and give him due credit.

Sources

Bliss, Michael. 1982. *The Discovery of Insulin.* Toronto: McClelland & Stewart.

——. 1984. *Banting: A Biography.* Toronto: McClelland & Stewart.

——. 1993. Rewriting Medical History. *Journal of History of Medicine and Allied Sciences, Inc.* 48: 253–74.

Canadian Diabetes Association. 1997. Diabetes Timeline.

Williams, Michael, J. 1993. J. J. R. Macleod: The Co-discoverer of Insulin: *Proceedings of the Royal College of Physicians of Edinburgh* 23, 3 (July).

Resources

Note: This list was compiled from dozens of sources. Because of the nature of many health and nonprofit organizations, some of the addresses and phone numbers below may have changed since this list was compiled. Many of these organizations have e-mail addresses as well. Please review "Diabetes Online" at the end of this list.

American Association of Diabetes Educators
500 North Michigan Avenue, Suite 1400
Chicago, IL 60611
1-800-388-DMED or (312) 661-1700
http://www.aadenet.org

The American Diabetes Association
ADA National Service Center
1660 Duke Street
Alexandria, VA 22314
(703) 549-1500

American Foundation for the Blind
11 Penn Plaza, Suite 300,
New York, NY 10001
(212) 502-7661, fax (212) 502-7777

American Heart Association
7320 Greenville Pike
Dallas, TX 75231
(214) 373-6300

American National Kidney Foundation
30 East 33rd Street
New York, NY 10016
(212) 889-22101
1-800-622-9010

Canadian Diabetes Association
15 Toronto Street, Suite 800
Toronto, Ontario M5C 2E3
(416) 363-3373
fax (416) 363-3393
http://www.diabetes.ca

The Diabetes Research and Wellness Foundation (provides free
    medical alert ID necklaces and diabetes self-management
    diaries)
P.O. Box 3837
Merrifield, VA 22116
(202) 298-9211
http://www.charities.org/dirs/health/drwf/index.html

International Diabetes Center
3800 Park Nicollet Boulevard
St. Louis Park, MN 55416
(612) 993-3393

The International Diabetes Federation
International Association Center
40 Washington Street B-1050
Brussels, Belgium
32-2-647- 44 14
http://www.idf.org

International Diabetic Athletes Association
1647-B West Bethany Home Road
Phoenix, AZ 85015
(602) 433-2113

Joslin Diabetes Center
1 Joslin Place
Boston, MA 02215
(617) 732-2415
http://www.joslin.org

MedicAlert Foundation
2323 Colorado Avenue
Turlock, CA 95382
1-800-825-3785

National Diabetes Information Clearinghouse
Box NDIC
Bethesda, MD 20892
(301) 468-2162

National Diabetes Outreach Program
One Diabetes Way
Bethesda, MD 20892-3600
1-800-438-5383

National Federation of the Blind
1800 Johnston Street
Baltimore, MD 21230
(410) 659-9314
http://www.nfb.org

National Osteoporosis Foundation
1150 17th Street NW, Suite 500
Washington, DC 20036-4603
(202) 223-2226,
1-800-223-9994

FOOD/NUTRITION

American Anorexia/Bulimia Association, Inc.
133 Cedar Lane
Teaneck, NJ 07666
(201) 836-1800

Anorexia Nervosa and Related Eating Disorders, Inc.
P.O. Box 5102
Eugene, OR 97405
(503) 344-1144

Bulimia, Anorexia Self-Help (BASH)
6125 Clayton Avenue, Suite 215
St. Louis, MO 63139
1-800-BASH-STL
(314) 991-BASH

Grocery Manufacturers of America
1010 Wisconsin Avenue, NW
Suite 900
Washington, DC 20007
(202) 337-9400
fax (202) 337-4508

National Anorexic Aid Society
5796 Karl Road
Columbus, OH 43229
(614) 436-1112

National Food Safety Database
(U.S. Department of Agriculture)
Dr. Mark Tamplin
University of Florida
Old Dairy Science Building 120, Room 105
Box 110365
Gainesville, FL 32611-0365
E-mail: mlt@gnv.ifas.ufl.edu

Organic Trade Association
50 Miles Street
P.O. Box 1078
Greenfield, MA 01302
(413) 774-7511
E-mail: ota@igc.apc.org

Overeaters Anonymous
P.O. Box 44020
Rio Rancho, NM 87174-4402
(505) 891-2664

TOLL-FREE HOTLINES

American Dietetic Association and National Center for Nutrition
   and Dietetics (NCND)
Consumer Nutrition Hotline 1-800-366-1655

American Podiatric Medical Association
1-800-FOOTCARE

Pharmaceutical Company Customer Care Lines

Bayer Diagnostics Division
1-800-348-8100

Boehringer Mannheim Corporation
1-800-858-8072

Cascade Medical
1-800-525-6718

Lifescan, a Johnson & Johnson Company
1-800-227-8862, 663-5521

Medisense, Inc.
1-800-527-3339

Novo-Nordisk Pharmaceuticals
1-800-727-6500

WOMEN'S HEALTH RESOURCES

American Medical Women's Association (AMWA)
801 North Fairfax, Suite 400
Alexandria, VA 22314
(703) 838-0500

Black Women's Health Project of the National Women's Health
    Network
450 Auburn Avenue, #157
Atlanta, GA 30312
(404) 659-3854

Center for Medical Consumers and Health Care Information
237 Thomson Street
New York, NY 10012
(212) 674-7105

People's Medical Society
14 E. Minor Street
Emmaus, PA 18049
(215) 967-2136

Women's Health Information Center
Boston Women's Health Book Collective
47 Nichols Avenue
Watertown, MA 02172
(617) 974-0271

MENOPAUSE (NATURAL AND SURGICAL)

Hysterectomy Educational Resources and Services (HERS)
422 Bryn Mawr Avenue

Bala Cynwyd, PA 19004
(215) 667-7757

North American Menopause Society (NAMS)
P.O. Box 94527
Cleveland, OH 44101
(216) 844-8748
www.menopause.org

Women's Midlife Resource Center
1825 Haight Street
San Francisco, CA 94117
(415) 221-7417

PREGNANCY AND CHILDBIRTH

ALACE (Association of Labor Assistance and Childbirth
    Educators)
P.O. Box 382724
Cambridge, MA 02238
(617) 441-2500
fax (617) 441-3167

ALACEHQ@aol.com
C/Sec, Inc. (Cesareans/Support, Education, and Concern)
22 Forest Road
Framingham, MA 01701
(508) 877-8266

Doulas of North America (DONA)
1100-23rd Avenue East
Seattle, WA 98112
(206) 324-5440
AskDONA@aol.com
The NAPSAC Directory (National Association of Parents and
    Professionals for Safe Alternatives in Childbirth)

Route 1, Box 646
Marble Hill, MO 63764
(314) 238-2010

National Association of Childbirth Assistants (NACA)
219 Meridian Avenue
San Jose, CA 95167
(408) 225-9167

PREGNANCY HOTLINES

Brewer Prenatal Nutrition Hotline: (802) 388-0276

Calcium Information Line: 1-800-321-2681
(Established in 1991 by the Calcium Information Center, a
    component of the Clinical Nutrition Research Units of the
    New York Hospital–Cornell Medical Center and Memorial
    Sloan-Kettering Cancer Center and Oregon Health Sciences
    University.)

Healthy Mothers, Healthy Babies: (703) 836-6110

National Maternal & Child Health Clearinghouse: (703) 821-8955

Pregnancy Riskline: 1-800-822-2229

DIABETES ONLINE

Through the Internet, you can participate in newsgroups and bulletin boards (public forums) on diabetes information. These can be accessed through either independent Internet providers, or through an interactive computer service, such as CompuServe, Prodigy, or America Online (AOL).

Literature searches are great ways of getting specific information. Medline is the best search service for medical journal articles (many of which are extremely technical). CompuServe, Prodigy, or America Online all give you access to Medline. Medline is also available through many public and university libraries all over Canada and the United States.

Another way of accessing good information is through a Web browser, such as Netscape. By browsing, you can go to various sites in cyberspace to find your information. When you don't know the World Wide Web (www) address, you can use a search engine, such as Yahoo or Webcrawler, to search for what you want by simply typing in your topic. The more specific you can be in your search, the better. For example, if you want information on nerve damage, don't type "nerves" but "diabetes nerve damage" or "diabetic neuropathy." A search engine is essentially an index to the Internet. When you go to a site, you can save or print the information. Flashing text (called hypertext) is a sign that you'll get more information when you click on it. This may even link you to other sites on the Internet. A good resource is *Internet for Dummies*, which will walk you through Internet access step by step.

A FEW SITES TO GET YOU STARTED

The American Diabetes Association
http://www.diabetes.org

The Canadian Diabetes Association
http://www.diabetes.ca

Diabetes Association of Greater Cleveland
http://www.dagc.org/

The British Diabetic Association
http://www.diabetes.org.uk/

The National Diabetes Education Initiative (NDEI)
http://www.ndei.org/

Diabetes Well (sponsored by the Pacific Medical Research Foundation)
http://www.diabeteswell.com/

The Diabetic Retinopathy Foundation
http://retinopathy.org/

The National Institute of Diabetes and Digestive and Kidney
    Disease
http://www.niddk.nih.gov/health/diabetes/diabetes.htm

The Diabetes Database of the National Institute of Diabetes
    and Digestive and Kidney Diseases (NIDDK)
http://www.aerie.com/nihdb/ndic/dmdbase.html

Americans with Disabilities Act Information on the Web
    (covers individuals with diabetes)
http://www.usdoj.gov/crt/ada

The Diabetes Prevention Program
http://www.preventdiabetes.com

The Indian Health Service Diabetes Program
http://www.tucson.ihs.gov/healthcare/professions/diabetes/

Eli Lilly and Company's Web site, Managing Your Diabetes
    Patient Education Program
http://www.lilly.com/diabetes

BIBLIOGRAPHY

Abbott Hommel, Cynthia. 1994. PHEC, The SUGAR Group. *Diabetes Dialogue* 41, 3 (fall): 38.

The Ad Hoc Technical Committee Working Group on Development of Management Principles and Guidelines for Subsistence Catches of Whales by Indigenous (Aboriginal) Peoples. 1981. International Whaling Commission and aboriginal/subsistence whaling: April 1979 to July 1981, special issue 4. Cambridge, England: International Whaling Commission.

Advocacy in Action. 1996. *Diabetes Dialogue* 43, 3 (fall): 50–52.

Allard, Johane P. 1996. Excerpts from International Conference on Antioxidant Vitamins and Beta-Carotene in Disease Prevention: A Canadian Perspective. Special publication of the Vitamin Information Program, Hoffman-LaRoche.

Allegheny General Hospital and Voluntary Hospitals of America, Inc. 1990. Blood Pressure: Check It Out. In *Countdown USA: Countdown to a Healthy Heart*. Pittsburgh: Allegheny General Hospital and Voluntary Hospitals of America, Inc.

——. 1990. Double Trouble. In *Countdown USA: Countdown to a Healthy Heart*. Pittsburgh: Allegheny General Hospital and Voluntary Hospitals of America, Inc.

——. 1990. The Fat Trap. In *Countdown USA: Countdown to a Healthy Heart*. Pittsburgh: Allegheny General Hospital and Voluntary Hospitals of America, Inc.

——. 1990. Flick Your Risk: By Tossing Out Those Cigarettes, You Can Slash Your Chances of Heart Disease. In *Countdown USA:*

Countdown to a Healthy Heart. Pittsburgh: Allegheny General Hospital and Voluntary Hospitals of America, Inc.

———. 1990. Get Off the Diet Rollercoaster. In *Countdown USA: Countdown to a Healthy Heart.* Pittsburgh: Allegheny General Hospital and Voluntary Hospitals of America, Inc.

———. 1990. The Heart Healthy Kitchen. In *Countdown USA: Countdown to a Healthy Heart.* Pittsburgh: Allegheny General Hospital and Voluntary Hospitals of America, Inc.

———. 1990. Oats Are In. In *Countdown USA: Countdown to a Healthy Heart.* Pittsburgh: Allegheny General Hospital and Voluntary Hospitals of America, Inc.

———. 1990. We're Winning: By Changing Lifestyles, We're Proving Every Day That Coronary Disease Can Be Beaten. In *Countdown USA: Countdown to a Healthy Heart.* Pittsburgh: Allegheny General Hospital and Voluntary Hospitals of America, Inc.

Allsop, Karen F., and Janette Brand Miller. 1996. Honey Revisited: A Reappraisal of Honey in Preindustrial Diets. *British Journal of Nutrition* 75: 513–20.

American Diabetes Association. 1995. [Online: http://www.diabetes.ca. Cited July 1997.] Document ID: ADA035.

———. 1998. Standards of Medical Care for Patients with Diabetes Mellitus. *Diabetes Care* 21 (supplement 1): [Online: http://www.diabetes.org. Cited January 1999].

———. 1999. Carbohydrate Counting: A New Way to Plan Meals. [Online: http://www.diabetes.org. Cited January 1999.]

———. 1999. An Introduction to Oral Medications for Diabetes. [Online: http://www.diabetes.com. Cited January 1999.]

———. 1999. The United Kingdom Prospective Diabetes Study (UKPDS) for Type 2 Diabetes: What You Need to Know about the Results of a Long–Term Study. [Online: http://www.diabetes.org. Cited January 1999.]

American Dietetic Association. 1993. Position of the American Dietetic Association: Use of Nutritive and Nonnutritive Sweeteners. *Journal of the American Dietetic Association* 93: 816–22.

American Dietetic Association and National Center for Nutrition and Dietetics (NCND). 1994. 10 Tips to Healthy Eating. Chicago: NCND.

Anderson, Pauline. 1995. Researchers Predict Beginning of The End of Diabetes. *The Medical Post* (22 August).

The Antioxidant Connection: Visiting Speakers Discuss Immunity, Diabetes. 1995. Toronto: Vitamin Information Program of Hoffman-La Roche Ltd.

Antonucci, T., et al. 1997. Impaired Glucose Tolerance Is Normalized by Treatment with the Thiazolidinedione. *Diabetes Care* 20, 2 (February): 188–93.

Appavoo, Donna, Rayanne Waboose, and Stuart Harris. 1994. Dialogue, Sioux Lookout Diabetes Program. *Diabetes Dialogue* 41, 3 (fall): 19–20.

Armstrong, David G., Lawrence A. Lavery, and Lawrence B. Harkless. 1996. Treatment-Based Classification System for Assessment and Care of Diabetic Feet. *Journal of the American Podiatric Medical Association* 87, 7 (July): 303–38.

Associated Press wire service. 1997. FDA Approves Drug to Reduce Insulin Needs for Some Diabetics. 30 January.

———. 1997. Study Finds That Teens Who Had Less Salt as Infants Have Lower Blood Pressure. 8 April.

———. 1997. Study Ranks Cities by Pudginess of Residents. 4 May.

Augustine, Freda. 1994. Helping My People. *Diabetes Dialogue* 41, 3 (fall): 42–43.

Badley, Wendy. 1994. Across the Country. *Diabetes Dialogue* 41, 3 (fall): 32.

Baker Cummins Inc.1997. Zbar clinical product information.

Barnie, Annette. 1994. At Risk in Northern Ontario: Looking for Answers in the Sioux Lookout Zone. *Diabetes Dialogue* 41, 3 (fall): 18–20.

Barwise, Kim, and Danielle Sota. 1996. Two Views. *Diabetes Dialogue* 43, 3 (fall): 42–43.

Bayer Inc. Healthcare Division. 1996. How Adults are Learning to Manage Diabetes with Their Lifestyle. *The Globe and Mail* (1 November).

———. 1996. Practical Advice for the Prandase Patient. Booklet. Toronto: Bayer Inc. Healthcare Division.

———. 1997. Bayer Launches Major International Research Project into Prevention of Diabetes. Media release (5 March).

———. 1997. Blood Glucose Monitoring: Guidelines to a Healthier You. Patient information pamphlet.

———. 1997. Dextrolog: For Recording Blood and Urine Glucose Test Results. Booklet.

——. 1997. Diabetes and Non-Prescription Drugs: Guidelines to a Healthier You. Patient information pamphlet.

——. 1997. Exercise: Guidelines to a Healthier You. Patient information pamphlet.

——. 1997. Food and Exercise: Guidelines to a Healthier You. Patient information pamphlet.

——. 1997. Insulin: Guidelines to a Healthier You. Patient information pamphlet.

——. 1997. Ketone Testing: Guidelines to a Healthier You. Patient information pamphlet.

——. 1997. Prandase (Acarbose) Tablets. Product monograph.

——. 1997. Prandase: A New Approach to NIDDM Therapy. Patient information booklet. Toronto: Bayer Inc. Healthcare Division.

——. 1997. Preventing the Complications of Diabetes: Guidelines to a Healthier You. Patient information.

——. 1997. Taking Care of Your Feet: Guidelines to a Healthier You. Patient information.

——. 1997. Understanding Type 2 Diabetes: Guidelines for a Healthier You. Patient information pamphlet.

Becton Dickinson and Co. Canada Inc.1997. Safety First. Patient information pamphlet.

Becton Dickinson Consumer Products. 1996. Blood Sugar Testing Diary. Patient information pamphlet.

Bequaert Holmes, Helen, and Laura M. Purdy (eds.). 1992. *Feminist Perspectives in Medical Ethics.* Bloomington, Ind.: Indiana University Press.

Berndl, Leslie. 1995. Understanding Fat. *Diabetes Dialogue* 42, 1 (spring): 17–20.

Best, Henry. 1996. Charles Herbert Best: 1899–1978. *Diabetes Dialogue* 43, 4 (winter):

Beyers, Joanne. 1995. How Sweet It Is! *Diabetes Dialogue* 42, 1 (spring): 6–8.

Bierman, June, and Barbara Toohey. 1992. *The Diabetic's Book.* New York: Pedigree Books.

A Bill of Health for the IUD: Where Do We Go From Here? 1994. *Advances in Contraception* 10: 121–31.

Bliss, Mic. 1982. *The Discovery of Insulin.* Toronto: McClelland & Stewart.

——. 1984. *Banting: A Biography.* Toronto: McClelland & Stewart.

———. 1993. Rewriting Medical History. *Journal of History of Medicine and Allied Sciences* 48: 253–74.

Boctor, M. A., G. Carson, A. Kenshole, and R. Turnell. 1997. Gestational Diabetes Debate: Controversies in Screening and Management. *Canadian Diabetes* 10, 2 (June): 5–7.

Bonen, Arent. 1995. Fueling Your Tank. *Diabetes Dialogue* 42, 4 (winter): 13–16.

Bril, Vera. 1994. Diabetic Neuropathy—Can It Be Treated? *Diabetes Dialogue* 41, 4 (winter): 8–9.

British Columbia Women's Hospital and Health Centre Society. 1995. *The Challenges Ahead for Women's Health.* British Columbia Women's Community Consultation Report. Vancouver: British Columbia Women's Hospital and Health Centre Society.

Britt, Beverley. 1991. Pesticides and Alternatives. Paper delivered at conference, Gardening without Chemicals, of the Canadian Organic Growers Toronto Chapter, 6 April, in Toronto, Ontario.

Brubaker, Patricia L. 1994. Glucagon-like Peptide-1. *Diabetes Dialogue* 41, 4 (winter): 17–18.

Bureau of Human Prescription Drugs. 1994. *Drugs Directorate Guidelines, Directions for Use of Estrogen-Progestin Combination Oral Contraceptives.* Ottawa: Drugs Directorate, Health Protection Branch, Health Canada.

Canadian Diabetes Association. 1991. Guidelines for the Nutritional Management of Diabetes in Pregnancy. Position statement. 15, 3 (September).

———. 1995. You Have Diabetes. . . . Can You Have That? Booklet. Toronto: Canadian Diabetes Association.

———. 1996. The Agony of De-Feet. *Equilibrium* no. 1: 12–14.

———. 1996. Alcohol and Diabetes—Do They Mix? Booklet. Toronto: Canadian Diabetes Association.

———. 1996. Balancing Your Blood Sugars: A Guide for People with Diabetes. Booklet. Toronto: Canadian Diabetes Association.

———. 1996. Complications: The Long-Term Picture. *Equilibrium* no. 1: 8–10.

———. 1996. Diabetes: What is it? Equilibrium no. 1: 4.

———. 1996. Health . . .The Smoke-Free Way. *Equilibrium* no. 1: 26.

———. 1996. How to Cope with a Brief Illness: A Guide for the Person Taking Insulin. Patient information pamphlet.

———. 1996. Insulin and Type 2 Diabetes. *Equilibrium* no. 1: 29–30.

———. 1996. Low Blood Sugars: Your Questions Answered. *Equilibrium* no. 1: 31–32.

———. 1996. Monitoring Your Blood Sugar. *Equilibrium* no. 1: 33.

———. 1996. Physical Activity. *Equilibrium* no. 1: 22–23.

———. 1996. Pills for Diabetes? *Equilibrium* no. 1: 27–28.

———. 1996. Pills for Treating Diabetes. Pamphlet.

———. 1996. Seven Tips for Your Sick Day Blues. *Equilibrium* no.1: 38–41.

———. 1996. Travelling with Diabetes. Booklet.

———. 1996. Travelling with Diabetes. Patient information pamphlet.

———. 1996. What Is Diabetes? CDA Document ID: ADA037. Toronto: Canadian Diabetes Association, February 2.

———. 1996. You Are What You Eat. *Equilibrium* no. 1: 16–20.

———. 1996. Your Diabetes Healthcare Team. *Equilibrium* no. 1: 34–6.

———. 1997. Balancing Your Blood Sugar: A Guide for People with Diabetes. Patient information pamphlet.

———. 1997. Diabetes Education. Patient information pamphlet.

———. 1997. Get the Best Out of Life. Patient information pamphlet.

———. 1997. Health Record for People with Diabetes. Patient information.

———. 1997. Living Well. Patient information pamphlet.

———. 1997. Pocket Partner: A Guide to Healthy Food Choices. Booklet. Toronto: Canadian Diabetes Association.

———. 1997. Pocket Serving Sizer. Patient information pamphlet.

———. 1998. Clinical Practice Guidelines for the Management of Diabetes in Canada. *Canadian Medical Association Journal* 159 (supplement 8): S1–S29.

Canadian Diabetes Association and Lifescan Canada, Ltd., McNeil Consumer Products Company. 1996. Health Record for People with Diabetes. Patient information booklet.

Canadian Institute of Child Health. 1994. Aboriginal Children. In *The Health of Canada's Children: A CICH profile*, 2d ed., 131–48. Ottawa: Canadian Institute of Child Health.

Canadian Medical Association. 1994. CMA's submission to the Royal Commission on Aboriginal Peoples. In *Bridging the Gap: Promoting Health and Healing for Aboriginal Peoples in Canada*, 9–17. Ottawa: Canadian Medical Association

Canadian Task Force on the Periodic Health Examination. 1994. *The Canadian Guide To Clinical Preventive Health Care*. Ottawa: Health Canada.

Cattral, Mark. 1996. Pancreas Transplantation. *Diabetes Dialogue* 43, 4 (winter): 6–8.

Chabun, Roxanne, and Debbie Stiles. 1996. Bar None. *Diabetes Dialogue* 43, 3 (fall): 18–21.

Chaddock, Brenda. 1995. The Magic of Exercise. *Canadian Pharmacy Journal* (September): 45.

———. 1996. Blood-Glucose Testing: Keep Up with the Trend. *Canadian Pharmacy Journal* (September): 17.

———. 1996. Doing the Things that Make a Difference. *Canadian Pharmacy Journal* (July/August): 19.

———. 1996. Foul Weather Fitness: The Hardest Part Is Getting Started. *Canadian Pharmacy Journal* (March): 42.

———. 1996. The Right Way to Read a Label. *Canadian Pharmacy Journal* (May): 26.

———. 1997. Activity Is Key to Diabetes Health. *Canadian Pharmacy Journal* (March): 14.

The Challenge: Newsletter of the International Diabetic Athletes Association 6, 1 (spring 1997): Entire issue.

Christrup, Janet. 1991. Nuts About Nuts: The Joys of Growing Nut Trees. *Cognition* (July): 20–22.

Clarke, Bill. 1996. Action Figures. *Diabetes Dialogue* 43, 3 (fall): 14–16.

Clarke, Peter V. 1996. Hemoglobin A1c Test Helps Long-Term Diabetes Management. *Monitor* 1, 1: 1–3.

Cleave, Barbara. 1997.Viewpoint. *Diabetes Dialogue* 44, 2 (summer): 2.

Cooked Food Byproducts May Be Hazardous to Diabetics. 1996. *The Medical Post* 2 (July): 55.

Cox, Bruce Alan (ed.). 1988. *Native People, Native Lands: Canadian Indians, Inuit and Metis.* Ottawa: Carleton University Press.

Creighton, Donald. 1976. *The Forked Road: Canada 1939–1957.* Toronto: McClelland & Stewart, Ltd.

Cronier, Claire. 1997. Sweetest Choices. *Diabetes Dialogue* 44, 1 (spring): 26–27.

Cunningham, John J. 1995. Vitamins, Minerals and Diabetes. Paper presented at the 22d annual conference of the Diabetes Educators Section of the Canadian Diabetes Association.

Deutsch, Nancy. 1996. Vitamin C Stores Critical for Diabetics. *Family Practice* (11 November): 24.

Diabetes: An Undetected Time-Bomb. 1996. *CARP News.* April.

Diabetes Clinical Research Unit of Mount Sinai Hospital Toronto for Sherwood Medical Industries Canada Inc. 1997. What Is Intensive Diabetes Management? Patient information pamphlet.

Discovery of Insulin Marked Turning Point in Human History. 1996. *The Globe and Mail.* 1 November.

Doyle, Patricia. 1995. *Insulin—The Facts.* Toronto: Canadian Diabetes Association.

Drum, David, and Terry Zierenberg. 1998. *The Type 2 Diabetes Sourcebook.* Los Angeles: Lowell House.

Dutcher, Lisa. 1994. A Wholistic Approach to Diabetes Management. *Diabetes Dialogue* 41, 3 (fall): 42.

Eli Lilly and Company. 1997. Insulin Management Information. Patient information pamphlet.

——. 1997. Managing your diabetes with Humalog. Booklet. Toronto: Eli Lilly and Company.

Eli Lilly of Canada Inc. 1997. The Accu-Chek Advantage System. Patient information pamphlet.

——. 1997. Is Your Insulin as Easy to Use as Humulin? Patient information pamphlet.

——. 1997. What You Should Know About Humulin. Booklet. Toronto: Eli Lilly of Canada Inc.

——. 1997. Your Blood Sugar Level . . . What Does It Tell You? Patient information pamphlet.

Eli Lilly of Canada Inc./Boehringer Mannheim Canada. 1996. First New Insulin in 14 Years Approved for Use in Canada. Media release (9 October).

——. 1997. Micral-S Kidney Chek. Patient information.

Emanuel, Ezekiel J., and Linda L. Emanuel. 1992. Four Models of the Physician-Patient Relationship. *Journal of the American Medical Association* 267 (16): 2221–26.

Engel, June V. 1996. Beyond Vitamins: Phytochemicals to Help Fight Disease. *Health News* 14 (June).

Engel, June. 1997. Eating Fiber. *Diabetes Dialogue* 44, 1 (spring): 16–18.

Expert Committee on the Diagnosis and Classification of Diabetes Mellitus. 1998. Report of the Expert Committee on the Diagnosis and Classification of Diabetes Mellitus. [Online: http://www.diabetes.org.] American Diabetes Association.

Farquhar, Andrew. 1996. Exercising Essentials. *Diabetes Dialogue* 43, 3 (fall): 6–8.

Feig, Denice S. 1997. The Fourth International Workshop Conference on Gestational Diabetes Mellitus. *Canadian Diabetes* 10, 2 (June): 2.

Final Report on Royal Commission on Aboriginal Peoples. 1997. In *Health And Healing, Inroads Of Chronic Disease* Vol. 3 [Online: http://www.libraxus.com. Cited July 1997.]

Findlay, Deborah, and Leslia Miller. 1994. Medical Power and Women's Bodies. In *Women, Medicine and Health*, B. S. Bolaria and R. Bolaria, eds. Halifax, Canada: Fernwood.

First Nations Health Commission, Assembly of First Nations. 1993. Report on the Second International Conference on Diabetes and Native Peoples. Honolulu: First Nations Health Commission, Assembly of First Nations.

Following the Patient with Chronic Disease. 1996. *Patient Care Canada* 7, 5 (May): 22–38.

Following the Patient with Stable Chronic Disease: Type II Diabetes Mellitus. 1996. *Patient Care Canada* 7, 5 (May): 22–41.

Fox, Mary Lou. 1994. Zeesbakadapenewin: Words of an Elder Grandmother about the Sugar Disease. *Diabetes Dialogue* 41, 3 (fall): 22–24.

Foxman, Stuart. 1996. Human vs. Beef/Pork Insulin. Toronto: Canadian Diabetes Association. Adapted from Nahla Aris-Jilwan, Pierre Malheux, Tina Kader, Alain Boisvert, DPH, and Sara Meltzer, *The Report of the Ad Hoc Committee on Beef-Pork Insulins* (Toronto: Canadian Diabetes Association, 1995).

Fraser, Eliabeth, and Bill Clarke. Loafing Around. *Diabetes Dialogue* 44, 1 (spring): 32–33.

Gabrys, Jennifer. 1996. Ask the Professionals. *Diabetes Dialogue* 43, 4 (winter): 60–61.

Gauthier, Serge G., and Patricia H. Coleman. 1993. Nutrition and Aging. *The Lederle Letter* 2, 2 (April): 1–2.

Gerth Mulvad, Gerth, and Orsoq Henning Sloth Pedersen Mulvad. 1992. Eat Meat and Blubber from Sea Mammals and Avoid Cardiovascular Disease. *Inuit Whaling* (special June issue).

Glory Enough For All: The Discovery of Insulin. 1988. Film. Toronto: Gemstone Productions Ltd. and Primedia Productions, Ltd.

Gordon, Dennis. 1997. Acarbose: When it Works/When it Doesn't. *Diabetes Forecast* (February): 25–28.

Graham, Joan. 1995. Impotence—The Complication No One Wants To Talk About. Toronto: Canadian Diabetes Association.

Graham, Peg. 1997. Rising Expectations. *Diabetes Dialogue* 44, 2 (summer): 32–33.

Grieving Necessary to Accept Diabetes. 1994. *Diabetes Dialogue* 41, 3 (fall): 35–36.

Guillebaud J. 1993. *Contraception: Your Questions Answered.* New York: Churchill-Livingston.

Guthrie, Diana, and Richard A. Guthrie. 1996. *The Diabetes Sourcebook.* Los Angeles: Lowell House.

Harrison, Pam. 1996. Rethinking Obesity. *Family Practice* (11 March): 24.

Hatcher, Robert A., et al. 1994. *Contraceptive Technology,* 16th ed. (rev.). New York: Irvington Publishers.

Halvorson, Mary, Francine Kaufman, and Neal Kaufman. 1996. A Snack Bar Containing Uncooked Cornstarch to Diminish Hypoglycaemia. Paper delivered at the American Diabetes Association 56th Scientific Sessions.

Health Watch/Shoppers Drug Mart. 1997. Mature Lifestyles: High Blood Pressure. Patient information pamphlet. Toronto: Health Watch/ Shoppers Drug Mart.

The Heart and Stroke Foundation of Ontario. 1997. Heart Disease and Stroke. Patient information.

——. 1997. How Do I Choose a Healthy Diet? Patient information.

Helwick, Caroline. 1996. Apnea, Diabetes Linked. *The Medical Post.* 28 May.

Ho, Marian. 1996. Learning Your ABCs, Part Two. *Diabetes Dialogue* 43, 3 (fall): 38–40.

Hot Flashes and Hormone Pills. 1994. *Macleans.* 7 February.

Houlden, Robyn. 1994. Health Beliefs in Two Ontario First Nations Populations. *Diabetes Dialogue* 41, 4 (winter).

How Adults Are Learning to Manage Diabetes with their Lifestyle. 1996. *The Globe and Mail* (1 November).

Hunt, John A. 1994. Fueling Up. *Diabetes Dialogue* 41, 4 (winter).

Hunter, J. E., and T. H. Applewhite. 1991. Reassessment of Trans Fatty Acid Availability in the U.S. Diet. *American Journal of Clinical Nutrition* 54: 363–69.

Hurley, Jane, and Stephen Schmidt. 1994. Going with the Grain. *Nutrition Action* (October): 10–11.

Improving Treatment Outcomes in NIDDM: The Questions and Controversies. 1996. *The Diabetes Report* 2, 1: 1–2.

International Food Information Council. 1991. *What You Should Know About MSG.* Washington, D.C.: International Food Information Council.

———. 1994. What You Should Know About Sugars. Washington, D.C.: International Food Information Council, May.

———. 1995. IFIC Review: Intense Sweeteners: Effects on Appetite and Weight Management. Washington, D.C.: International Food Information Council, November.

———. 1995. IFIC Review: Uses and Nutritional Impact of Fat Reduction Ingredients. Washington, D.C.: International Food Information Council.

———. 1996. What You Should Know About Aspartame. Washington, D.C.: International Food Information, 4 November.

———. 1997. Antibiotics in Animals: An Interview with Stephen Sundlof, D.V.M., Ph.D. Washington, D.C.: International Food Information Council.

———. 1997. Putting Fun Back into Food. Washington, D.C.: International Food Information Council.

———. 1997. Q&A about Fatty Acids and Dietary Fats. Washington, D.C.: International Food Information Council.

———. 1997. Sorting Out the Facts about Fat. Washington, D.C.: International Food Information Council.

Jeffrey, Susan. 1996. Uncooked Cornstarch Snacks Aid Diabetics. *The Medical Post.* 12 November.

Jelly Beans Offer Sweet Relief. 1997. *Diabetes Dialogue* 44, 2 (summer): 52–53.

Jovanovic-Peterson, Lois, June Biermann, and Barbara Toohey. 1996. *The Diabetic Woman: All Your Questions Answered.* New York: G.P. Putnam's Sons.

Joyce, Carol. 1996. What's New in Type 2. *Diabetes Dialogue* 43, 3 (fall): 32–36, 63.

Kaptchuk, Ted, and Micheal Croucher. 1986. *The Healing Arts: A Journal Through the Faces of Medicine.* Documentary. London: The British Broadcasting Corporation.

Kea, David. 1992. Herd Health: The Biggest Reward of Ecological Dairy Farming. *Cognition* 93 (winter): 26–27.

Kelly, Catherine. 1997. Hormone Replacement Therapy. *Diabetes Dialogue* 44, 2 (summer): 28–30.

Kenshole, Anne. 1997. To Be or Not To Be Pregnant. *Diabetes Dialogue* 44, 2 (summer): 6–8.

Kermode-Scott, Barbara. 1996. NIDDM Affecting Huge Numbers, Says Expert. *Family Practice* (11 March): 21.

Kewayosh, Alethea. 1994. The Way We Are: The Eye of the Storm—A First Nations Perspective on Diabetes. *Diabetes Dialogue* 41, 3 (fall): 56–57.

The Kidney Foundation of Canada. 1993.Your Kidneys. Patient information.

——. 1995. Diabetes and Kidney Disease. Patient information pamphlet.

——. 1995. High Blood Pressure and Your Kidneys. Patient information pamphlet.

——. 1995. Kidney Stones. Patient information pamphlet.

——. 1995. Organ Donation: Have You Thought about It? Patient information.

——. 1995. Treating Kidney Failure. Patient information.

——. 1995. Urinary Tract Infections. Patient information.

Kock, Henry. 1991. Restoring Natural Vegetation as Part of the Farm. In *Gardening without Chemicals '91.* Toronto: Canadian Organic Growers Toronto Chapter.

Korytkowski, Mary. 1996. Something Old, Something New. *Diabetes Spectrum* 9 (4 November): 211–12.

Kra, J. Siegfried. 1996. *What Every Woman Must Know About Heart Disease.* New York: Warner Books.

Kuczmarski R. J., K. M. Flegal, S. M. Campbell, and C. L. Johnson. 1994. Increasing Prevalence of Overweight among U.S. Adults: The National Health and Nutrition Examination Surveys, 1960 to 1991. *Journal of the American Medical Association* 272: 205–11.

Kumar, S., et al. 1996. Troglitazone, An Insulin Action Enhancer, Improves Metabolic Control in NIDDM Patients. *Diabetologia* 30, 6 (June): 701–9.

Kushi, Mishio. 1993. *The Cancer Prevention Guide.* New York: St. Martin's Press.

Lebovitz, Harold E. 1996. Acarbose, an Alpha-Glucosidase Inhibitor, in the Treatment of NIDDM. *Diabetes Care* 19 (supplement 1): 554–61.

Leiter, Lawrence A. 1996. Acarbose: New Treatment in NIDDM Patients. Paper sponsored by Bayer, Inc.

Levine, R. J. 1988. *Ethics and Regulation of Clinical Research.* New Haven, Conn.: Yale University Press.

Lichtenstein, A. H., et al. 1993. Hydrogenation Impairs the Hypo-lipidemic Effect of Corn Oil in Humans. *Arteriosclerosis and Thrombosis* 13:154–61.

Lichti, Janice, C. 1996. Mind Boosters. *Healing Arts Magazine* (March): 14–15.

LifeScan Canada Inc. 1997. How to Choose Your New Blood Glucose Meter. Patient information pamphlet.

——. 1997. One Touch Profile: For Complete Diabetes Management. Patient information.

——. 1997. Surestep. Patient information pamphlet.

LifeScan Education Institute. 1996. Spring at Last! *The Diabetes News* (spring): 1–2.

Lilly Diabetes Care. 1997. Your Blood Sugar Level . . . What Does It Tell You? Patient information pamphlet.

Linden, Ron. 1996. Hyperbaric Medicine. *Diabetes Dialogue* 43, 4 (fall): 24–26.

Little, Linda. 1996. Vitamin E May Help Cut Diabetics' Risk of Heart Disease. *The Medical Post* (14 May).

Little, Margaret. 1996. Step Right Up. *Diabetes Dialogue* 43, 3 (fall): 24–26.

Los Angeles Daily News. 1997. Diabetes Implants Tested (23 January).

Ludwig, Sora. 1997. Gestational Diabetes. *Canadian Diabetes* 10, 2 (June): 1, 8.

Macdonald, Jeanette. 1997. The Facts about Menopause. *Diabetes Dialogue* 44, 2 (summer): 24–26.

MacMillan, Harriet L., Angus B. MacMillan, David R. Offord, and Jennifer L. Dingle. 1996. Aboriginal Health. *Canadian Medical Association Journal* 155: 1569–78.

Maltman, Grant. 1994. Banting: Co-discoverer of Insulin and . . . Artist. *Diabetes Dialogue* 41, 4 (winter): 41–42.

——. 1995. The Birth of an Idea. *Diabetes Dialogue* 42, 4 (winter): 40–43.

Marliss, Errol B., and Rejeanne Gougeon. 1993. Focus on Women: Dieting as a Possible Risk Factor for Obesity. *The Lederle Letter* 2, 4 (August): 1–2.

Marliss, Errol B., Rejeanne Gougeon, and Sandra Schwenger. 1992. Weight-Reducing Diets May Compromise Nutrition. *The Lederle Letter* 1, 3 (August): 1–2.

Martin, Cheryl. 1996. Acarbose (Prandase). *Communication* (March/April): 38.

Mastroianni, Anna C., Ruth Faden, and Daniel Federman (eds.). 1994. *Women and Health Research: Ethical and Legal Issues of Including*

Women in Clinical Studies, Vol. 1. Washington, D.C.: National Academy Press.

McCarten, James. 1995. Toxic or Not, Inuit Stand by Whale Meat. *The Edmonton Journal.* 28 December.

Medisense Canada Inc. 1995. MediSense Blood Glucose Sensor. Product mongraph.

———. 1996. Real World Factors That Interfere With Blood-Glucose Meter Accuracy. Patient information pamphlet.

———. 1997. Reducing Your Risk of Diabetes Complications. Patient information pamphlet.

———. 1997. Seven Key Factors for Real World Accuracy in the Real World. Patient information pamphlet.

———. 1997. Seven Key Steps to Control Your Diabetes. Patient information pamphlet.

Mihill, Chris. 1996. New Fears Over Link Between Cow's Milk And Diabetes. *The Guardian.* 4 October.

Monoject Diabetes Care Products. 1997. How To Take Insulin. Patient information.

Morrison, Bruce R., and C. Roderick Williams. 1986. *Native Peoples Canadian Experience.* Toronto: McClelland & Stewart, Ltd.

Musgrove, Lorraine. 1997. Ask the Professionals. *Diabetes Dialogue* 44, 1 (spring): 60–61.

National Pharmacy Continuing Education Program. 1997. Non-Insulin-Dependent Diabetes Mellitus. Booklet. Toronto: National Pharmacy Continuing Education Program.

National Pharmacy Continuing Education Program and Bayer Inc. 1997. Non-Insulin Dependent Diabetes Mellitus. Patient information pamphlet. February.

Neergaard, Lauran. 1997. Study Finds Low Hormone Levels May Encourage Weight Gain. Associated Press wire service. 14 May.

Neuschwander-Tetri, B. A., et al. 1998. Troglitazone-Induced Hepatic Failure Leading to Liver Transplantation. A Case Report. *Annals of Internal Medicine* 129 (1 July): 38–41.

New Developments in the Management of Type II Diabetes. 1995. *The Diabetes Report* 1, 2.

New Perspectives in the Management of NIDDM. 1996. *The Diabetes Report* 1, 3.

Novolin. 1997. Product monograph.

———. 1996. All About Insulin. Booklet. Toronto: Novo Nordisk Canada Inc.

——. 1996. Keeping Well with Diabetes: Novolin Care. Patient information pamphlet.

——. 1996. Nutrition for Diabetes. Patient information manual.

——. 1996. Watch your step. Booklet. Toronto: Novo Nordisk Canada Inc.

——. 1997. Novolin ge: Insulin, Human Biosynthetic Antidiabetic Agent. Product monograph.

Nutrition News. 1996. *Diabetes Dialogue* 43, 4 (winter): 57.

——. 1997. *Diabetes Dialogue* 44,1 (spring): 56.

Nutrition Principles for the Management of Diabetes and Related Complications. 1994. Technical review. *Diabetes Care* 17: 490–518.

Olestra: Yes or No? 1996. *Diabetes Dialogue* 43, 3 (fall): 44.

Ontario College of Pharmacists Drug Information Service. 1996. Acarbose (Prandase). *New Drugs/Drug News* 14, 2 (March/April): 1–2.

Orbach, Susie. 1990. *Fat is a Feminist Issue.* New York: Berkeley Books.

Ortho-McNeil Inc. 1993. *The History of Contraception Museum.* Toronto: Ortho-McNeil Inc.

Orton, David. 1995. Rethinking Environmental-First Nations Relationships. *Canadian Dimension* 29, 1 (February/March). [Online: Greenweb bulletin #3, http://www.indians.org. Cited April 1997.]

——. 1995. Some Limitations of a Left Critique and Deep Dilemmas in Environmental-First Nations Relationships. Presentation at the Learned Societies Conference on the environment and the relations with First Nations, cosponsored by the Society for Socialist Studies and the Environmental Studies Association of Canada, 5 June, in Montreal, Canada.

Pharmacia and Upjohn. 1997. It Takes Two: A Couple's Guide to Erectile Dysfunction. Patient information booklet.

Pharma Plus. 1997. Diabetes. Patient information pamphlet.

Postl, B., J. Irvine, S. MacDonald, and M. Moffatt. 1994. Background Paper on the Health of Aboriginal Peoples in Canada. In *Bridging the Gap: Promoting Health and Healing for Aboriginal Peoples in Canada,* 19–56. Ottawa: Canadian Medical Association.

Prevention and Treatment of Obesity: Application to Type 2 Diabetes. 1997. Technical review. *Diabetes Care* 20: 1744–66.

Prochaska, James O. 1995. A Revolution in Diabetes Evaluation. Paper presented at the 22d annual conference of the Diabetes Educators Section of the Canadian Diabetes Association.

Proper Knowledge of a Healthy Diet Makes Huge Difference. 1996. *The Globe and Mail* (1 November): 3.

PROSWEET Canada. 1997. Choosing Your Sweetener. Product information.

———. Canada. 1997. PROSWEET: The Low Calorie Pure Sugar Taste Sweetener. Product information.

Protein Content of the Diabetic Diet. 1994. Technical review. *Diabetes Care* 17: 1502–13.

Purdy, Laura M. 1996. *Reproducing Persons: Issues in Feminist Bioethics.* Ithaca, N.Y.: Cornell University Press.

Q&A on Low-Calorie Sweeteners. 1997. *The Diabetes News* 1, 2 (spring): 3.

The Receptor 7, 3 (fall/winter 1996): Entire issue.

Reddy, Sethu. 1995. Smoking and Diabetes. *Diabetes Dialogue* 42, 4 (winter): 33–35.

Research, Improvement in Products Never Stops in Health Industry. 1996. *The Globe and Mail.* 1 November.

Reuters Health Summary. 1997. Hostility and Heart Risk. 22 April.

———. 1997. Obese Children May Lack Antioxidants. 22 April.

———. 1997. Obesity Hormone May Prevent Diabetes. 29 April.

Reuters wire service. 1997. Diabetes Raises Dementia Risk. 13 February.

———. 1997. Diets Slow Reaction Times. 8 April.

———. 1997. Feeding Your Child for a Lifetime. 10 April.

———. 1997. High-Carbohydrate Diet Not for Everyone. 16 April.

———. 1997. Study: You Can Lose Weight and Cigarettes. 19 June.

Rifkin, Jeremy. 1995. Playing God with the Genetic Code. *Health Naturally* (April/May): 40–44.

Rosenthal, M. Sara. 1996. *The Breast Sourcebook.* Los Angeles: Lowell House.

———. 1997. *The Gynecological Sourcebook,* 2d ed. Los Angeles: Lowell House.

———. 1997. *The Pregnancy Sourcebook,* 2d ed. Los Angeles: Lowell House.

———. 1998. *The Breastfeeding Sourcebook,* 2d ed. Los Angeles: Lowell House.

———. 1998. *The Fertility Sourcebook,* 2d ed. Los Angeles: Lowell House.

Rowlands, Liz, and Denis Peter. 1994. Diabetes—Yukon Style. *Diabetes Dialogue* 41, 3 (fall): 32–33.

Ruggiero, Laura. 1997. Helping People with Diabetes Change: Practical Applications of the Stages of Change Model. Professional information. LifeScan Education Institute.

Ryan, David. 1996. At the Controls. *Diabetes Dialogue* 43, 3 (fall).

Schoepp, Glen. 1996. What Is the Role of Acarbose (Prandase) in Diabetes Management? *Pharmacy Practice* 12, 4 (April): 37–38.

Schwartz, Carol. 1996. An Eye-Opener. *Diabetes Dialogue* 43, 4 (winter): 20–22.

Selected Vitamins and Minerals in Diabetes. 1994. Technical review. *Diabetes Care* 17: 464–79.

Seto, Carol. 1995. Nutrition Labelling—U.S. style. *Diabetes Dialogue* 42, 1 (spring): 32–34.

Sherwin, Susan. 1984. *Patient No Longer: Feminist Ethics and Health Care.* Philadelphia: Temple University Press.

Sherwood Medical Industries Canada Inc. 1997. Monoject: Diabetes Care Products. Patient information pamphlet.

Sinclair, A. J. 1993. Rational Approaches to the Treatment of Patients with Non-Insulin-Dependent Diabetes Mellitus. *Practical Diabetes Supplement* 10, 6 (November/December): 515–20.

Spicer, Kay. 1994. Traditional Foods of Aboriginal Canadians. *Diabetes Dialogue* 41, 3 (fall): 44–47.

Splenda (brand sweetener) Information Centre. 1997. Sucralose Overview. Product information.

Stehlin, Dori. 1999. A Little Lite Reading. [Online: http://www.fda.gov/fdac/foodlabel/diabetes.html. Cited January 1999.]

Sweet Promise from Sugar Substitute? 1996. *The Medical Post* (2 July): 55.

Tetley, Deborah. 1997. Fish Farmer Hopes to Tame Diabetes on Akwesasne. *The Toronto Star.* 12 April.

Thompson, John Herd, with Allen Singer. 1985. *Canada 1922–1939: Decades of Discord.* Toronto: McClelland & Stewart, Ltd.

Todd, Robert. 1996. The Sporting Life. *Diabetes Dialogue* 43, 3 (fall): 28–29.

Tookenay, Vincent F. 1996. Improving the Health Status of Aboriginal People in Canada: New Directions, New Responsibilities. *Canadian Medical Association Journal* 155: 1581–83.

Toronto and Region Organic Directory. 1991. Toronto: Canadian Organic Growers, Toronto Chapter.

Trapped by Furs. 1997. Presentation at the symposium on conflicting interests of animal welfare and indigenous peoples, 17 January, at Erasmus University, Rotterdam, Finn Lynge.

Type II Diabetes. 1997. Shoppers Drug Mart Education Series NIDDM, vol. 95, p. 11.

U.S. Food and Drug Administration (FDA). 1999. *Nutrient Claims Guide for Individual Foods.* Special report. Focus on Food Labeling series. FDA publication no. 95-2289. Washington, D.C.: FDA.

Vegetarian Resource Group. 1997. Getting to the Roots of a Vegetarian Diet. Baltimore, Md.: Vegetarian Resource Group.

Vitamin Information Program, Fine Chemicals Division of Hoffman-La Roche Ltd. Diabetes: Facts and Figures. 1995. *News from the VIP* no. 2 (fall): 1–4.

——. 1995. Folic Acid Surveys Say Consumer Awareness Is Low. *News from the VIP* no. 2 (fall): 3.

——. 1995. VIP Conference on Elderly Attracts Canadian Media. *News from the VIP* no. 2 (fall): 1.

——. 1995. What's Your Type? *News from the VIP* no. 2 (fall): 2.

Wanless, Melanie. 1997. The Weight Debate. *Diabetes Dialogue* 44, 1 (spring): 22–25.

Whitcomb, Randall. 1996. The Key to Type 2. *Diabetes Dialogue* 43, 4 (winter): 16–18.

White, John R., Jr. 1996. The Pharmacologic Management of Patients with Type II Diabetes Mellitus in the Era of New Oral Agents and Insulin Analogs. *Diabetes Spectrum* 9, 4: 227–34.

Willett, W. C., et al. 1993. Intake of Trans Fatty Acids and Risk of Coronary Heart Disease Among Women. *Lancet* 341: 581–85.

Williams, Michael J. 1993. Macleod: The Co-discoverer of Insulin. *Proceedings of the Royal College of Physicians of Edinburgh* 23, 3 (July).

World Wide Fund For Nature. 1991. *Combining the Old and the New.* Caring for the Earth: A Strategy for Sustainable Living IUCN—The World Conservation Union, United Nations environment programme. Gland, Switzerland: World Wide Fund For Nature.

Wormworth, Janice. 1995. Toxins and Tradition: The Impact of Food-Chain Contamination on the Inuit of Northern Quebec. *Canadian Medical Association Journal* 152, 8 (15 April):

Yale, Jean-François. Glucose Results: Plasma or Whole Blood? *Monitor* 1, 2: 1–4.

Yankova, Diliana. 1997. Diabetes in Bulgaria. *Diabetes Dialogue* 44, 1 (spring): 36–39.

Zinman, Bernard. 1996. Insulin Analogues. *Diabetes Dialogue* 43, 4 (winter): 14–15.

('b' indicates boxed material; 't' indicates a table)

A

"Abdominal delivery," 135

Aboriginal people
   GDM screening, 138
   morbidity in, 19
   term, 16

ACE inhibitors, kidney disease, 268

Acesulfame potassium (Ace-K)

Acromegaly, 16

"Active living," 178

Adult-onset diabetes, Type 2
   diabetes, 3

Aerobic exercise, 175

Aerobic, term, 173

African Americans
   GDM screening, 138
   hypertension risk, 9
   Type 2 diabetes, 4, 5, 15

Age, Type 2 diabetes risk factor, 13

Agricultural sector, animal-food
   production, 280b, 292–295

Alcohol
   abuse and pancreatitis and, 20

bone loss and, 159
hypertension risk factor, 9
use, diabetic diet, 205–208

Allen Diet, 187–188

Allylic sulphides, 289

Alpha-glucosidase inhibitors,
   234–236

Alphalinolenic acid, 289

Alzheimer's disease, diabetes
   induced, 256

"Ambulance cells," 274

American Association of
   Advancement of Science,
   diet, 290

American Association of Diabetes
   Educators, 47

American Diabetes Association,
   47, 217
   DCCT, 275
   dietary guidelines, 189,
      194–195, 197–198, 198t
   self-testing, 27, 214–215,
      223–224

American National Health and Nutrition Examination Survey III, 184–185

American Society for Clinical Nutrition, 47

Amputations, diabetes induced, 269–270

Androgen-related side effects, OCs and, 80–81

Androgens, ERT/HRT, 111, 121–122

Anemia, OCs and, 80

Animal-food production, 280b, 292–295

Anorexia nervosa, 51, 52

Antioxidants, 12, 287

Arcarbose, 234–236

Arching Spring, diaphragm, 95

Arteriosclerosis, diabetes induced, 261

Artificial sweeteners, 202–204

Asian Americans, Type 2 diabetes in, 5, 16

Aspartame, 202, 203

Autoimmune disease, Type 1 diabetes, 2–3

Autonomic neuropathy, diabetes induced, 256–257

B

"Bad" cholesterol, 7, 77, 103, 174, 230, 237, 283, 286

Barbasco Roota, 78

Barrier methods, birth control, 76, 93–100

Beef/pork insulin, 242, 243b

Beer, diabetic diet, 206

Beta cells, role of, 2

Betaglucan, 289

Beverly Hills Diet, 50

Biguanides, OHAs, 230, 231, 233

Bilateral oophorectomy, 152–153

Binge eating disorder, 59–61

Bingeing, 51, 52, 53, 59, 75

Birth control, methods of, 76–77

Birth defects, diabetes induced, 128–129, 134

Blindness, diabetes induced, 257–258

Blood clots, OCs risk of, 80

Blood fat disorders, 77

Blood pressure
  description of, 8–9
  lowering of, 10

Blood pressure test, 228

Blood sugar level
  bone loss and, 160
  estrogen and, 71, 72, 78
  exercise and, 178, 179–180
  maintaining good, 130b
  menopause and, 75, 142, 151–152, 154–156
  menstruation and, 74
  oral contraceptives and, 77–78
  oxygen and, 174
  PMS, 74–76
  progestin, 77–78
  self-testing of, 21t, 27, 28b–29b, 31, 32–34, 214–215, 223–224, 277

Bone densitometry (DEXA) test, 161–162

Bone loss, 156, 158–160

"Borderline diabetes," 19, 26

Borg Scale of Perceived Exertion, 176, 177t

Bovine somatotropin (BST), 293

Bovine spongiform encephalopathy (BSE), 293–295

Bread and Circus supermarket, 298
Breakthrough bleeding, 109
Breast cancer
    HRT, 101, 163–164
    menstrual history, 164
    postmenopausal, 162–163
    pregnancy history, 164–165
Breastfeeding, maternal diabetes, 138–139
Breastfeeding Sourcebook, The, 129, 139
Breast Sourcebook, The, 162
British Diabetes Association, dietary guidelines, 189, 194–195
Bulimia nervosa, 51, 52
Burdock root, phytoestrogen, 114

C

Caffeine, bone loss and, 159
Calcitonin, 159
Calcium
    foods rich in, 161
    loss of, 158–159
Calcium and Common Sense, 161
California Institute of Technology, 290, 292
Calories, 199t, 200
Caprenin, 55
Carbohydrate counting (Carb counting), 198
Carbohydrates
    diabetic diet, 187, 188, 189, 190t, 192
    exercise and, 180–181, 181t
Cardiologist, 221
Cardiovascular disease, Type 2 diabetes, 4
Caucasians, 4, 123
Ceiling level, heart beat, 175

Certified diabetes educator (CDE), diabetes care team, 211–212, 227, 242
Cervical cap, barrier method, 76, 98–100
Cesarean section (C-section), 135, 136–137
    macrosomia, 128, 134–136
    obesity and, 119–120
"Change of life," 145
Chemotherapy, and menopause, 154
Childhood onset, Type 1 diabetes, 3
Cholesterol
    fat types and, 281, 282
    nutritional claim, 199t
    role of, 7
    Type 2 diabetes risk factor, 7, 77–78
Cholesterol test, 8, 228
Cigarette smoking
    bone loss and, 159
    eye disease, 260
    hypertension risk factor, 9
    kidney disease, 267
    macrovascular complications, 253
    obesity and, 67–68
    Type 2 diabetes risk factor, 11
Clomiphene citrate, 123–124
Coalition for Excess Weight Risk Education, 47
Coil Spring Rim, diaphragm, 95–96
Cola test, GDM, 132–133
Community Health Representative, diabetes care team, 212
Companion planting, 297

Complications
    prevention of diabetic, 275–276
    Type 1 diabetes induced,
        253–254
    Type 2 diabetes induced,
        251–252
Compulsive overeating, 59–61
Condoms, barrier method, 76
Conjunctivitis, diabetes induced,
    260
Contraindication, term, 71
Conventional treatment, diabetes,
    275
Copper, wound healing, 288
Corpus albicans, 74
Corpus luteum, menstrual cycle,
    73–74
Cortical bones, 156, 157
Corticosteroid, 125
"Country food," 18
"Crash and burn" diet, 49
Crohn's disease, bone loss and, 159
Cushing disease, Type 2 diabetes
    and, 16
Cyclamate, 202, 203–204
Cystocele, falling bladder, 168

D

Dalkon Shield, 91
Dental problems, diabetes
    induced, 260
Depo-Provera, 78
Depression, impact on diet, 44
DES daughters, 210
Diabetes
    symptoms of, 22–23
    types of, 1–3, 21t. *See also*
        Type 1 diabetes, Type 2
        diabetes

Diabetes Control and
    Complications Trial (DCCT),
    26–27, 29, 254, 275, 276
Diabetic ID card, 35, 36t, 40
Diabetic ketoacidosis (DKA), 31
Diabetic nephropathy, 266
Diaphragm, barrier method, 76,
    94–98
Diet, compulsive eating, 61
Dietary guidelines, diabetic, 189,
    190t
Diethylstilbestrol (DES), 210
Dieting, chronic, 48–50
Dietitian, diabetes care team, 212
Doctor's rights, 217
Dong quai (*Angelica sinensis*),
    phytoestrogen, 114
Dowager's hump, 156
Down's syndrome, Type 2 diabetes
    and, 16
D-tagatose, 204

E

Eating disorders, 50–53
    bone loss and, 159
Electrolysis, hirsutism, 126
Endocrinologist, medical care
    team, 211, 218–219
Endometrial cancer, hormonal
    birth control, 77, 80
Endometrial hyperplasia, 103, 122
Endorphins, eating and, 53
End-stage renal disease (ESRD),
    Type 2 diabetes and, 17, 264
Enterocele, falling small intestine,
    168
Estrogen
    function of, 102–103
    levels, PCO, 123

loss, during menopause, 146, 147, 150–151, 154–156
production of, 72–74
side effects of, 83t
synthetic forms of, 107
Type 2 diabetes and, 71, 78
urinary incontinence treatment, 166
Estrogen replacement therapy (ERT), 101–102, 104, 110–114
contraindications, 113
surgical menopause, 153
"Estrogen toxic," 103
Estrone, 103
Exchange list, ADA, 194–195, 197–198, 198t
Exchange Lists for Meal Planning, 198
Exercise, 10–11, 30, 41, 150, 171–178, 173t
Type 2 diabetes, 182–184, 188
Exercise/fitness instructor, diabetes care team, 212
Eye disease, diabetes induced, 257–260, 276
Eye examination, 228

F

Fat cells, function of, 64
"Fat genes," 7, 64
Fat, psychological role of, 56–59. *See also* Obesity
Fat substitutes, 285–286
Fats
consumption of, 53, 54, 56
in diabetic diet, 189, 190t, 199t, 281
tips for using, 291b
types of, 281–286

Fatty acids, 281
Female condom, birth control, 76
Female-factor infertility, 126
Fenfluramine, 67
Fen/Phen, 67
Fertility Sourcebook, The, 124, 126, 268
Fertility treatments, PCO, 123–124
Fiber, diabetic diet, 286–288
Fibrocystic breast disorder, OCs and, 80
Fibroids, HRT, 107
Flat Spring Rim, diaphragm, 96
Foam, birth control, 76
Follicle stimulating hormone (FSH), 73, 75, 121
during menopause, 145, 146, 147
surgical menopause, 153
Follicles, menstrual cycle, 73–74
Food addiction, twelve step program for, 61–63, 62b
Food additives, 46
Food and Drug Administration, toxin residues, 293
Food cravings, PMS, 75
Food labels, nutrient claims, 199–201, 199t
Foot disorders, diabetes induced, 269–274
Foot examination, 228
"Fracture risk estimate," 161
Fractures, osteoporosis-linked, 151
Fructosamine test, 226
Fruits, eating more, 292b
"Full-blown Type 2" diabetes, 4–5
Functional foods, 289–290

G

"Gaining muscle," 171

Gallbladder disease
  cholesterol and, 282
  ERT/HRT, 107

Gastroenterologist, 221

Gastrointestinal Sourcebook, The, 264

Gender difference
  heart disease, 210, 262–263
  Type 2 diabetes, 210–211

Genetic inheritance, Type 2 diabetes risk factor, 14

Gerontologist, 221–222

Gestational diabetes mellitus (GDM), 24, 118, 119, 129, 131–135

Glucagon kit, 40

Glucose, conversion to, 196b

Glucose meter, 31–33, 214, 245, 249

Glucose meter checkup, 227–228

Glucose screening, GDM diagnosis, 132–134

Glyburide, OHAs, 233

Glycemic index, 196b

Glycohemoglobin (HbA$_{1c}$) test, 33, 119, 215, 225–227, 227t

Glycosylated hemoglobin, 33, 119, 215, 225

Gonadotropin releasing hormone (GnRH), 72–73

"Good" cholesterol, 7, 13, 77, 84, 102–103, 174, 205, 283

"Good time disease," 44

Grain, diabetic diet, 288

Grocery Manufactures of America, pesticides, 298

Guar gum, 238

Gynecologist, 222

H

Health diary, keeping, 223

Heart disease
  diabetes induced, 261–264
  estrogen and, 104–105
  fen/phen and, 67
  gender difference, 210, 262–263
  HRT, 163
  Type 2 diabetes, 4, 11, 101, 162

High blood pressure. *See* Hypertension

"High blood sugar," 2. *See also* Hyperglycemia

High-density lipoproteins (HDL), "good" cholesterol, 7, 13, 77, 84, 102–103, 174, 205, 283

Hip fractures, senile osteoporosis, 157

Hirsutism, 82, 121, 125–126

Hispanics
  GDM screening, 138
  Type 2 diabetes, 4, 5, 15

Honeymoon cystitis, 266

Hormone replacement therapy (HRT), 101–109, 102b, 111–114
  breast cancer and, 101, 163–164
  common questions about, 114
  contraindications, 113
  surgical menopause, 153
  Type 2 diabetes and, 71, 100–101, 253

Hot flashes, 144, 145, 147–150

Human chorionic gonadotropin (HCG) hormone, 74, 124, 145

Human insulin, 242

Human menopausal gonadotropin (HMG), 124

Hydrogenation, process of, 283–284

Hydrolysis, process of, 48
Hydrolyzed proteins, 48
Hyperbaric Oxygen Therapy (HBO), 274
Hyperglycemia, 30–31, 129
Hyperinsulinemia, 1–2, 25–26
Hyperpigmentation, 158
Hyperprolactenemia, 125
Hypertension, 8–10
    as diabetic symptom, 23
Hypertrophy, 247
Hypoglycemia, 20, 23, 29, 35–40
    alcohol use and, 207
    diabetic pregnancy and, 135
    OHAs, 232–234
Hypothalamus, weight gain and, 65, 72–74, 148
Hypothyroidism, 64

I

Impaired fasting glucose (IFG), 20, 21t
Impaired glucose tolerance (IGT), 19–20, 21t, 26, 48
Infertility, Type 2 diabetes, 117, 121–123
Inheritance, Type 2 diabetes, 2
Injections, insulin, 246–247
Insoluble fiber, 286–287
Insulin
    equipment with, 245, 248–249
    estrogen and, 71, 72
    role of, 2
    types of, 240–242, 243b, 244t, 245
Insulin-dependent diabetes mellitus (IDDM), Type 1 diabetes, 3, 24
Insulin lispro, 240–241

Insulin pens, 245, 248–249
Insulin-requiring Type 2 diabetes, 4, 26
Insulin resistance, 2, 3, 24–26, 71, 77, 229
    exercise and, 178–179
    PCO, 122–123, 125
    weight gain and, 64
Insulin shock, 37
Insulin therapy, Type 2 diabetes, 3, 25–26, 239–242, 243b, 244t, 245, 246–249
Intensive therapy, diabetes, 275
International Food Information Council, sugar consumption, 194
Internist, primary care physician, 213, 221
Intrauterine devices (IUD), 76, 89–93
Involuntary urination, 165
Irritable bladder, 165, 166
Islets of Langerhans, 2
Isoflavones, 289
Isothiocyanates, 289

J

Jaundice, neonatal, 129
Jelly bean test, GDM, 132–133
Juvenile diabetes, Type 1 diabetes, 3
Juvenile-onset diabetes, Type 1 diabetes, 3

K

Kegel exercise, urinary incontinence treatment, 166–167
Ketones, formation of, 31

Kidney disease
 diabetes induced, 121, 252–253, 264–268, 276
 hypertension and, 9–10
Kidney test, 228
Kidneys, function of, 265

L

Lactoovovegetarians, 295
Lactovegitarians, 295
Lancets, 33, 245, 249
Lancing devices, 33, 245
Laproscopic surgery, PCO, 125
Leg cramps, 181–182
Leisure diet, 45–48
Leptin, weight gain and, 65–66
Lesbians, breast cancer, 164
Levonorgestrel, 86–87
Licorice, phytoestrogen, 114, 115
Lipid disorder, 77
Lipodystrophy, 247
Lippes Loop, 91
Liver, role of, 2, 282
"Low calories," nutritional claim, 199t, 200
"Low cholesterol," nutritional claim, 199t
Low-density lipoproteins (LDL), "bad" cholesterol, 7, 77, 103, 174, 230, 237, 283, 286
Low-fat products, impact of, 54–56
"Low fat," nutritional claim, 199t, 200
Luteinizing hormone (LH), menstrual cycle, 73, 121

M

Macrosomia, 128, 134
Macrovascular complications, diabetes, 251–252, 253, 254–256, 257–260, 261–264, 265–266, 269–274
Macular edema, diabetes induced, 258
Mad cow disease, 293–295
Mature-onset diabetes in the young (MODY), Type 2 diabetes, 3
Mature-onset diabetes, Type 2 diabetes, 3
Meal plan, diabetic, 187, 191–192, 195b, 198–199, 279, 286–288
Meal planning, 29–30, 41
Meat, 291b
Medical care team, Type 2 diabetes, 211–215, 221–222, 224–225
Medical norms, determination of, 209
Medical team, prenatal, 130b
Medication
 antidiabetic, 229–239
 drug complicating diabetic treatment, 22b
 hypertension and, 10
 obesity and, 66–67
 self-testing and, 33
 Type 2 diabetes risk factor, 21
Medroxyprogesterone, 108
Melasma, 112
Mellitis, term, 3
Menarche, 80, 141, 143, 164
"Menopausal mood swings," 141, 152
Menopause
 blood sugar level, 75, 142, 151–152, 154–156
 HRT, 1–3, 104
 menopausal stage, 144
 metabolism slowdown, 64
 short-term symptoms, 145

stages of, 143–145
term, 141
tests for, 145
Type 2 diabetes, 13–14, 253
Menstrual cycle, description of, 72–74
Menstruation
erratic, 145, 146–147
first day of, 74
Type 2 diabetes and, 74
Metformin, OHAs, 231
Metrodin, 124
Microvascular complications, diabetes, 252, 253–254, 257–261, 264, 266, 269–274
Milk fat, 291b
Mini-pill, 76, 77, 79–80, 85
Monosodium glutamate (MSG), 48
Monounsaturated fats, 282
Moss, Kate, 52
Motherwort, phytoestrogen, 114
"Mouth hunger," 61, 67
Mouth orgasm, 53
Multiracial Americans, Type 2 diabetes in, 16
Muscles, exercise and, 176–177

N

National Cancer Institute, 164
National Institute of Diabetes and Digestive and Kidney Diseases (NIDDK), 276
National Institutes of Health Consensus Panel on Osteoporosis, 161
National Osteoporosis Foundation, 162, 179
National Weight Report, 47–48
Native Americans, Type 2 diabetes in, 4, 5, 15, 17–19

Native people, term, 16–17
Natural progesterone, 108
Nature Medicine, leptin, 65
Navajo Indians, ESRD in, 17
Nephrologist, 221
Neurologist, 221
Newborns, maternal diabetes and, 128–129
Non-insulin-dependent diabetes mellitis (NIDDM), Type 2 diabetes, 3
Norplant, 76, 77, 78, 79, 85–89
North American Society for the Study of Obesity, 47
Nothing in Common, 269
Nutritive sweeteners, 202

O

Obesity. *See also*, Fat
childhood, 184
cigarette smoking and, 11, 67–68
definition of, 5, 29, 43
drug treatment for, 66–67
hypertension risk factor, 9
insulin resistance and, 25
pregnancy and, 119–120
Type 2 diabetes risk factor, 5, 7, 43, 253
urinary incontinence, 167
Obesity rates, American cities, 47–48
Obstetrician, 222
Olestra, fat substitute, 55, 285, 286
Omega-3 oils, 282, 283
Oophorectomy, 141–142, 152–153
Opthamologist, 221
Oral contraceptives (OC), 76, 77–85
Type 2 diabetes and, 71, 77–79

Oral hypoglycemic agents (OHAs), 37
Type 2, diabetes, 230–236
Organic Trade Association, 298, 299
Orlistat (Xenical), 66–67
Orthopedist, 222
Osteoporosis, 104, 156–157, 160–162
weight-bearing activity, 179
Ovarian cancer, hormonal birth control, 77, 80
Ovarian cysts, hormonal birth control, 77, 80
Ovaries, 72–74
Overeaters Anonymous, twelve step program, 62b, 63
Overexercising, 51
Overflow incontinence, 165, 166
"Overnutrition," 17
Ovovegetarians, 295
Ovulation, 72–73
"Oxidative stress," 12
Oxygen
body's need for, 174–175
disabled and, 176–177

P

Pacific Islanders, Type 2 diabetes in, 17
Pancreas
healthy, 223, 224
Type 1 diabetes, 3
Type 2 diabetes, 2
Pancreatectomy, 21
Pancreatitis, 20
Patient's rights, 216–217
Pelvic inflammatory disease (PID), IUDs and, 93

Pergonal, 124
Perimenopausal, menopausal stage, 144
Peripheral vascular disease (PVD)
diabetes induced, 261
Type 2 diabetes, 4
Pescovegitarians, 295
Pessary, 167
Pesticides, use of, 297–298
Pharmacist, diabetes care team, 212–213, 217
Phentermine, 67
Phenylketonuria, 203
Photocoagulation, eye disease, 259
Phytoechemicals, 289
Phytoestrogens, 114–115, 286
Pima Indians, 17, 65
Pituitary gland, menstrual cycle role, 72
Pollution, impact on diet, 18–19
Polycystic Ovarian Syndrome (PCO), 121–123
Polyneuropathy, diabetes induced, 256
Polyunsaturated fats, 282, 284
Postmenopausal, menopausal stage, 144
Postmenopausal osteoporosis, 156
"Postmenopausal pregnancy," 117
Postmenopausal urinary incontinence, 165–167
Postpartum depression, maternal diabetes and, 140
Posture, importance of, 172
Prader-Willi disease, Type 2 diabetes and, 16
Pregestational diabetes, 126, 128
Pregnancy
hyperglycemia and, 30, 129

hypertension risk factor, 9–10
Type 1 diabetes, 127–129, 131
Type 2 diabetes, 117–119,
    127–129, 131
Type 2 diabetes risk factor, 5, 24
Pregnancy Sourcebook, The, 140
Premarin, 107, 108
Premenopause, menopausal stage,
    143–144
Premenstrual syndrome, Type 2
    diabetes and, 74–76
Prentif cavity-rim cervical cap,
    99–100
Primary care physician, medical
    care team, 211, 213–215
Progesterone
    HRT and, 101, 108
    menstrual cycle, 73, 74
Progestin, blood sugar levels,
    77–78, 80–83, 82t, 122
Proliferatory phase, menstrual
    cycle, 73
Protein, diabetic diet, 189, 190t
Proximal motor neuropathy, dia-
    betes induced, 257
Pulse rate, exercise, 176
Purging, 51, 75

R

Radiation, and menopause, 154
Rapid eye movement (REM) sleep,
    11–12
Rectocele, falling rectum, 168
Reduced sugar, nutritional claim,
    201
Redux, 67
Remodeling, bones, 158
Retina, diabetes induced disorders
    of, 259

Rezulin, 236–238
Risk factors
    hypertension, 9–10
    modifiable/ Type 2 diabetes,
        6–12, 21–22
    nonmodifiable/Type 2 diabetes,
        13–16
    Type 2 diabetes, 5–6
"Rubber tipping," 260–261

S

Saccharin, 202–203
Saf-T-Coil, 91
Salatrim, 55
Salt, hypertension risk factor, 9
Saponins, 289
Saturated fat, 281–282, 284–285
Scrapies, 294
Second opinion, 217, 222–223
Secondary amenorrhea, 122
Secondary diabetes, 21
Secondary osteoporosis, 156, 157
Secretory phase, menstrual cycle,
    73
Sedentary life style, Type 2 dia-
    betes risk factor, 10–11
Self-testing, blood sugar levels,
    21t, 27, 28b–29b, 31, 32–34,
    214–215, 223–224, 277
Semivegitarians, 295
Senile osteoporosis, 156, 157
Seniors, vitamin deficiency in, 12
Sexual activity, Type 2 diabetes,
    120, 268–269
Sexual desire, menopause and, 150
Sexual dysfunction, diabetes
    induced, 268–269
Shoes, shopping for healthy, 273b,
    273

Side effects
  Alpha-glucosidase inhibitors (Arcarbose), 236
  diaphragm, 96
  ERT/HRT, 111–112
  estrogen, 83t, 111
  insulin therapy, 247
  IUDs, 92–93
  Norplant, 88–89
  OCs, 79, 80–81
  OHAs, 232
  progestin, 80–83, 82t
  thiazoladinediones, 237, 238–239
"Side-effect diabetes," 21
Simplesse, fat substitute, 285
Skin, changes during menopause, 155–156
Skin disorders, diabetes induced, 274
Sleep disorders, Type 2 diabetes risk factor, 11–12
Soluble fiber, 286
Southeast Asians, Type 2 diabetes in, 16
Steel Magnolias, 121
Steroids, discovery of, 78
Stomach disorders, diabetes induced, 264
Stress incontinence, 165–166
Stress, hypertension and, 10
Stroke, Type 2 diabetes, 4, 254–255
Subdermal implants, birth control, 76, 85–89
Sucralose, 202, 2033
Sugar, 192–194, 193b, 201–202
  role in diabetes, 2
Sugar alcohols, 202, 204–205
"Sugar free," nutritional claim, 201

"Sugar shows," 68
Sulphonylureas, OHAs, 230–231, 232t, 233–234
Sunblock, use of, 155–156
Surgical menopause, 104, 141–142, 152–154, 159
Sustainable farming, 296–297

T

"Talk test," exercise, 176
Target zone, heart beat, 175, 176
Television, impact on diet, 45, 68
Thalidomide, 210
Thiazoladinediones, 236–238
Threshold level, heart beat, 175
"Thrifty gene," 15, 16
Torcar, 86
Toxic shock syndrome (TSS), 94, 96
Trabecular bones, 156, 157
Trans-fatty acids, 281, 283–284
Travel, insulin therapy, 248–249
Trigger foods, hot flashes, 149
Triglyceride, 282
Troglitazone, 236–238
Tubal ligation, 100
Turner's syndrome, Type 2 diabetes and, 16
Type 1 diabetes, disease of, 2–3, 21t, 24, 26–27, 31
Type 2 diabetes, disease of, 1–2, 21t, 23–24
  prevalence of, 4, 6
  question to ask, 219–220
  signs and symptoms, 22–23

U

United King Prospective Diabetes Study (UKPDS), 27, 29, 276–277

"Unopposed estrogen therapy,"
103, 106, 142
Unsaturated fat, 281, 284–285
Urethrocele, falling urethra, 168
Urge incontinence, 165, 166
Urinary incontinence, 165–167
Urinary tract infection (UTI),
266–267, 268
Uterine cancer
HRT and, 106–107
risk of, 106
Uterine prolapse, 167–168

V

Vaginal birth after cesarean
(VBAC) , 136
Vaginal dryness, 144, 145, 150–151,
156
Vaginal sponge, barrier method,
76, 94
Vaginal yeast infection, 216, 268
Vegans, 295
Vegetables, eating more, 292b
Vegetarian diet, 295
Vision, blurred, 22

Vitamin deficiency, Type 2 diabetes risk factor, 12
Vitamin E, hot flashes, 149

W

Weight-bearing activities, 178–179
Weight, determining normal, 53
Weight gain, as diabetic symptom,
22
Weight loss, Type 2 diabetes, 29
Wild yams, phytoestrogen, 114
Withdrawal bleeding, 79, 109
Women's Health Initiative (WHI),
101
Women
fat as issue, 56–59, 60b
heart disease and, 262
medical research exclusion,
209–210
Wounds, treatment for, 273–274, 288

X-Y-Z

Xenical, 66–67
Yo-Yo diet syndrome, 49
Zinc, wound healing, 288